Neurodevelopmental Disorders Across the Lifespan

A Neuroconstructivist Approach

Oxford Series in Developmental Cognitive Neuroscience

Series Editor

Mark H. Johnson, Centre for Brain and Cognitive Development
Birkbeck College, University of London, UK

Neuroconstructivism Volume I: How the brain constructs cognition
Denis Mareschal, Mark H. Johnson, Sylvain Sirois, Michael W. Spratling,
Michael S. C. Thomas, and Gert Westermann

Neuroconstructivism Volume II: Perspectives and Prospects
Edited by Denis Mareschal, Sylvain Sirois, Gert Westermann, and Mark H. Johnson

*Toward a Unified Theory of Development: Connectionism and Dynamic Systems
Theory Re-Considered*
Edited by John P. Spencer, Michael S. C. Thomas, and James L. McClelland

The Making of Human Concepts
Edited by Denis Mareschal, Paul C. Quinn, and Stephen E. G. Lea

Attention, Genes, and Developmental Disorders
Kim Cornish and John Wilding

Neurodevelopmental Disorders Across the Lifespan

A Neuroconstructivist Approach

Edited by

Emily K. Farran

Reader,
Psychology and Human Development,
Institute of Education,
University of London,
London, UK

Annette Karmiloff-Smith

Professorial Research Fellow,
Birkbeck Centre for Brain and
Cognitive Development,
University of London,
London, UK

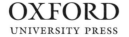

OXFORD
UNIVERSITY PRESS

OXFORD

UNIVERSITY PRESS

Great Clarendon Street, Oxford ox2 6DP

Oxford University Press is a department of the University of Oxford.
It furthers the University's objective of excellence in research, scholarship,
and education by publishing worldwide in

Oxford New York

Auckland Cape Town Dar es Salaam Hong Kong Karachi
Kuala Lumpur Madrid Melbourne Mexico City Nairobi
New Delhi Shanghai Taipei Toronto

With offices in

Argentina Austria Brazil Chile Czech Republic France Greece
Guatemala Hungary Italy Japan Poland Portugal Singapore
South Korea Switzerland Thailand Turkey Ukraine Vietnam

Oxford is a registered trade mark of Oxford University Press
in the UK and in certain other countries

Published in the United States
by Oxford University Press Inc., New York

British Library Cataloguing in Publication Data
Data available

Library of Congress Cataloging in Publication Data
Library of Congress Control Number: 2011943535

Typeset in Minion by Cenveo, Bangalore, India
Printed and bound by
CPI Group (UK) Ltd, Croydon, CR0 4YY

ISBN 978–0–19–959481–8

10 9 8 7 6 5 4 3 2 1

Whilst every effort has been made to ensure that the contents of this book are as complete,
accurate and up-to-date as possible at the date of writing, Oxford University Press
is not able to give any guarantee or assurance that such is the case. Readers are
urged to take appropriately qualified medical advice in all cases. The information
in this book is intended to be useful to the general reader, but should not be used
as a means of self-diagnosis or for the prescription of medication.

Acknowledgements

We have many people to warmly thank for their contributions to this book. First and foremost, our greatest appreciation goes to all our chapter contributors, who all did their utmost to follow our editorial guidelines so that the book was not a mere juxtaposition of albeit interesting chapters but conveyed a common cohesive approach. Not only did they take all our detailed comments on board, but they also revised their chapters with amazing promptness, which meant that we actually met our planned deadline—an incredible feat! Second, all authors as well as May Tassabehji also generously commented alongside the editors on other chapters, again contributing to the book's cohesiveness. Third, we would particularly like to thank Charlotte Green and Abigail Stanley of Oxford University Press and freelance copyeditor Martina Habeck, who made our task much smoother at multiple levels. Finally, we thank our partners, John Willoughby and Mark Johnson, for their patience while we inundated every home tabletop surface with chapters, reference lists and Post-it notes!

Chapter 1 (Michael S. C. Thomas, Harry R. Purser and Jo Van Herwegen)

This research was supported by Economic and Social Research Council grants RES-062-23-2721 and RES-062-33-0005, and a Leverhulme Study Abroad Fellowship to MT held at the University of Chicago.

Chapter 2 (Annette Karmiloff-Smith)

Thank you to Karen Berman, Brian Haas and Allan Reiss for very useful comments on this manuscript and to Lauren Willmott for help in preparing references. We also thank Allan Reiss and Paul Thompson for providing Figures 2.1 and 2.2.

Chapter 3 (Lucy R. Osborne)

Thank you to Elizabeth Fisher for reviewing this chapter.

Chapter 6 (Kate Breckenridge, Janette Atkinson and Oliver Braddick)

The research described in this chapter was supported by grants G0601007 and G7908507 from the Medical Research Council to JA and OB, a studentship from the Biotechnology and Biological Sciences Research Council to KB, and grants from the Economic and Social Research Council (RES-000-22-2659) and the Williams Syndrome Foundation to KB and JA. We thank Professor Margaret Woodhouse of Cardiff University for collaboration in testing the Down syndrome group; John Wattam-Bell, Shirley Anker, Dee Birtles, Marko

Nardini, Dorothy Cowie and many other past members of the Visual Development Units at University College London and the University of Oxford for their help and support in our programme; and Harriet Hallas for help in preparation of this manuscript. Lastly, we thank the many families who have willingly taken part in our studies.

Chapter 9 (Kerry D. Hudson and Emily K. Farran)

The preparation of this chapter and the authors' current research is supported by a Collaborative Awards in Science and Engineering PhD studentship from the Economic and Social Research Council (ESRC) and the Williams Syndrome Foundation, UK and by an ESRC grant (grant number RES-062-33-0005).

Chapter 10 (Carolyn B. Mervis and Angela E. John)

We are very grateful to the individuals with Williams syndrome and their families who have participated so enthusiastically in research studies throughout the world. It is only through their participation that researchers are able to document the language and cognitive strengths and weaknesses of individuals with Williams syndrome and to address their implications both for developmental theory and for the design of language intervention programs targeted for individuals with this syndrome. The authors' research on Williams syndrome and the preparation of this chapter were supported by the National Institute of Child Health and Human Development (grant number R37 HD29957) and the National Institute of Neurological Disorders and Stroke (grant number R01 NS35102).

Chapter 12 (Emily K. Farran and Susan C. Formby)

The preparation of this chapter and the authors' current research is supported by an Economic and Social Research Council grant (grant number RES-062-33-0005) and a PhD studentship from the University of Reading.

Chapter 13 (Janette Atkinson and Oliver Braddick)

The research described in this chapter was supported by grants G0601007 and G7908507 from the Medical Research Council to Janette Atkinson and Oliver Braddick and John Wattam-Bell. We thank John Wattam-Bell, Shirley Anker, Dee Birtles, Marko Nardini, Dorothy Cowie and many other past members of the Visual Development Units at University College London and the University of Oxford for their help and support in our programme, and Harriet Hallas for help in preparation of this manuscript. Lastly, we thank the many families who have willingly taken part in our studies.

Chapter 16 (Joanne S. Camp, Emily K. Farran and Annette Karmiloff-Smith)

The preparation of this chapter and the authors' current research is supported by a Bloomsbury Colleges PhD studentship and Economic and Social Research Council grant number RES-062-33-0005. Thank you to Lauren Willmott for help at the preparation stage, and to Daniel Ansari for helpful comments on this chapter.

Chapter 18 (Ann Steele, Janice Brown and Gaia Scerif)

We are extremely grateful to Sarah Paterson for generosity with her data. Kim Cornish and Annette Karmiloff-Smith contributed to all aspects of the data reported in sections 4 and 5, in addition to their ongoing intellectual input to our work. Of course, none of these findings could have been achieved without the continuing support of children, families, schools and the national support associations that are so critical to all of what we do. We cannot thank them enough.

Contents

List of Contributors *xi*

Introduction: **Williams syndrome: A model for the neuroconstructivist approach** *1*
Annette Karmiloff-Smith and Emily K. Farran

Part 1 **Cognition, Brain, Genes**

1 Cognition: The developmental trajectory approach *13*
Michael S. C. Thomas, Harry R. Purser and Jo Van Herwegen

2 Brain: The neuroconstructivist approach *37*
Annette Karmiloff-Smith

3 Genes: The gene expression approach *59*
Lucy R. Osborne

Part 2 **Clinical and Practical Outcomes**

4 Clinical profile: Diagnosis and prognosis *85*
Kay Metcalfe

5 Adult outcomes and integration into society *103*
Chris Stinton and Patricia Howlin

Part 3 **Domain-General Processes**

6 Attention *119*
Kate Breckenridge, Janette Atkinson and Oliver Braddick

7 Sleep-related learning *135*
Dagmara Annaz and Anna Ashworth

8 Memory *149*
Stefano Vicari and Deny Menghini

9 Executive function and motor planning *165*
Kerry D. Hudson and Emily K. Farran

Part 4 **Domain-Specific Processes**
Part 4a **Verbal Domain**

10 Precursors to language and early language *187*
Carolyn B. Mervis and Angela E. John

11 Later language *205*
Vesna Stojanovik

Part 4b **Visual Domain**

12 Visual perception and visuospatial cognition *225*
Emily K. Farran and Susan C. Formby

13 Spatial cognition, visuomotor action and attention *247*
Janette Atkinson and Oliver Braddick

Part 4c **Social Domain**

14 Face processing and social interaction *265*
Deborah M. Riby

15 Mental state understanding and social interaction *279*
Ruth Campos and María Sotillo

Part 4d **Numeracy and Literacy**

16 Numeracy *299*
Joanne S. Camp, Emily K. Farran and Annette Karmiloff-Smith

17 Literacy *313*
Yvonne M. Griffiths

Part 5 **The Neuroconstructivist Approach to Domain-General and Domain-Specific Processes**

18 Integrating domain-general and domain-specific developmental processes: Cross-syndrome, cross-domain dynamics *339*
Ann Steele, Janice Brown and Gaia Scerif

Conclusion: **Future theoretical and empirical directions within a neuroconstructivist framework** *363*
Annette Karmiloff-Smith and Emily K. Farran

Author Index *373*

Subject Index *383*

List of Contributors

Dagmara Annaz
Department of Psychology
Middlesex University
London, UK

Anna Ashworth
Department of Psychology
Middlesex University
London, UK

Janette Atkinson
Visual Development Unit
Division of Psychology and
Language Sciences
University College London
London, UK

Oliver Braddick
Visual Development Unit
Department of Experimental Psychology
University of Oxford
Oxford, UK

Kate Breckenridge
Division of Psychology and
Language Sciences
University College London
London, UK

Janice Brown
Department of Psychology
London South Bank University
London, UK

Joanne S. Camp
Department of Psychology and
Human Development
Institute of Education
University of London
London, UK

Ruth Campos
Department of Basic Psychology
Faculty of Psychology
Autónoma University of Madrid
Madrid, Spain

Emily K. Farran
Department of Psychology and Human
Development
Institute of Education
University of London
London, UK

Susan C. Formby
Department of Psychology and Clinical
Language Science
University of Reading
Reading, UK

Yvonne M. Griffiths
Department of Psychology and Human
Development
Institute of Education
University of London
London, UK

Patricia Howlin
Institute of Psychiatry
London, UK

Kerry D. Hudson
Department of Psychology and
Clinical Language Science
University of Reading
Reading, UK

Angela E. John
Department of Psychological and
Brain Sciences
University of Louisville
Louisville, Kentucky, USA

Annette Karmiloff-Smith
Birkbeck Centre for Brain and Cognitive
Development
Department of Psychological Sciences
University of London
London, UK

Deny Menghini
Department of Neuroscience
Children's Hospital Bambino Gesù
Rome, Italy

Carolyn B. Mervis
Department of Psychological and
Brain Sciences
University of Louisville
Louisville, Kentucky, USA

Kay Metcalfe
Department of Genetic Medicine
Central Manchester University Hospital
Manchester, UK

Lucy R. Osborne
Department of Medicine
University of Toronto
Toronto, Ontario, Canada

Harry R. Purser
Department of Psychology and Human
Development
Institute of Education
University of London
London, UK

Deborah M. Riby
School of Psychology
Newcastle University
Newcastle, UK

Gaia Scerif
Department of Experimental Psychology
University of Oxford
Oxford, UK

María Sotillo
Department of Basic Psychology
Faculty of Psychology
Autónoma University of Madrid
Madrid, Spain

Ann Steele
Department of Experimental Psychology
University of Oxford
Oxford, UK

Chris Stinton
Cerebra Centre for
Neurodevelopmental Disorders
School of Psychology
University of Birmingham
Birmingham, UK

Vesna Stojanovik
Department of Psychology and
Clinical Language Science
University of Reading
Reading, UK

Michael S. C. Thomas
Centre for Brain and Cognitive
Development
Department of Psychological Sciences
Birkbeck, University of London
London, UK

Jo Van Herwegen
Department of Psychology
Kingston University
Kingston upon Thames, UK

Stefano Vicari
Department of Neuroscience
Children's Hospital Bambino Gesù
Rome, Italy

Science is not a collection of truths. It is a continuing exploration of mysteries.

Freeman Dyson

Williams syndrome: A model for the neuroconstructivist approach

Annette Karmiloff-Smith and Emily K. Farran

Introduction: why Williams syndrome?

There was a time when most of the research into neurodevelopmental syndromes was merely based on a brief clinical assessment and a few standardised tests. However, with the huge technological advances in subtle in-depth phenotyping at the cognitive level as well as in genetics and brain imaging, multidisciplinary research into neurodevelopmental disorders is now the rule rather than the exception. This book provides just such an approach, taking the neurodevelopmental disorder Williams syndrome (WS) as a model syndrome, with the aim that the book will serve as a paradigm for multidisciplinary, neuroconstructivist approaches to a wide range of other syndromes.

But why WS as our model disorder? After all, it is a rather rare, sporadic disorder occurring in only 1 in 15 000-20 000 births (although a Norwegian study [Stromme et al., 2002] yielded an estimate of 1 in 7500 births). Although WS was first described by two cardiology groups (Williams et al., 1961; Beuren et al., 1962), both identifying the association of several clinical features in affected individuals, it took another couple of decades before the syndrome started to be extensively investigated by cognitive psychologists and neuroscientists. Our choice for this book of such a rare syndrome as a model for studying neurodevelopmental disorders from a neuroconstructivist viewpoint was based on two crucial reasons. The first is the fact that WS has been extensively researched from multiple levels of description: genes and gene expression, brain structure and function, the electrophysiology of the brain, brain chemistry, cognitive processing across multiple domains as well as the social and everyday practical problems of growing up with WS. The second is the fact that WS has been studied across the lifespan, with now a growing number of studies on infants and toddlers with WS as well as a large bulk of research on children, adolescents and adults.

The neuroconstructivist approach to neurodevelopmental disorders

Given its rarity, what made the study of WS so popular in the research community? Interestingly, the reasons were initially rooted in a theoretical debate about whether domain-specific abilities were modular, that is, whether they functioned independently of one another (e.g. number having nothing to do with language, face processing having nothing to do with navigation), and could be shown to be dissociated in cases of adult neuropsychological patients but also in neurodevelopmental syndromes.

The initial descriptions of WS (e.g. Bellugi et al., 1988) highlighted the seemingly extraordinary language abilities of adolescents and adults with WS, their extreme social friendliness and their normal scores on standardised face-processing tasks. These proficiencies sat alongside serious impairments in visuospatial cognition and number processing. So, the claims went, the uneven profile in WS was the perfect example of cognitive modules operating independently of one another, as can be seen in the following quotations:

> For instance, children with Williams syndrome have a barely measurable general intelligence and require constant parental care, yet they have an exquisite mastery of syntax and vocabulary. They are, however, unable to understand even the most immediate implications of their admirably constructed sentences.
>
> (Piattelli-Palmarini, 2001)

> The linguistic performance of [individuals with] WS can be explained in terms of selective deficits to an otherwise normal modular system.
>
> (Clahsen & Temple, 2003)

> . . . overall the genetic double dissociation is striking . . . The genes of one group of children [specific language impairment] impair their grammar while sparing their intelligence; the genes of another group of children [WS] impair their intelligence while sparing their grammar.
>
> (Pinker, 1999)

Contrast these with the following neuroconstructivist-inspired quotations, which, surprisingly, are describing the same syndrome, but this time with a focus on the dynamics of development:

> In sum, brain volume, brain anatomy, brain chemistry, hemispheric asymmetry, and the temporal patterns of brain activity are all atypical in people with WS. How could the resulting system be described as a normal brain with parts intact and parts impaired, as the popular view holds? Rather, the brains of infants with WS develop differently from the outset, with subtle, widespread repercussions . . .
>
> (Karmiloff-Smith, 1998)

> We argue that rather than being the paradigm case for the independence of language from cognition, Williams syndrome provides strong evidence of the interdependence of many aspects of language and cognition.
>
> (Mervis & Becerra, 2007)

The striking difference between these sets of quotations not only encapsulates early research into WS, but also continues to illustrate the theoretical differences guiding current research into this fascinating syndrome. There is no doubt that debates will continue to rage over the extent to which WS is a direct window on the nature–nurture debate.

WS is not alone in having quite opposing theoretical positions that guide cognitive and neural research. Autism spectrum disorders (ASDs) are another set of neurodevelopmental syndromes for which researchers either abide by a strictly modular view or take the neuroconstructivist stance, as the following quotations nicely illustrate.

Autism is due to a deficit in an innately-specified module that handles theory-of-mind computations only.

(Leslie, 1992)

. . . a module that is localized in the orbito-frontal cortex.

(Baron-Cohen, 1999)

Again, contrast these with the following three neuroconstructivist-inspired quotations:

Autism affects the interconnectivity among and within various cognitive systems.

(Carpenter et al., 2001)

In autism, functional brain development goes awry such that there is increased intra-regional specialization and less inter-regional interaction.

(Johnson et al., 2002)

. . . examine the crucial role of unbalanced excitatory-inhibitory networks . . . leading to ASD through altered neuronal morphology, synaptogenesis and cell migration.

(Persico & Bourgeron, 2006)

It quickly becomes obvious that the nativist, modular view of the mind/brain of WS and ASD differs radically from the neuroconstructivist view of the mind/brain. The former calls upon the existence of uneven cognitive profiles to support a static view based solely on the end state and the assumption that the brain is modularised from the start, whereas the latter focuses on the uneven profile being the resultant product of dynamic processes of development over time.

Although the neuroconstructivist approach argues against the strictly modular, nativist view, it is important to stress that neuroconstructivism does not imply that the neonate brain is a blank slate with no structure, as empiricists would claim. Nor does it entertain the possibility that just any part of the brain can process any and all inputs. On the contrary, neuroconstructivism maintains that the neonate cortex has some regional differentiation in terms of neuron types, density of neurons, firing thresholds and so on. These differences are not domain-specific, aimed at the sole processing of proprietary inputs, but nor do they amount to simple domain-general constraints. Rather, they are 'domain-relevant', meaning that different parts of the brain have small differences that turn out to be more appropriate/relevant to certain kinds of processing over others. However, initially, brain activity is widespread for processing all types of input, and competition between regions gradually settles which domain-relevant circuits actually become domain-specific over time (Karmiloff-Smith, 1998). So, starting out with tiny differences across brain regions in terms of the patterns of connectivity, the balance of neurotransmitters, synaptic density, neuronal type/orientation and the like, some areas of the brain are somewhat more suited (i.e. more relevant in terms of their computational properties) than others to the processing of certain kinds of input, and over time they ultimately win out. In other words, the computational properties of a particular brain circuit may be more relevant to certain types of processing (e.g. holistic versus componential processing) than to others, although they are initially not specific to that type of processing alone. It is only after developmental time and repeated processing that such a circuit becomes domain-specific as ontogenesis proceeds (Karmiloff-Smith, 1992, 1998). There is thus a gradual process of recruitment of particular pathways and structures for specific functions (Elman et al., 1996), such that brain pathways that were previously partially activated in a wide range of task contexts increasingly confine their activation to a narrower range of inputs and situations (Johnson et al., 2002).

The neuroconstructivist position is supported by neuroimaging research showing that the functional specialisation of brain regions is highly context-sensitive and depends on interactions with other brain regions through feedback processes and top-down modulation (Mechelli et al., 2001). This process becomes most evident in brain organisation in people who lack one sensory modality. For example, in individuals who have been blind from an early age, the visual cortex is recruited for the tactile modality (Braille reading) instead (Sadato et al., 1996). Moreover, the use of transcranial magnetic stimulation to block processing in this area affects tactile identification of Braille letters in the blind, but not in seeing people, who instead display impaired visual processing when stimulated in this area (Cohen et al., 1997). It therefore seems that the functional development of cortical regions is strongly constrained by available sensory inputs and that the final organisation of the cortex is an outcome of interactive processes such as competition for space.

Multilevel analyses

Another issue that arises with respect to the study of neurodevelopmental disorders is the distinction that must be drawn between the behavioural, cognitive and neural levels of description. It is entirely possible that individuals may reveal scores in the normal range on a given test and yet may be achieving that success via different cognitive-level and neural-level processes compared with typically developing controls. This is certainly the case, for instance, for the good face-processing scores identified in adolescents and adults with WS, which turn out to be sustained by different cognitive and neural processes than healthy controls. Equally, cross-syndrome comparisons can reveal an association at the behavioural level that is not mirrored at the neural level. Compare attention deficit hyperactivity disorder and WS; both groups show impaired inhibitory processes, but in attention deficit hyperactivity disorder this is associated with increased activation of the dorsolateral prefrontal cortex and dorsal anterior cingulate cortex, whereas in WS these same areas show an associated decrease in activation (see Chapter 9).

Moreover, there is a frequent slippage in the literature from relative differences to absolute ones. For example, when comparing two domains (A and B), with individuals showing levels of performance that are consistent with those seen in mental-age-matched controls in domain A but that are well below those levels in domain B, researchers tend to conclude that ability A is intact and B impaired, despite the fact that performance in A is still several years behind that of the typical child of equivalent chronological age. The neuroconstructivist view that focuses on interactions between domains across developmental time would never simply dismiss delay as irrelevant or count a relative advantage of one system over another as an absolute one, leading to claims of intactness (see discussions in Karmiloff-Smith, 1998; Karmiloff-Smith et al., 2003). A process that is vital, say, at Time 2 may no longer play a role at Time 5. Yet, its presence at Time 2 may have been crucial to a healthy developmental trajectory and outcome; delay can alter subsequent multilevel interactions, with cascading effects on developmental outcome.

The very notion of 'intactness/preservation' has a static connotation and implies genetic determinism, as if states in the brain were entirely hard-wired, unchanging and unaffected by developmental or environmental factors. The neuroconstructivist view, by contrast, considers the brain as a self-structuring, dynamically changing organism over developmental time as a function of multiple interactions at multiple levels, including gene expression (e.g. Casey & Durston, 2006; Johnson, 2001). Research on birds and mammals eloquently illustrates this point. Extensive evidence from studies of the neural and epigenetic consequences of song listening and song production in passerine birds (Bolhuis et al., 2000) shows how gene expression changes over developmental time and may be significantly more important during learning than during final production (see Chapter 3). Rather than something fixed and predetermined, gene expression in the birds turned out to be a function of how many elements the bird copied from its tutor. A second example comes from early mammalian development and also underlines the potential role of the environment in shaping long-term patterns of gene expression (Kaffman & Meaney, 2007). These authors studied brain development in rodent pups and traced how differences in maternal grooming behaviour influence patterns of gene expression in their pups, with lifelong effects. Rather than supporting the concept that gene expression is preprogrammed, the research showed that differences in the amount of postnatal pup grooming and stroking change the amount of expression of genes involved in the body's responses to stress, and that these changes last the pup's lifetime. These kinds of dynamic environment–gene relations are likely to be a pervasive feature of mammalian brain development, including that of humans. In general, epigenesis is not deterministic under tight genetic control. Rather, as Gottlieb (2007) stressed, epigenesis is probabilistic and only under very broad genetic control.

Neuroconstructivism does not rule out domain specificity; it argues that it cannot be taken for granted and must always be questioned. Unlike the nativist perspective, neuroconstructivism—like Piaget's constructivism—offers a truly developmental approach that focuses on change and emergent outcomes. Moreover, every aspect of development turns out to be dynamic and interactive. Genes do not act in isolation in a predetermined way. Even the *FOXP2* gene, about which there was much excitement regarding its role in human language, must be thought of in terms of the downstream gene targets to which the *FOXP2* gene product binds. The profiles of those downstream genes suggest roles in a wide range of general, not domain-specific, functions including morphogenesis, neurite growth, axon guidance, synaptic plasticity and neurotransmission (Teramitsu & White, 2007). This is very different from theorising at the level of cognitive modules and making claims about 'a gene for language', and points to the multilevel complexities of understanding human development in any domain.

The importance of full developmental trajectories

Neuroconstructivism argues that if the adult brain is in any way modular, this is the product of an emergent developmental process of modularisation, not its starting point (Karmiloff-Smith, 1992, 1998, 2006, 2009; Elman et al., 1996; Johnson et al., 2002; Westermann et al., 2010). A crucial error is to conflate the specialised brains of adults that have developed normally prior to damage in later life with those of infants and children, which are still in the process of developing (Karmiloff-Smith et al., 2002). Infancy studies have highlighted the fact that we cannot use the phenotypic outcome in adults to simply assume the pattern of abilities and impairments in the start state. In other words, researchers should not directly relate the effects of deleted genes to cognitive-level outcomes in adults. In fact, as we shall see in this book, genetic mutations are more likely to affect low-level basic processes that will have differing, cascading effects on different domains as developmental trajectories emerge over time. Indeed, timing plays a critical role in normal development, and its effects on atypical development must be centre stage when we endeavour to build a comprehensive theory of WS in particular and of neurodevelopmental disorders in general. Moreover, genetic mutations contributing to neurodevelopmental disorders in infants are likely to affect widespread systems within the brain (Karmiloff-Smith, 1998; Chapters 2 and 3). This does not preclude that the outcome of the dynamic developmental process could end up with some areas being more impaired than others. However, this would not be the pattern necessarily apparent at the outset, but would be the result of processing demands of certain kinds of inputs to those areas and to differences in synaptogenesis across various cerebral regions (Huttenlocher, 2002). By contrast, the nativist modular view seriously underestimates the dynamics of the changing patterns of connectivity within and across different brain areas during development.

Another important issue to bear in mind is that typical development also of course involves change, so matching on mental age can at times be very misleading. Indeed, a neurodevelopmental disorder might show a pattern of performance that seems to be atypical when compared with a matched control group. However, this kind of comparison—with a static point in development—neglects the possibility that the performance of the atypical group might resemble a pattern observed somewhere along the developmental trajectory of typical children. A clear illustration of this comes from the visual domain. As will be discussed in Chapter 13, many neurodevelopmental disorders show a relative deficit in dorsal visual stream processing relative ventral visual stream processing. However, this is the case in typical development, too, in that when young (<5 years), children also show poorer dorsal-stream than ventral-stream processing. Care must therefore be taken to determine whether the pattern of performance in an atypical group is delayed or atypical, as this has important implications for our understanding of the constraints on atypical developmental trajectories. This can only be achieved by sampling the whole developmental trajectory in both the typical and the atypical case.

Recent technological advances are now enabling us to take the same cautions in research at the neural level. Imaging of brain activation in children has begun to characterise the developmental trajectories of emerging brain networks. For instance, we will see in

Chapter 16 that the brain network activated during number processing in young children is different from that activated in adults. This questions whether it is appropriate that we rely on what we know about the brain of typical adults to determine whether atypical groups show typical brain activation (Karmiloff-Smith, 2010; Chapter 2). It is entirely possible that the pattern of activation observed in a neurodevelopmental disorder is present somewhere along the typical developmental trajectory of emerging brain networks. Currently, knowledge of the development of typical brain networks remains quite limited, but there is an emerging body of work to suggest that during the next decade we will be in the position to take developmental trajectories into account, not only in terms of behaviour but also in terms of the development of neural networks.

A neuroconstructivist view of remediation

Rather than invoking 'intact' and 'impaired' modules, assessing atypical development in terms of cascading developmental effects of tiny perturbations early in the developmental trajectory should result in a better understanding of genetic disorders in children. However, perhaps the notion of impaired versus intact brain systems in uneven cognitive profiles might be useful for clinical practice, even if theoretically it underplays the role of development. If a patient has scores in the normal range in a specific domain, surely there is no need to consider remediation in that domain? The nativist would probably agree and focus solely on the domains of deficit. However, the neuroconstructivist would not rule out intervention also in a proficient domain. For instance, take a patient who presents with a serious deficit in, say, number but scores in the normal range for all other domains. It would be tempting in such a case to tailor remediation solely to the domain of number. However, that misses the very point of the neuroconstructivist framework. First, the scientist would need to trace back to infancy the origins of the number deficit, which might not be in the number domain directly; it could be a deficit in the visual system in scanning arrays of objects. A scanning deficit might affect other domains but to a lesser degree, meaning that these other domains could look normal in subsequent development but may camouflage subtle deficits. Once one explores multiple, low-level interacting processes that underpin early development, this leads to a more dynamic, neuroconstructivist view of remediation also.

Conclusions

It is clear that development—whether typical or atypical, whether human or nonhuman—is fundamentally characterised by plasticity for learning, with the infant brain dynamically structuring itself over the course of ontogeny. The infant brain is not a collection of static, built-in modules handed down by evolution. Rather, the infant brain follows developmental trajectories that are the emergent property of dynamic multidirectional interactions between biological, physical and social constraints.

About the book

This book places the neuroconstructivist approach to developmental disorders at its very heart. We start in Part 1 with three chapters that take WS as a model syndrome (all studies discussed refer to individuals with the classic WS deletion unless otherwise stated) for the discussion of cognition, brain and genes. The Cognition chapter focuses on the critical issue of building task-specific developmental trajectories for typical development and then judging whether and how atypical developmental trajectories fit or diverge from this trajectory, as well as pinpointing how this approach differs from the usual method of matching on the basis of chronological or mental age. The Brain chapter examines how the WS brain in particular and atypically developing brains in general differ from the typical brain in terms of structure, function, physiology and biochemistry. It particularly stresses the multidirectional interactions between genes, cognition, behaviour and brain, raising such questions as whether, in WS, the parietal cortex starts out smaller or whether it becomes smaller over developmental time because of atypical processing in that region. It bemoans the fact that almost everything we know about the WS brain emanates from studies of adult brains and stresses the need to trace brain anatomy, brain biochemistry and brain function across developmental time, that is, to study the developing brain across time from infancy to adulthood. The chapter also highlights the need for in-depth cross-syndrome comparisons at the cerebral level. The Genes chapter goes well beyond the identification of mutated genes that contribute to syndromic outcomes and focuses mainly on the crucial topic of gene expression. It shows how genes cannot be thought of in terms of static one-to-one mappings between gene function and cognitive outcome, because the temporal and spatial expression of genes changes over developmental time.

The first part is followed by two chapters specifically on WS (Part 2), describing the clinical profile as well as the adult outcomes and the daily problems individuals have in integrating into society. Their fluent language and friendly demeanour is frequently misjudged by others as this can mask their real disabilities. It is clear that a detailed syndrome-specific clinical profile is crucial both for research and for life decisions for individuals with neurodevelopmental disorders, whose problems are not only apparent in early infancy but continue throughout life and into old age. These are concerns of the individuals themselves but also of parents, teachers and policy makers.

Parts 3 and 4 tackle the important issues of how domain-general and domain-specific processes operate in neurodevelopmental disorders. In Part 3, we cover the development of attention, sleep-related learning, memory, executive function and motor planning in WS and other neurodevelopmental disorders. These processes affect specific domains of cognition to varying degrees. Part 4 goes into the details of specific domains such as language, visual perception, visuospatial cognition and visuomotor action, as well as looking at face processing and mental state understanding as they relate to social interaction. One of the particularly interesting cross-syndrome comparisons is between WS and ASD in the social domain, because superficially these conditions seem to present with such different profiles, with people with WS being overly friendly and fascinated by faces, whereas ASD is characterised by aloofness and a distaste for faces. Yet, in reality there are many overlaps between the syndromes, which both culminate in atypical social interaction. We end Part 4 with an account of the domain-specific processes involved in numeracy and literacy.

Part 5 offers a very timely account of how domain-general and domain-specific processes are integrated over developmental time, pointing to numerous important issues about the dynamics of developmental integration processes. Finally, the editors round off the book with a concluding discussion of how a neuroconstructivist, multidisciplinary approach enriches our understanding of neurodevelopmental disorders.

References

Baron-Cohen, S. (1999). Does the study of autism justify minimalist innate modularity? *Learning and Individual Differences*, **10**, 179–91.

Bellugi, U., Marks, S., Bihrle, A.M., & Sabo, H. (1988). Dissociation between language and cognitive functions in Williams syndrome. In D. Bishop, & K. Mogford (Eds), *Language Development in Exceptional Circumstances* (pp. 177–89). Edinburgh: Churchill Livingstone.

Beuren, A.J., Apitz, J., Harmjanz, D. (1962). Supravalvular aortic stenosis in association with mental retardation and a certain facial appearance. *Circulation* **26**, 1235–40.

Bolhuis, J.J., Zijlstra, G.G.O., den Boer-Visser, A.M., & van der Zee, E.A. (2000). Localized neuronal activation in the zebra finch brain is related to the strength of song learning. *Proceedings of the National Academy of Sciences of the USA*, **97**, 2282–85.

Carpenter, P.A., Just, M.A., Keller, T.A., Cherkassky, V., Roth, J.K., & Minshew, N.J. (2001). Dynamic cortical systems subserving cognition: fMRI studies with typical and atypical individuals. In J.L. McClelland & R.S. Siegler (Eds), *Mechanisms of Cognitive Development: Behavioral and Neural Perspectives* (pp. 353–83). Mahwah, NJ: Lawrence Erlbaum.

Casey, B.J., Durston, S. (2006). From behavior to cognition to the brain and back: what have we learned from functional imaging studies of ADHD? *American Journal of Psychiatry*, **163**, 957–60.

Clahsen, H., & Temple, C. (2003). Words and rules in children with Williams syndrome. In Y. Levy & J. Schaeffer (Eds), *Towards a Definition of Specific Language Impairment in Children* (pp. 323–52). Dordrecht: Kluwer.

Cohen, L.G., Celnik, P., Pascualleone, A., Corwell, B., Faiz, L., Dambrosia, J., et al. (1997). Functional relevance of cross-modal plasticity in blind humans. *Nature*, **389**, 180–83.

Elman, J., Bates, E., Johnson, M., Karmiloff-Smith, A., Parisi, D., & Plunkett, K. (1996). *Rethinking Innateness: A Connectionist Perspective on Development*. Cambridge, MA: MIT Press/Bradford Books.

Gottlieb, G. (2007). Probabilistic epigenesis. *Developmental Science*, **10**, 1–11.

Huttenlocher, P.R. (2002). *Neural Plasticity: The Effects of the Environment on the Development of the Cerebral Cortex*. Cambridge, MA: Harvard University Press.

Johnson, M.H. (2001). Functional brain development in humans. *Nature Reviews Neuroscience*, **2**, 475–83.

Johnson, M.H., Halit, H., Grice, S.J., & Karmiloff-Smith, A. (2002). Neuroimaging and developmental disorders: a perspective from multiple levels of analysis. *Development and Psychopathology*, **14**, 521–36.

Kaffman, A. & Meaney, M.J. (2007). Neurodevelopmental sequelae of postnatal maternal care in rodents: clinical and research implications of molecular insights. *Journal of Child Psychology and Psychiatry*, **48**, 224–44.

Karmiloff-Smith, A. (1992). *Beyond Modularity: A Developmental Approach to Cognitive Science*. Cambridge, MA: MIT Press.

Karmiloff-Smith, A. (1998). Development itself is the key to understanding developmental disorders. *Trends in Cognitive Sciences*, **2**, 389–98.

Karmiloff-Smith, A. (2006). The tortuous route from genes to behaviour: a neuroconstructivist approach. *Cognitive, Affective and Behavioural Neuroscience*, **6**, 9–17.

Karmiloff-Smith, A. (2009). Nativism vs neuroconstructivism: rethinking developmental disorders. special issue on the interplay of biology and environment. *Developmental Psychology*, **45**, 56–63.

Karmiloff-Smith, A. (2010). Neuroimaging of the developing brain: taking "developing" seriously. *Human Brain Mapping*, **31**, 934–41.

Karmiloff-Smith, A., Scerif, G., & Ansari, D. (2003). Double dissociations in developmental disorders? Theoretically misconceived, empirically dubious. *Cortex*, **39**, 161–63.

Karmiloff-Smith, A., Scerif, G., & Thomas, M.S.C. (2002). Different approaches to relating genotype to phenotype in developmental disorders. *Developmental Psychobiology*, **40**, 311–22.

Leslie, A.M. (1992). Pretense, autism, and the "theory-of-mind" module. *Current Directions in Psychological Science*, **1**, 18–21.

Mechelli, A., Price, C.J., & Friston, K.J. (2001). Nonlinear coupling between evoked rCBF and BOLD signals: a simulation study of hemodynamic responses. *NeuroImage*, **14**, 862–72.

Mervis, C.B., & Becerra, A.M. (2007). Language and communicative development in Williams syndrome. *Mental Retardation and Developmental Disabilities Research Reviews*, **13**, 3–15.

Persico, A.M., & Bourgeron, T. (2006). Searching for ways out of the autism maze: genetic, epigenetic and environmental clues. *Trends in Neuroscience*, **29**, 349–58.

Piattelli-Palmarini, M. (2001). Speaking of learning. *Nature*, **411**, 887–88.

Pinker, S. (1999). *How the Mind Works*. London: Penguin Books.

Sadato, N., Pascual-Leone, A., Grafman, J., Ibanez, V., Deiber, M.-P., et al. (1996). Activation of the primary visual cortex by Braille reading in blind subjects. *Nature*, **380**, 526–28.

Stromme, P., Bjornstad, P.G., & Ramstad, K. (2002). Prevalence estimation of Williams syndrome. *Journal of Child Neurology*, **17**, 269–71.

Teramitsu, I. & White, S.A. (2007). FoxP2 regulation during undirected singing in adult songbirds. *Journal of Neuroscience*, **26**, 7390–94.

Westermann, G., Thomas, M.S.C., & Karmiloff-Smith, A. (2010). Modelling typical and atypical cognitive development. In U. Goswami (Eds), *Handbook of Childhood Development* (pp. 723–48). Oxford: Wiley-Blackwell.

Williams, J.C., Barratt-Boyes, B.G., & Lowe, J.B. (1961). Supravalvular aortic stenosis. *Circulation*, **24**, 1311–18.

Part 1

Cognition, Brain, Genes

Cognition: The developmental trajectory approach

Michael S. C. Thomas, Harry R. Purser
and Jo Van Herwegen

Introduction

One emphasis of the current volume is on the use of developmental trajectories in the study
of developmental disabilities. This chapter is intended for the reader who wants to find out
about the developmental trajectory approach, and why it can be advantageous for investigating neurodevelopmental disorders such as Williams syndrome (WS). The chapter
focuses on theoretical, methodological and analytical issues surrounding trajectories, but it
is grounded in examples drawn from one aspect of research on WS, that of figurative language development (e.g. understanding the intended meaning of the metaphor 'your hair
is a bird's nest today'). Figurative language is relevant to everyday communication skills,
and it is of theoretical interest because it lies at the interface of language, cognition and
social skills. It therefore brings to the fore issues surrounding the uneven cognitive profile
frequently observed in WS and considered at length elsewhere in this volume (e.g. Chapters
11 and 15). In particular, we consider how the development of figurative language fares in
WS, given the apparent strengths in language and social skills whereas the overall IQ indicates moderate levels of learning disability. The methods we describe are more general,
however, and could be applied to a variety of neurodevelopmental disorders.

The developmental trajectory approach involves constructing functions of task performance against age, thereby allowing developmental change to be compared across typically
and atypically developing groups. Trajectories that link performance to measures of mental
age can be used to ascertain whether any performance difference compared with controls is
commensurate with the developmental state of other measures of cognition in the disorder
group, that is, to reveal the developmental relations that exist within disorders that show
uneven cognitive profiles. Conceptually, the trajectory approach we consider here is very
similar to standard analyses of variance (ANOVA). However, instead of testing the difference
between group means, one evaluates the difference between the straight lines used to depict
the developmental trajectory in each group.

We discuss two applications of this approach in studies of WS. The first is in the domain
of figurative language comprehension, where research indicates that individuals with WS
may access different, less abstract knowledge in figurative language comparisons, despite
the relatively strong verbal abilities found in this disorder. The second is an investigation

of whether lexical-semantic knowledge in WS is in line with receptive vocabulary, where data suggest conventional vocabulary measures may overestimate lexical-semantic knowledge in WS. We discuss the trajectory approach in the context of Karmiloff-Smith's (1998) view that a good understanding of neurodevelopmental disorders depends upon an understanding of the developmental process itself.

The origin of the WS cognitive profile

WS is notable for the uneven cognitive profile observed in the disorder (Karmiloff-Smith, 1998; Mervis et al., 2003). Broadly speaking, language and social skills are a relative strength, whereas visuospatial skills are a relative weakness and overall cognitive ability is below the normal range. But note that these are relative statements. The disorder is caused by a now well-characterised genetic mutation: a significant number of genes are lost from one copy of chromosome 7, which may then have knock-on effects on the expression of multiple other genes across the genome. With respect to cognition, these effects may alter brain development and/or affect ongoing neural function. Certainly, both global and local differences have been observed in brain structure using magnetic resonance imaging measures (Meyer-Lindenberg et al., 2004; Meyer-Lindenberg et al., 2006; see Chapter 2 for a review). The eventual explanation of the WS cognitive profile will involve links between the genetic abnormalities, the differential effects on brain structure and function, the particular cognitive profile as inferred from a battery of behavioural tests, and a characterisation of how the structure of the subjective physical and social environment may be different for the individual with WS, potentially exaggerating the effects of the genetic mutation across development.

Let us consider the WS cognitive profile in more detail. Researchers began their investigation of the disorder by running a battery of standardised tests (e.g. Bellugi et al., 1994; Wang & Bellugi, 1994). Standardised tests are carefully designed to focus on particular cognitive skills. Part of the test construction involves giving the test to a large sample of typically developing (TD) children and adults. This allows for the formulation of tables indicating what performance level on the test should be expected at a given age and to what extent any given performance level is above or below average for that age. Standardised tests have several origins: they are used in education to identify children who are delayed or gifted; they are used with adults for purposes of job recruitment, to identify skill sets; and they are used with adults who have suffered acquired brain damage, to identify whether certain skills have been lost.

When the battery of tests was run on individuals with WS, there were some surprising differences in ability levels. Almost none of the cognitive abilities were at the level one would expect given the individual's chronological age. Initially, it was remarked how language skills (assessed, for example, by a receptive-vocabulary test) seemed to be better than nonverbal abilities, particularly those involving visuospatial construction (such as drawing, or copying designs by arranging coloured blocks). The ability to recognise faces was also a relative strength and seemed linked to the social skills (or at least the overt friendliness) exhibited by individuals with WS (e.g. Bellugi et al., 1994; Pinker, 1994, 1999). The profile was particularly highlighted by using comparisons with other neurodevelopmental disorders. For example, language ability in WS seemed to be better than that in Down syndrome (DS) despite comparable results on a full IQ test (e.g. Wang & Bellugi, 1994). Some language skills seemed to be stronger in individuals with WS than in those with specific language impairment, despite the higher IQs in the latter group (e.g. Ring & Clahsen, 2005). Social skills in WS contrasted with those found in autism, where individuals appear socially withdrawn. Figure 1.1 depicts data from Annaz (2006), who compared test results from TD children with those from children with WS, DS, high-functioning autism or low-functioning autism.

Figure 1.1 reflects the different uneven profiles evident in the four disorders. For children with WS, receptive-vocabulary scores were a little below those for TD children and face recognition was at the same level, but there were marked deficits in the two visuospatial-construction tasks. In children with high-functioning autism, performance was similar to that of TD children and none of the tasks here picked up their difficulty in the autistic diagnostic triad of socialisation, communication and a restricted repertoire of interests. For the children with low-functioning autism, performance on pattern construction was strong,

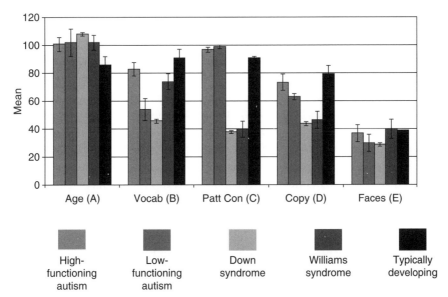

Fig. 1.1 (See also Plate 1) Cross-syndrome comparison of cognitive profiles on four tasks. (A) Mean chronological age (in months). (B) Age equivalent (in months) according to the British Picture Vocabulary Scale. (C) Age equivalent (in months) according to the Pattern Construction subtest of the British Abilities Scales II. (D) Age equivalent (in months) according to the Copying subtest of the British Abilities Scales II. (E) Raw test scores on the Benton Facial Recognition Test. Results are shown for children with high-functioning autism (n=16, 5-11 years of age), low-functioning autism (n=17, 5-11 years of age), Down syndrome (n=15, 6-13 years of age), or Williams syndrome (n=15, 5-12 years of age) and for typically developing children (n=25, 3-12 years of age). Note that the typically developing group had a lower mean chronological age than the disorder groups. The error bars show the standard error of the mean. Data from Annaz (2006).

a little less so for copying, but now there were marked deficits for vocabulary and face recognition. The group with DS, by contrast, scored poorly across all the tasks.

Where do these different uneven cognitive profiles come from? How are they related to the different genetic and environmental causes of each disorder? This is one of the principal questions considered in this book. One way to address this question would be to repeat the same set of tests at progressively younger ages. The data in Figure 1.1 represent a snapshot at a single point in time. If snapshots at younger ages demonstrated the same relative profiles right back into infancy, we might conclude that the underlying causes of the profiles were there from the start. Perhaps they result from the atypical development of parts of the brain responsible for each aspect of the cognitive profile. Perhaps the relevant genetic causes in each disorder only act on these brain mechanisms during development?

There are some practical difficulties in using this method to investigate the origins of the uneven profiles. For example, behavioural tests are often only appropriate over a certain age range. If we want to examine a given behaviour in an 18-month-old versus a 4-year-old versus a 12-year-old, we may have to use different tests. However, this creates the risk that differences in cognitive profiles at different ages may arise from the different tasks we are using. Moreover, tests have different levels of sensitivity in their relation to cognitive processes. If individuals are given a long time to generate their response in, say, pointing to the correct picture out of a set of four that corresponds with a target word, it is possible the individual may use a different strategy to get to the correct answer. The behaviour may look the same even though the process is different. So there might be concerns whether our behavioural measures are necessarily telling us about the nature of the underlying cognitive processes.

Relatedly, there are some theoretical concerns stemming from the fact that many of the behaviours we are measuring from infancy onwards are products of experience-dependent learning processes. There is no vocabulary or grammar system at 6 months. At 18 months, there might be a small vocabulary in typical development, but still little in the way of grammar. Visuospatial construction requires a combination of visual perception, planning and motor control that is not apparent until early childhood. The earlier we get, then, in generating our snapshots, the more we may be looking for 'proto' or seed versions of the systems we are measuring at later ages. And a worry may register at the back of our minds: what is the contribution of the learning process to the cognitive profile we see at later ages?

Even if we manage to generate a set of profile snapshots back to early infancy, there are also theoretical issues to address when attempting to marry up these cognitive-level data to the brain level and genetic level. Current views are that no single brain area is responsible for generating a high-level behaviour; rather, a network of brain areas act together. The relationship of brain areas to behaviour is thus a many-to-one relationship (see Chapter 2). Moreover, genes tend to be involved in the development and maintenance of multiple brain regions: the relationship of genes to brain areas is a many-to-many relationship (Kovas & Plomin, 2006; Chapter 3). Such issues are beyond the scope of this chapter, but they clearly pose a challenge for linking behaviour to cognition, brain and genome.

Perhaps more to the point, however, is that early snapshot data like these have indeed been collected, and the answer is that the cognitive profile of a given disorder does not always look the same at different ages. For example, in WS, when the 'proto' systems for vocabulary and number in toddlers were compared with the developed systems in adulthood, the relative patterns were different. For numerosity judgements, individuals with WS did well in infancy but poorly in adulthood, whereas for language they performed poorly in infancy but well in adulthood (Paterson et al., 1999). In other words, if we use a snapshot of cognitive profiles, these profiles may look different at different ages. An alternative approach is needed.

Developmental trajectories

The main drawback of the snapshot approach is one that has bedevilled many theories of typical development, in particular those that characterise cognitive development as a set of stages through which children pass on their way to adulthood. Such theories raise a difficult question: what are the transitional mechanisms that move a child from one snapshot/stage to the next? Stipulating the nature of these mechanisms lies at the heart of any theory of development, whether it concerns typical or atypical development. To understand development is to understand the causes of change over time. Moreover, the cognitive system comprises many components that continually interact with each other in order to generate behaviour. These components do not develop in isolation but in the context of these interactions. Across development, components become more fine-tuned and sometimes new components are fashioned (e.g. the reading and number systems develop through the protracted, structured experience provided by education). Problems with the development of one component are likely to impact on the other components with which it interacts. Networks of components that interact to deliver function may provide opportunities for better-developing components to compensate for more poorly developing components, offering multiple pathways to developmental success (Thomas, 2010). Together, these factors suggest that developmental theories are best informed by assessing how behaviour changes with age, and such theories will comprise an understanding of the multiple constraints that shape increases in the complexity of behaviour over time. These constraints will include the (possibly atypical) learning properties of cognitive components, the wider network of components in which any one component operates, the structure of the physical and social environment (including the rewards and discouragements it offers) and the motivation of the child.

Instead of snapshots of behaviour, then, the aim of experimental designs should be to construct a function that links changes in task performance with age. Ideally, such designs should assess multiple areas of cognition; they should use measures that are sensitive across a wide age range; they should follow a group of children longitudinally; and they should contrast multiple disorders to reveal which behavioural strengths and weaknesses are specific to that disorder. For practical reasons, many approaches begin with cross-sectional studies, measuring children of different ages. Trajectories generated from cross-sectional studies can later be validated by longitudinal work to see if individual children indeed follow the trajectory predicted by the initial cross-sectional sample. Figure 1.2 (Annaz, 2006) replots the data from Figure 1.1 in the form of developmental trajectories for just two of the standardised tests, the British Picture Vocabulary Scale (BPVS; Dunn et al., 1997) and the Pattern Construction subtest of the British Abilities Scales Second Edition (Elliot et al., 1997). These tests mark one of the strongest and one of the weakest skills in WS, respectively. Age-equivalent score (or 'test age') is one of the scores derived from a standardised test; it indicates the age of the average child who achieves a given score (e.g. on a certain test, a score of 80% correct might be achieved by the average 10-year-old). For TD children, by definition, their test age should be much the same as their chronological age, and this is what is shown on both standardised tests in Figure 1.2. For receptive vocabulary, the WS group shows a developmental trajectory running underneath and parallel to the TD group: in WS, there is a small deficit but development is occurring at the same rate. For pattern construction, by contrast, development is poor: it is at 'floor' (the lowest level of sensitivity for the measure) and only starting to increase after around 8 years of age. The two autistic groups are indistinguishable from the TD group on pattern

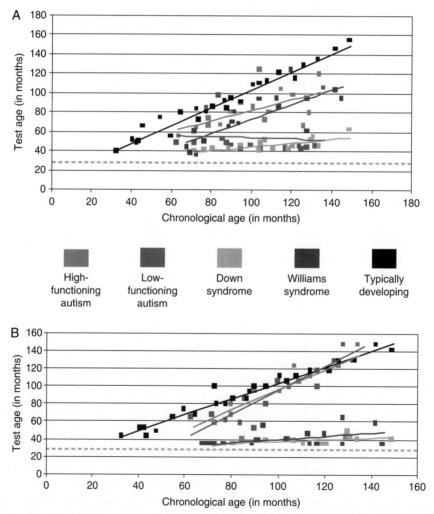

Fig. 1.2 (See also Plate 2) Developmental trajectories for the five groups described in Figure 1.1. (A) British Picture Vocabulary Scale. (B) Pattern Construction subtest of the British Abilities Scales II. The dashed line depicts 'floor' performance on the task. Data from Annaz (2006).

construction, but the low-functioning group reveals floor performance on vocabulary, with the odd notable exception in the group. Lastly, children with DS show floor performance and very slow rates of development for both tasks.

Along with a change in research methodology, the developmental trajectory approach employs a different family of analytical techniques, including analysis of covariance, hierarchical regression and structural equation modelling (Thomas et al., 2009). In this chapter, we focus on the first of these techniques, a relatively straightforward method for comparing group developmental trajectories instead of the group means that are compared in the snapshot approach, usually via ANOVA (see Thomas et al., 2009, for a detailed discussion of the linear trajectories analytic technique, and http://www.psyc.bbk.ac.uk/research/DNL/stats/Thomas_trajectories.html for worked examples).

Comparing linear developmental trajectories

The data in Figure 1.2 demonstrate how straight lines can be used to model the function linking age and task performance. In some cases, nonlinear data can be transformed so that linear methods can be used (e.g. a log-log transformation can be used to linearise the relationship between response time and age). A linear function is defined by two parameters, the intercept (task performance at the earliest age measured) and the gradient (the rate of change in performance with age). When comparing a trajectory for a disorder group with the trajectory for typical development or with the trajectory for another disorder group, linear trajectories may differ in three ways: the intercepts may differ, the gradients may differ or both may differ. When only the intercepts differ (as is the case for receptive vocabulary in WS and typical development), the difference between groups remains the same whatever the age at which a comparison is made. If the gradients differ, then the relationship between the groups will depend on the age at which the comparison is made.

The use of trajectories to compare development across groups allows for a richer vocabulary to describe group differences. In addition to showing different types of delay, groups may differ in the shapes of their trajectories. For example, a disorder group may show a nonlinear trajectory, whereas the typical group shows a linear trajectory. This would happen if performance in the disorder group were to asymptote (reach a ceiling) at a premature level. Relatedly, a group might show a flat trajectory across the age range, suggesting that performance had achieved its maximum level given the developmental constraints of the system. Or there may be no systematic relationship between age and task performance in one of the groups. Comparisons between groups that collapse performance across wide age ranges, such as those shown in Figure 1.1, discard the opportunity to characterise developmental trajectories using this richer vocabulary.

Comparing two groups on a single measure provides a simple between-participants design. The use of two or more tasks per group allows for more complex comparisons, including repeated-measures and mixed designs (analogous to those used in ANOVA). For example, one might use a receptive and a productive language task. The TD group provides an indication of the performance difference one might expect between these two tasks at different ages. Using this information, one can examine whether any individual with a disorder demonstrates the difference one would expect for his or her chronological age. Or indeed, one can ask whether the task difference found in that individual is present at any age in the TD sample, providing the opportunity to identify markers of atypicality on an individual basis.

The above methods consider building a trajectory that links task performance to chronological age, but in many cases we do not expect individuals with disorders to exhibit performance in line with chronological age. In WS, for example, strengths and weaknesses tend to be relative, with almost all skills falling below chronological-age expectations, the Benton face recognition task (Benton, 1983) being one exception (Annaz et al., 2009a). In these cases, the more interesting comparison depends on building trajectories that link task performance to mental age. The logic here is that, since we know that development is occurring more slowly in a given cognitive domain in a group of individuals with a disorder, task performance might be just what you would expect for the developmental stage that the relevant cognitive system has achieved. Standardised tests are the usual way to measure the developmental stage of a cognitive domain. The standardised test is selected for whether the experimental task relates to, say, language or visuospatial skills or reasoning or motor skills. For example, a task requiring an individual to describe the meaning of words relates to the domain of lexical semantics within language. One might then use a standardised test of receptive language, such as the BPVS, to assess the developmental stage of each individual's language system. For each individual, one would then have three scores: task performance on word definitions, the test (mental) age on receptive vocabulary and the child's chronological age. From these data, one can then generate two plots for the group: one that relates task performance to chronological age and one that relates task performance to mental age. The heuristic here is then as follows: if ability A is developing at the same rate as some other (also delayed) ability B, then plotting a trajectory between performance on A and the mental age on ability B will normalise the developmental pattern. That is, if the ability to provide word definitions is delayed, there will be a difference between TD and disorder trajectories when plotted against the chronological age, but the trajectories will lie on top of each other when they are plotted against the mental age according to the receptive-vocabulary test.

Of course, there is no requirement that trajectories are only plotted against mental ages derived from standardised tests. Trajectories can be used to link performance on any pair of tasks and to examine whether an identical relationship exists in the TD and disorder groups. This begins to get us closer to the constraints that are shaping development in disorder and TD groups. For example, if a relationship exists between two tasks A and B in a disorder group but not in the TD group (and assuming neither group is at floor or ceiling on the tasks), one inference is that A is providing a limit on (or support for) the development of B in the disorder group but not in the TD group. If a relationship exists between two tasks A and B in the TD group but not in the disorder group, one inference is that the relevant cognitive systems are not causally interacting in the disorder group. When allied with cross-syndrome comparisons, the developmental trajectory approach provides a powerful source of information on the atypical constraints that can shape the emergence of impaired performance, and in doing so the approach provides a perspective on the constraints that shape typical development. For example, Annaz et al. (2009a) compared the face recognition skills of the children whose data are shown in Figures 1.1 and 1.2. All of the four disorder groups showed impaired task performance compared with the TD group. However, trajectory analyses revealed that development was atypical in *different ways* in the four disorders, and together these disorders shed light on the constraints that must operate in normal development.

We now turn to consider the application of the trajectory approach to one domain of behaviour in WS, that of figurative language development.

Application of the trajectory approach to figurative language development

Figurative language is a good illustration of the point that high-level behaviours require the integration of a number of cognitive systems. For example, let us say that one day while drawing pictures with her mother, a child draws lots of fantastic shapes. Her mother compliments her using a metaphor: 'Your mind is on fire today.' To understand the message (that the child is being very creative), the child must perceive the speech, integrate the meanings of the words with the syntactic structure, know that the sentence is literally false given the context (there are no flames!), juxtapose the two concepts (how thinking and fire can be similar) and so infer the communicative intent (of creativity). Such an integration between systems is particularly relevant for WS because both receptive vocabulary and social skills are viewed as relative strengths, whereas conceptual thinking is viewed as a relative weakness. Which abilities will determine performance: the strongest or the weakest? We will find, perhaps unsurprisingly, that the developmental trajectory approach reveals a more complex picture. In this section, we present three worked examples of the developmental trajectory approach applied to WS, where developmental trajectories were constructed using receptive-vocabulary age.

Development of understanding of nonliteral similarity

The first example is an investigation of the development of understanding of nonliteral similarity, which is a component of metaphor comprehension: in order to understand a metaphorical utterance, one must construe a similarity between two terms yet also realise that those terms belong to separate conventional categories, as in 'thinking' and 'fire' in the example above (e.g. Bowdle & Gentner, 2005). Thus, assessing the ability to understand nonliteral similarity statements is an initial step in investigating metaphor comprehension because such understanding necessitates knowing that entities can be similar to each other despite belonging to different semantic or conceptual categories.

Comprehension of nonliteral similarity is also involved in other types of figurative language, such as irony, analogy, idioms and proverbs, which together constitute a significant component of everyday communicative interactions. To investigate nonliteral similarity, Thomas and colleagues (2010) began by administering a simple picture-based categorisation task to individuals with WS, TD children aged 4–11 years and TD adults. In a paradigm adapted from Vosniadou and Ortony (1983), the participants were required to complete similarity comparison statements and categorisation statements (e.g. 'Eyes are like . . .?' or 'Eyes are the same kind of thing as . . .?') by choosing one of two response words. The pairs

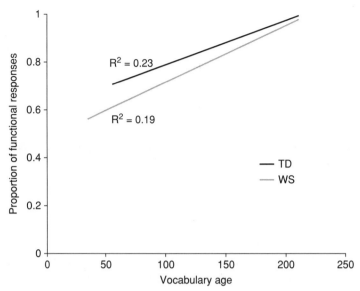

Fig. 1.3 Proportion of functional responses plotted against verbal mental age in the comparison task: functional–anomalous contrast (e.g. responses to the question 'Are eyes like a camera or like a wall?'). R^2 is the proportion of variance in the data points accounted for by the best-fit trajectory. Abbreviations: TD = typically developing, WS = Williams syndrome. Data from Thomas et al. (2010).

of response words were formed from items that were literally, perceptually or functionally similar to the target word or else anomalous (e.g. 'ears', 'buttons', 'camera' or 'wall', respectively). Participants' justifications of responses were also recorded to gain an insight into how responses were selected. The logic of the study (after Vosniadou & Ortony, 1983) was that selecting nonliteral or literal responses to similarity statements ('like') instead of anomalous responses justified attributing the ability to recognise similarity across categories. For categorisation statements ('same kind of thing'), the response given was taken as evidence of having conceptual categories organised on the basis of the type of response, i.e. selecting literal responses over anomalous ones reflected knowledge of literal categories.

For the purposes of illustrating the developmental trajectory approach, we will focus on functional similarity. Eyes and a camera perform the same function of processing images, even though they may be perceived as looking quite different. A pair of buttons, by contrast, may look perceptually similar to eyes without sharing any similar function. Figure 1.3 shows that the proportion of functional responses over anomalous ones tended to increase with increasing vocabulary age (as measured by the BPVS; Dunn et al., 1997). This relationship was very similar for both groups, indicating that individuals with WS develop an understanding of functional similarity in the typical way. In tandem with this emerging understanding of functional similarity, the TD group also showed an increasing preference for functionally related responses over perceptually related ones with increasing vocabulary age in the comparison task, depicted in Figure 1.4. We call this a preference because an understanding of perceptual similarity was clearly demonstrated by even the

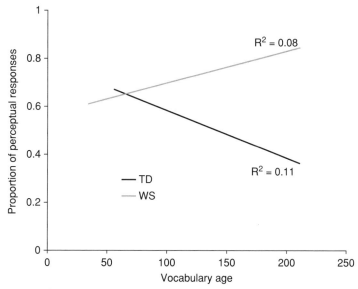

Fig. 1.4 Proportion of perceptual responses plotted against verbal mental age in the comparison task: functional/perceptual contrast (e.g. responses to the question 'Are eyes like a camera or a [pair of] buttons?'). Abbreviations: TD = typically developing, WS = Williams syndrome. Data from Thomas et al. (2010).

youngest TD participants. However, Figure 1.4 also shows that such an increasing preference for functionally similar items with increasing vocabulary ability was absent from the WS group. In view of the finding that people with WS clearly do learn about functional similarity, this group difference in functional responding, even given receptive vocabulary, cannot be attributable to a lack of understanding of functional relations in the WS group. The implication is that although TD children develop a grouping of concepts on the basis of functional nonliteral similarity in addition to literal similarity, individuals with WS may not, despite acquiring the requisite knowledge to do so (i.e. assimilation rather than accommodation). The results of this study are consistent with the notion that where individuals with WS use figurative language, they may do so without fully understanding the abstract relations that underlie it (see Bertrand et al., 1994).

Development of lexical-semantic knowledge

For our second example, additional evidence for a dissociation between language use and language knowledge in WS was found in a related study by Thomas and colleagues (Purser et al., 2011). This study investigated the development of lexical-semantic knowledge using the developmental trajectory approach. Lexical-semantic knowledge was assessed with the definitions task (in which participants are asked to define words; e.g. 'What is an elephant?') and also with a novel categorisation task that involved sorting toy animals into semantic categories (participants were asked questions such as 'Which live in the sea?' and 'Which lay eggs?'). The latter task was designed to avoid the metacognitive demands of the definitions task, such as knowing what a definition is and understanding

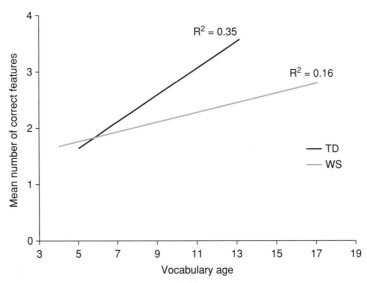

Fig. 1.5 Mean number of features given by participants in the definitions task plotted against verbal mental age in years. Abbreviations: TD = typically developing, WS = Williams syndrome. Data from Purser et al. (2011).

that the task requires listing features or attributes of the target concept in descending order of salience and diagnosticity. The domain of animals was chosen to make the tasks as easy as possible for participants with WS, because it has been shown that individuals with WS as young as 10 years have similar basic knowledge in this area as controls matched for verbal mental age (Johnson & Carey, 1998). Verbal mental age was once more assessed via the BPVS (Dunn et al., 1997).

Figure 1.5 shows the two groups' performances on the definitions task. The WS group's performance began at a level appropriate for vocabulary age, but then the TD group improved more steeply than the WS group. The gradients of the trajectories rather than the intercepts differed. In the categorisation task (Figure 1.6), the WS group's performance developed at a similar rate to that of the TD group, but was markedly poorer on average than predicted by vocabulary age. Here the intercepts differed but not the gradients. This pattern of results suggests that individuals with WS have a lower level of lexical-semantic knowledge than expected given their receptive vocabulary (an area, remember, that tends to be a relative strength in WS), although this knowledge increases with advancing vocabulary age at a similar rate to that seen in typical development. Of potential importance is the implication that vocabulary tests such as the BPVS might overestimate lexical-semantic knowledge in individuals with WS, so that the use of other more general tests is recommended for assessing language ability in this population.

Considering these two studies together, the importance of attempting to measure development rather than using matching methods is clear: some differences between groups that are marked at one point in development are not apparent at another point. The preference for functional similarity is something that emerges across typical development,

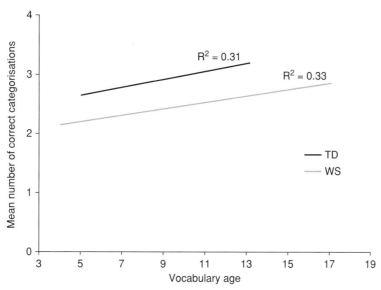

Fig. 1.6 Mean number of correct categorisations plotted against verbal mental age in years. Abbreviations: TD = typically developing, WS = Williams syndrome. Data from Purser et al. (2011).

whereas there is no sign of it ever appearing for individuals with WS. The disparity between WS and TD lexical-semantic knowledge is stable across development, whereas the meta-cognitive demands of the definitions task increasingly disadvantage the WS group at higher ability levels. This kind of information is not only unavailable in matched designs, but such designs discourage a developmental scientific vocabulary; they discourage us from thinking developmentally.

Development of metaphor and metonym comprehension

Compared with vocabulary and grammar, pragmatic skills have been less explored in WS. Pragmatic skills relate to the ability to use language within a social context. Because fluent communication skills and the overly social behavioural profile are often found in WS, pragmatics has sometimes been assumed not to be a weakness (Rice et al., 2005). However, when Laws and Bishop (2004) investigated pragmatic skills in 19 children and young adults with WS and compared their outcome on the Children's Communication Checklists with that of individuals with DS or specific language impairment and with TD children, participants with WS showed poorer social relationships, restricted interests and overall pragmatic language impairments. These included stereotyped conversation, inappropriate initiation of conversation and use of conversational rapport (Laws & Bishop, 2004). Karmiloff-Smith and colleagues (1995) carried out an early study with 11 adults with WS and asked them to explain what the protagonist meant by sarcastic and metaphorical statements in stories. Half of the adults failed to explain the meaning of the metaphors and sarcastic expressions used in their study (Karmiloff-Smith et al., 1995). Sullivan and colleagues (2003) investigated the understanding of ironic jokes in older children and adults with WS, in comparison with those with Prader–Willi syndrome and nonspecific learning disability. In this study, the participants were presented with four stories, after which they were asked a question about what the speaker had meant by an ironic joke or sarcastic statement and were also asked to give a justification of their answer. Adolescents with WS failed to classify the ironic jokes as such and judged them to be lies. The participants with Prader–Willi syndrome and nonspecific mental retardation showed similar deficits. The participants with WS differed in that they justified their answer by looking at the facts of what happened in the scenarios, whereas the other two groups focused on the mental states of the characters. This study thus showed that participants with WS have difficulty in distinguishing lies from jokes, which sits uncomfortably with claims about good language abilities and social skills in WS (Sullivan et al., 2003).

Idioms are figurative expressions established by usage in which the meaning cannot be deduced from the individual words, such as 'kick the bucket'. Mervis and colleagues (2003) investigated the understanding of idioms in adolescents and adults with WS in relation to conservation abilities. Conservation relates to the logical understanding that some properties of an object remain constant even though the object has undergone some transformation – for example the realisation that even though a fixed amount of water looks more in a small, thin glass than in a low, fat glass, the amounts are the same in each case. The ability to conserve has been linked to the understanding of idioms because for these expressions, the listener has to ignore the surface meaning but keep deeper underlying meanings active. It therefore relates the linguistic phenomenon to the underlying conceptual skills. In total, Mervis et al. (2003) tested 37 adults and adolescents with WS on the comprehension of idioms using the Familiar and Novel Language Comprehension Test from Kempler and Van Lancker (1996). In this task, the participant is asked to select the meaning of the sentence produced by the researcher from four pictures. In the participants with WS, the understanding of idioms was significantly poorer (mean of correct answers 5.95 out of 16) than the understanding of literal language (mean 12.95 out of 16). Furthermore, the performance on the comprehension of idioms correlated strongly with the number of conservation problems solved. Conceptual abilities therefore appeared to be the limiting factor in idiom comprehension.

This brings us to our third example. These studies provided snapshots of performance in adults. Although they indicated that figurative language is a problem domain for individuals with WS, there is no insight into the developmental origins of the difficulty. Metaphor and metonymy are two types of figurative expressions in which a topic is linked to a vehicle based upon the fact that they share some common ground (to use the terminology in that literature). In a metaphor (e.g. 'your hair is a bird's nest'), the topic (hair) and vehicle (bird's nest) belong to different conceptual domains (i.e. a body feature versus an animal's abode) but are linked by a shared feature (physical appearance of spiky untidiness). In a metonym (e.g. 'the policeman directed the bus, meaning the policeman instructed the driver of the bus where to go'), the two terms belong to the same conceptual domain (i.e. the term 'bus' is used here to refer to the bus driver, not the bus itself). Figure 1.7 demonstrates the development of metaphor and metonym comprehension in children with WS compared with TD children, using a developmental trajectory approach (Annaz et al., 2009b). As shown in Figure 1.7, although there was a reliable relationship between

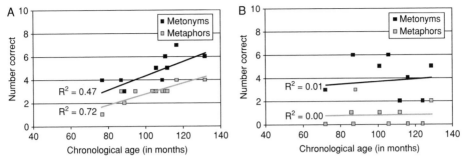

Fig. 1.7 Developmental trajectories linking performance on the metonym and metaphor comprehension tasks with chronological age. (A) Typical development. (B) Williams syndrome. Data are shown from 10 participants with Williams syndrome and 10 typically developing children between the ages of 6 and 10 years. In this task, the children were read 20 short stories that incorporated a metaphor or metonymy and were then asked to explain what the expression referred to. Abbreviations: TD = typically developing, WS = Williams syndrome. Data from Annaz et al. (2009b).

performance and increasing chronological age in TD children for both metaphors and metonyms, performance in children with WS did not improve with increasing chronological age for either metaphor or metonymy. Group comparisons showed that overall performance in the WS group was lower compared with the TD group: performance in children with WS was not at the level expected for their chronological age. Nevertheless, there was an advantage for metonymy comprehension over metaphors in both groups, indicating that comprehension of metonyms is easier than metaphor.

Performance on metaphors and metonymy comprehension between the two groups was then compared using trajectories built either against receptive-vocabulary mental age (once more, as measured by the BPVS; Dunn et al., 1997) or visuospatial-construction mental age (as measured by the Pattern Construction subtest of the British Ability Scales (BAS-II; Elliot et al., 1997) shown in Figures 1.8 and 1.9. These analyses showed that participants with WS performed at a similar level to TD children when performance on metonymy was plotted against their vocabulary comprehension abilities, but was worse than

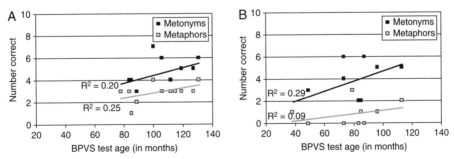

Fig. 1.8 Developmental trajectories linking performance on the metonym and metaphor comprehension tasks with receptive-vocabulary mental age as measured by the British Picture Vocabulary Scale. Abbreviations: TD = typically developing, WS = Williams syndrome. Data from Annaz et al. (2009b).

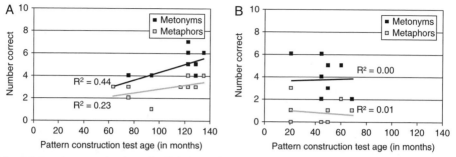

Fig. 1.9 Developmental trajectories linking performance on the metonym and metaphor comprehension tasks with visuospatial-construction mental age as measured by the Pattern Construction subtest of the British Abilities Scales II. Abbreviations: TD = typically developing, WS = Williams syndrome. Data from Annaz et al. (2009b).

expected on metaphors. Following the heuristic we outlined earlier, if replotting a trajectory against mental age instead of chronological age aligns the disorder trajectory with the TD trajectory, then development in the ability is in line with the developmental stage of the system measured by the standardised test. Metonymy was in step with the developmental stage of the language system but metaphor was not. By comparison, performance on neither metonymy nor metaphors was in line with the visuospatial abilities in WS.

The results from this study demonstrate that both metaphor and metonymy comprehension in children with WS were below the level expected for their chronological age, reflecting the difficulty that these children experience with figurative language. The facts that comprehension of metonymy developed earlier than metaphor in both groups and that metonymy comprehension but not metaphor was in line with receptive-vocabulary scores in children with WS suggest that these two types of expressions require at least partially separate sets of cognitive mechanisms (Annaz et al., 2009b; Rundblad & Annaz, 2010).

While the study from Annaz and colleagues (2009b) was the first to use the developmental trajectory approach to provide information on metaphor and metonymy comprehension in individuals with WS, the study only investigated lexicalised metaphors and metonyms. These are familiar expressions that might have been encountered before and thus their meaning might have been stored in the mental lexicon (Bowdle & Gentner, 2005). For example, after frequently encountering the phrase 'Karen is a cold woman', a person might store the term 'cold' as a polysemous word with two independent but conceptually related meanings, namely a literal meaning as in 'cold weather' and a nonliteral meaning as in 'a cold person', meaning an unemotional person (Geiger & Ward, 1999). Therefore, for lexicalised expressions a meaning can be derived in two ways: if an expression has been encountered before, the meaning can be directly retrieved from the mental lexicon (sense selection); alternatively, a meaning can be created (sense creation) upon encountering the expression similar to the way in which a meaning is created when making up novel expressions (Bowdle & Gentner, 2005; Glucksberg, 1989). However, it is unclear for which expressions children can directly access a meaning in the mental lexicon and for which ones the meaning needs to be created online, especially for children with neurodevelopmental disorders who show an overall language delay. Thus, examining trajectories for the comprehension of novel expressions will be more informative about the developmental processing generating behaviour in typical and atypical groups (Van Herwegen et al., in preparation).

Additionally, it is important to complement the use of standardised tests and investigate what other cognitive abilities are related to metaphor and metonymy comprehension in WS. In particular, there is a need for studies that use tests that are sensitive enough to measure variations in performance in both typical and atypical groups. For example, Annaz and colleagues (2009b) plotted performance against mental ages derived from the BPVS and Pattern Construction tests. However, individuals with WS generally score higher on receptive-vocabulary tasks than on other language tasks (Brock, 2007) and performance on pattern construction is very poor (indeed, as Figure 1.2 shows, perform-ance is sometimes at floor on this task; see also Farran & Jarrold, 2003). It is important to note that performance at floor and ceiling level can cause artefacts in the trajectory (Thomas et al., 2009). Thus, the fact that visuospatial abilities do not relate to metaphor and metonymy comprehension in WS might be explained by performance at floor level on pattern construction. The next step is to explore the developmental relationship between metaphor, metonymy and other potentially relevant cognitive abilities such as theory-of-mind abilities, semantic knowledge and inferencing abilities (Rundblad et al., in preparation).

Returning to the broader point, figurative language lies at the interface of language and cognition and therefore targets a key aspect of the uneven cognitive profile found in WS. Although some people with WS have been reported to make use of figurative conversa-tional devices, the relationship to conceptual understanding has been unclear. The use of such devices tends to be somewhat inappropriate to the social context or involve *non sequiturs* (Bertrand et al., 1994; Udwin & Yule, 1990). The results from the metaphor and metonymy study suggest that figurative language may be deployed as a kind of 'frozen' vocabulary, whereby each phrase is retrieved fully formed from memory rather than created by online processes. This would explain why metonymy was in line with receptive vocabu-lary, whereas metaphor, which is more cognitively demanding, was further delayed. The use of frozen language by people with WS may lead to an overestimation of language abilities by parents/carers, teachers and peers, resulting in people with WS meeting language that they do not understand. Such difficulties in language comprehension have clear ramifications for effective tuition and would contribute to the difficulties in social interaction identified in children and adolescents with WS (e.g. Gosch & Pankau, 1997).

Challenges to the developmental trajectory approach

Despite our emphasis that a developmental perspective is central to understanding the origins of neurodevelopmental disorders (see Karmiloff-Smith, 1998), it is fruitful to consider arguments that have been raised against the approach. There are simple practical reasons why a developmental trajectory approach might not be appropriate. If a behaviour appears over a very short period of time, then charting behavioural change over a wide age range will be of little benefit. Nevertheless, some researchers have also posed theoretical challenges about the need to adopt a developmental perspective at all, and we consider one such challenge in this section.

In 2002, Thomas and Karmiloff-Smith questioned the 'residual normality' assumption for neurodevelopmental disorders. The assumption entails that atypical development can produce selective deficits while the rest of the system develops in a normal manner. We have seen previously the suggestion that the interactivity of cognitive components across development makes it seem unlikely that components can develop in isolation, in either typical or impaired fashion. Thomas and Karmiloff-Smith (2002) employed connectionist simulations of development to show how the assumption of isolated atypical development against a background of typical development would be undermined by the process of compensation or deficit spread (see also Baughman & Thomas, 2008). Isolated impairment (or indeed typical development) would only occur under very particular developmental conditions. They therefore concluded that making inferences about what patterns of behavioural deficits imply about the underlying cognitive structures crucially depends on how the actual process of development works in the system.

Nevertheless, this conclusion has recently been questioned by Machery (2011). Machery argues that the critical test of residual normality is to compare end states of typical and atypical systems, rather than to consider development. This is because development is often robust in biological systems, with many pathways leading to the same end state or goal state. Deviant development may nevertheless lead to a typical mature system. Machery's view is tied up with a commitment to the massive-modularity hypothesis, in which every cognitive function is served by a distinct cognitive component (although this position need not be aligned to a commitment that these components are necessarily innate; see Fodor, 1983; Machery, 2011). Massive modularity entails a one-to-one mapping of function to neural substrate (see also Chapter 2 for criticism of the one-to-one mapping view). One striking difficulty with this view is the question of granularity: is there a module for language? One for syntax versus one for vocabulary? Separate modules for different aspects of syntax? Should we attribute a dedicated module to a given cognitive function as soon as we can dissociate it from other cognitive functions experimentally or statistically?

The theoretical picture is complicated by more nuanced hypotheses. For example, an alternative view is that aspects of language may be subserved by relatively independent component processes, and these components are available to and used by several experimentally dissociable language functions. There is multiplicity but there is also sharing. One reason for positing some degree of shared resources is the implausibility of positing a cognitive module for each cognitive function that is fractionated in WS. In 2006, Thomas argued that the recent history of research into cognition in WS had served to reveal ever-finer details of fractionation in the cognitive profile. To take one example, although Mervis and colleagues (Mervis et al., 1999) found a normal relationship between utterance length and syntactic complexity in WS, overall supposition of TD grammar in WS is not justified: closer inspection reveals inconsistent patterns within grammar itself. More errors are made in morphology than in syntax (Karmiloff-Smith et al., 1997); within morphology, more errors are found in irregular verbs than regular verbs (Clahsen

& Almazan, 1998; though see Thomas et al., 2001); within syntax, there is fractionated development yielding behaviours that are appropriate for neither chronological nor mental age (Grant et al., 2002; Mervis et al., 1999). For example, Mervis et al. (1999) reported that performance on the Test for Reception of Grammar (Bishop, 1983) was particularly poor for complex constructions such as relative clauses and embedded sentences. Such fine-level differentiation could be resolved by the more nuanced position involving resource sharing: perhaps more complex grammatical forms rely more on short-term memory than simpler forms and it is the short-term memory system that is compromised.

Another reason for focusing on development rather than its end point is that we, as developmental psychologists, are trying to advance understanding of how language develops and functions and of the processes by which it can go awry. An appeal to modules is static and can lessen our theoretical understanding. For example, explaining the acquisition of complex syntactic rules by positing a complex syntactic grammar module that simply comes 'online' (i.e. is turned on) at some point in development sheds little light on the origins of behaviour. Mechanistic explanations are required to explain how cognitive functions come into existence. Indeed, one reasonable test of a snapshot or end state explanation is to attempt to couch it in developmental terms. Given the importance of comparing developmental versus snapshot accounts, in the following paragraphs we offer a worked example. What happens when we try to change a snapshot account into a developmental theory?

Machery (2011) cites a small study by Clahsen and Almazan (1998) as an example of how WS can be used to support the massive-modularity hypothesis. The relevant finding of the study is that the four participants with WS presented poorer performance on inflecting irregular past tenses (e.g. 'went' from 'go') than on inflecting regular ones ('walked' from 'walk'). The authors presented the following explanation: 'The common property shared by the unimpaired linguistic phenomena is that they involve computational knowledge of language, whereas the impaired phenomena involve (specific kinds of) lexical knowledge, i.e. the retrieval of subnode information from lexical entries. Thus, it seems that for children with WS, the computational system for language is selectively spared yielding excellent performance on syntactic tasks and on regular inflection, whereas the lexical system and/or its access mechanisms required for irregular inflection are impaired.' On this account, then, people with WS have problems accessing 'subnodes', but not in accessing the nodes themselves (because accessing nodes must be necessary in order to append an '-ed' to them in computing the regular past-tense form.)

Thomas and Karmiloff-Smith (2005) suggested that at least three learning mechanisms would be necessary to turn this snapshot explanation of the deficit into a developmental account: first, an ability to encode the relationship between present- and past-tense forms; second, a mechanism for storing lexical entries (nodes); and third, a mechanism for attaching subentries to these lexical items (subnodes; grammatically related forms of the main-node lexical entry). However, as soon as one imputes learning abilities to the static system, new questions are raised. Why can the node learning system not compensate for the impairment to the subnode learning system? It would merely need to store the errant subnodes as nodes in order to deliver normal-looking behaviour, for example by storing and accessing 'went' independently of 'go'. As Thomas and Karmiloff-Smith (2005) emphasised, such compensation *cannot* be available if there is to be a behavioural impairment with irregular past-tense formation. Why not? The end state account of the deficit is inadequate here because the most obvious developmental extension suggests that a compensatory route should be available. And if there were such a route, there would be no behavioural deficit in the first place. The snapshot model would need a more complicated developmental account attached to it, with ad-hoc reasons why particular modes of learning were not available. The implication is that once considered within a developmental framework, the initial snapshot characterisation of the behavioural deficit is itself incorrect.

Returning, then, to Machery's argument that the critical test of residual normality is to compare end states of typical and atypical systems, our worked example indicates that it is impossible to do so without considering developmental processes for the purpose of constraining our hypotheses about what those end states really are. Without considering how a cognitive process could develop and upon what simpler processes it could rely, our characterisation of the end state may remain superficial or be entirely incorrect. We may end up postulating an incorrect set of functional components, that is, with an implausible cognitive ontology.

Conclusion

We have argued that neurodevelopmental disorders need to be construed within a developmental framework, particularly when we wish to explain why some disorders display marked unevenness in their cognitive profiles. Such a construal is aided by the use of empirical designs that emphasise the dimension of development, that is, change over time. These designs in turn rely on particular analytical techniques, such as the construction of developmental trajectories. In this chapter, we considered the basics of one such analytical approach and illustrated the approach with the example of the development of figurative language abilities in Williams syndrome. This ability lies at the interface of language and cognition and thus targets a key aspect of the characteristic uneven cognitive profile observed in this neurodevelopmental disorder. The future will involve more complex use of developmental designs, complemented by longitudinal data, cross-syndrome comparisons and ultimately cross-level trajectories, as we begin to understand the developmental relationships between genes, brain, cognition, environment and behaviour.

Editor commentary (Emily K. Farran & Annette Karmiloff-Smith)

This chapter focused on the central question throughout this book, that is, the importance of the process of development itself for understanding neurodevelopmental disorders. Here, the chapter tackled head-on the issue of chronological-age and mental-age matching, and offered an alternative approach. The authors compare the commonly used 'snapshot' approach, in which level of ability is determined at a static time point in the developmental process, with the developmental trajectory approach, where changes in ability over developmental time are explored. This neuroconstructivist approach enables us to explore the constraints (in this case cognitive constraints) that shape the emergence of a particular skill and its rate of development, and how this compares with typical development or with development in other atypical groups. Using this technique, one can explore not only cross-syndrome dissociations but also the causes of cross-syndrome associations, which, as we will learn throughout this book, often differ for different syndrome groups. The chapter showed that seemingly similar levels of impairment can stem from very different patterns of atypical development. Knowledge about the specifics of the developmental process is critical for answering questions related to how behavioural functions develop and how other cognitive abilities, genes, brain development and the individual's environment influence that developmental process.

References

Annaz, D. (2006). *The Development of Visuospatial Processing in Children with Autism, Down Syndrome, and Williams Syndrome*. PhD thesis, University of London.

Annaz, D., Karmiloff-Smith, A., Johnson, M. H., & Thomas, M. S. C. (2009a). A cross-syndrome study of the development of holistic face recognition in children with autism, Down syndrome and Williams syndrome. *Journal of Experimental Child Psychology*, **102**, 456–86.

Annaz, D., Van Herwegen, J., Thomas, M., Fishman, R., Karmiloff-Smith, A., & Rundblad, G. (2009b). Comprehension of metaphor and metonymy in children with Williams syndrome. *International Journal of Language and Communication Disorders*, **44**, 962–78.

Baughman, F.D., & Thomas, M.S.C. (2008). Specific impairments in cognitive development: a dynamical systems approach. In B.C. Love, K. McRae, & V.M. Sloutsky (Eds), *Proceedings of the 30th Annual Conference of the Cognitive Science Society* (pp. 1819–24). Austin, TX: Cognitive Science Society.

Bellugi, U., Wang, P.P., & Jernigan, T.L. (1994). Williams syndrome: an unusual neuropsychological profile. In S. Broman, & J. Grafman (Eds), *Atypical Cognitive Deficits in Developmental Disorders: Implications for Brain Function* (pp. 23–56). Hillsdale, NJ: Lawrence Erlbaum.

Benton, A., Hamsher, K., Varney, N.R., & Spreen, O. (1983). *Benton Test of Facial Recognition*. New York, NY: Oxford University Press.

Bertrand, J., Mervis, C.B., Armstrong, S.C., Ayers, J. (1994). *Figurative Language and Cognitive Abilities of Adults with Williams Syndrome*. Presented at the 1994 National Williams Syndrome Professional Conference, La Jolla, CA.

Bishop, D.V.M. (1983). *The Test for Reception of Grammar*. Manchester: Age and Cognitive Performance Research Centre, University of Manchester.

Bowdle, B., & Gentner, D. (2005). The career of metaphor. *Psychological Review*, **112**, 193–216.

Brock, J. (2007). Language abilities in Williams syndrome: a critical review. *Development and Psychopathology*, **19**, 97–127.

Clahsen, H., & Almazan, M. (1998). Syntax and morphology in Williams syndrome. *Cognition*, **68**, 167–98.

Dunn, L.M., Dunn, L.M., Whetton, C., & Burley, J. (1997). *British Picture Vocabulary Scale Second Edition*. Windsor: NFER-Nelson.

Elliot, C.D., Smith, P., & McCulloch, K. (1997). *British Ability Scales Second Edition*. London: NFER-Nelson.

Farran, E.K., & Jarrold, C. (2003). Visuo-spatial cognition in Williams syndrome: Reviewing and accounting for the strengths and weaknesses in performance. *Developmental Neuropsychology*, **23**, 175–202.

Fodor, J.A. (1983). *Modularity of Mind: An Essay on Faculty Psychology*. Cambridge, MA: MIT Press.

Geiger, O., & Ward, L. (1999). Metaphors and the mental lexicon. *Brain and Language*, **68**, 192–98.

Glucksberg, S. (1989). Metaphors in conversation: How are they understood? Why are they used? *Metaphor and Symbol*, **4**, 125–43.

Gosch, A., & Pankau, R. (1997). Personality characteristics and behaviour problems in individuals of different ages with Williams syndrome. *Developmental Medicine and Child Neurology*, **39**, 527–33.

Grant, J., Valian, V., & Karmiloff-Smith, A. (2002). A study of relative clauses in Williams syndrome. *Journal of Child Language*, **29**, 403–16.

Johnson, S.C., & Carey, S. (1998). Knowledge enrichment and conceptual change in folkbiology: evidence from Williams syndrome. *Cognitive Psychology*, **37**, 156–200.

Karmiloff-Smith, A. (1998). Development itself is the key to understanding developmental disorders. *Trends in Cognitive Sciences*, **2**, 389–98.

Karmiloff-Smith, A., Grant, J., Berthoud, I., Davies, M., Howlin, P., & Udwin, O. (1997). Language and Williams syndrome: how intact is "intact"? *Child Development*, **68**, 246–62.

Karmiloff-Smith, A., Klima, E., Bellugi, U., Grant, J., & Baron-Cohen, S. (1995). Is there a social module? Language, face processing and Theory of Mind in individuals with Williams syndrome. *Journal of Cognitive Neuroscience*, **7**, 196–208.

Kempler, D., & Van Lancker, D. (1996). *Familiar and Novel Language Comprehension Test (FANL-C)* [unpublished manuscript] <http://blog.emerson.edu/daniel_kempler/fanlc.html> accessed 28 June 2011.

Kovas, Y., & Plomin, R. (2006). Generalist genes: implications for the cognitive sciences. *Trends in Cognitive Sciences*, **10**, 198–203.

Laws, G., & Bishop, D.V.M. (2004). Pragmatic language impairment and social deficits in Williams syndrome: a comparison with Down's syndrome and specific language impairment. *International Journal of Language and Communication Disorders*, **39**, 45–64.

Machery, E. (2011). Developmental disorders and cognitive architecture. In P.R. Adriaens & A. De Block (Eds), *Maladapting Minds: Philosophy, Psychiatry, and Evolutionary Theory* (pp. 91–116). Oxford: Oxford University Press.

Mervis, C.B., Morris, C.A., Bertrand, J., & Robinson, B.F. (1999). Williams syndrome: findings from an integrated program of research. In H. Tager-Flusberg (Ed.), *Neurodevelopmental disorders* (pp. 65–110). Cambridge, MA: MIT Press.

Mervis, C.B., Robinson, B.F., Rowe, M.L., Becerra, A.M., & Klein-Tasman, B.P. (2003). Language abilities in individuals with Williams syndrome. In L. Abbeduto (Ed.), *International Review of Research in Mental Retardation*, vol. 27 (pp. 35–81). Orlando, FL: Academic Press.

Meyer-Lindenberg, A., Kohn, P., Mervis, C.B., Kippenhan, S., Olsen, R.K., Morris, C.A., et al. (2004). Neural basis of genetically determined visuospatial construction deficit in Williams syndrome. *Neuron*, **43**, 623–31.

Meyer-Lindenberg, A., Mervis, C.B., & Berman, K.F. (2006). Neural mechanisms in Williams syndrome: a unique window to genetic influences on cognition and behaviour. *Nature Reviews Neuroscience*, **7**, 379–92.

Paterson, S., Brown, J.H., Gsödl, M., Johnson, M.H., & Karmiloff-Smith, A. (1999). Cognitive modularity and genetic disorders. *Science*, **286**, 2355–58.

Pinker, S. (1994). *The Language Instinct*. London: Penguin Books.

Pinker, S. (1999). *Words and Rules*. London: Weidenfeld & Nicolson.

Purser, H.R.M., Thomas, M.S.C., Snoxall, S., Mareschal, D., & Karmiloff-Smith, A. (2011). Definitions versus categorisation: assessing the development of lexico-semantic knowledge in Williams syndrome. *International Journal of Language and Communication Disorders*, **46**, 361–73.

Rice, M., Warren, S., & Betz, S. (2005). Language symptoms of developmental language disorders: an overview of autism, Down syndrome, fragile X, specific language impairment and Williams syndrome. *Applied Psycholinguistics*, **26**, 7–27.

Ring, M., & Clahsen, H. (2005). Distinct patterns of language impairment in Down's syndrome, Williams syndrome, and SLI: the case of syntactic chains. *Journal of Neurolinguistics*, **18**, 479–501.

Rundblad, G., & Annaz, D. (2010). Development of metaphor and metonymy comprehension: receptive vocabulary and conceptual knowledge. *British Journal of Developmental Psychology*, **28**, 547–63.

Rundblad, G., Annaz, D., & Van Herwegen, J. (in preparation). Comprehension of lexicalised metaphor and metonymy in Williams syndrome.

Sullivan, K., Winner, E., & Tager-Flusberg, H. (2003). Can adolescents with Williams syndrome tell the difference between lies and jokes? *Developmental Neuropsychology,* **23**, 85–103.

Thomas, M.S.C. (2006). Williams syndrome: fractionations all the way down? *Cortex,* **42**, 1053–57.

Thomas, M.S.C. (2010). Language acquisition in developmental disorders. In M. Kail & M. Hickmann (Eds), *Language Acquisition across Linguistic and Cognitive Systems* (pp. 67–87). Amsterdam: John Benjamins.

Thomas, M.S.C., Annaz, D., Ansari, D., Serif, G., Jarrold, C., & Karmiloff-Smith, A. (2009). Using developmental trajectories to understand developmental disorders. *Journal of Speech, Language, and Hearing Research,* **52**, 336–58.

Thomas, M.S.C., Grant, J., Gsodl, M, Laing, E., Barham, Z., Lakusta, L., Tyler, L.K., et al. (2001). Past tense formation in Williams syndrome. *Language and Cognitive Processes,* **16**, 143–76.

Thomas, M.S.C., & Karmiloff-Smith, A. (2002). Are developmental disorders like cases of adult brain damage? Implications from connectionist modelling. *Behavioral and Brain Sciences,* **25**, 727–88.

Thomas, M.S.C., & Karmiloff-Smith, A. (2005). Can developmental disorders reveal the component parts of the human language faculty? *Language Learning and Development,* **1**, 65–92.

Thomas, M.S.C., Van Duuren, M., Purser, H.R.M., Mareschal, D., Ansari, D., & Karmiloff-Smith, A. (2010). The development of metaphorical language comprehension in typical development and in Williams syndrome. *Journal of Experimental Child Psychology,* **106**, 99–114.

Udwin, O., & Yule, W. (1990). Expressive language of children with Williams syndrome. *American Journal of Medical Genetics, Supplement,* **6**, 108–114.

Van Herwegen, J., Annaz, D., & Rundblad, G. (in preparation). *Comprehension of Novel Metonymy and Metaphor in Williams Syndrome and Typically Developing Children.*

Vosniadou, S., & Ortony, A. (1983). The emergence of the literal-metaphorical-anomalous distinction in young children. *Child Development,* **54**, 154–61.

Wang, P.P., & Bellugi, U. (1994). Evidence from two genetic syndromes for a dissociation between verbal and visual-spatial short-term memory. *Journal of Clinical Experimental Neuropsychology,* **16**, 317–22.

Chapter 2

Brain: The neuroconstructivist approach

Annette Karmiloff-Smith

Introduction

The brain is by far the most complex organ in the human body and probably the most intricate system in the whole of the universe. Containing some 100 billion nerve cells (or neurons), each of which can make contact with tens of thousands of other neurons, our brain's connectivity is quite mind-blowing. Even in the typically developing (TD) population, no two brains are exactly alike, including those of monozygotic twins with identical genes, because our brains change the strengths and patterns of connectivity throughout our lives as a function of development and experience. At a more gross level of description, however, our brains are relatively similar in terms of anatomy, biochemistry and functional relations, although numerous developmental changes take place between infancy and adulthood (Huttenlocher, 2002; Johnson, 2001). But what happens when gene mutations and atypical experience affect neurogenesis and the development of connectivity, as in the case of Williams syndrome (WS) and other neurodevelopmental disorders?

The atypically developing brain

As with many other neurodevelopmental disorders, what is known about the brain of individuals with WS (over 30 articles published in 2008, see a review by Martens et al., 2008, and numerous other studies since) is predominantly from assessment of the adolescent and adult brain towards the end of its developmental trajectory. Although this is obviously useful information, it raises numerous questions. The majority of existing neural analyses seem to take the view that brain abnormality causes cognitive abnormality, a one-way arrow, rather than considering a more dynamic bidirectional, neuroconstructivist view of atypically developing brains. Take, for instance, the fact that the parietal cortex is small in WS adult brains and that individuals with WS are extremely poor at numerical tasks. Does this automatically imply that the reduction in the parietal grey matter causes the numerical deficits, as is the case when focal damage to the intraparietal sulcus impairs numerical reasoning in hitherto normal adult neuropsychological patients? Or should we raise rather different, neuroconstructivist questions, given that our focus is on a neurodevelopmental disorder and not on damage to an otherwise normally developed adult brain? Indeed, we should ask a developmental question: did the WS parietal region start out proportionally small in the neonate brain, or did it become small because consistently atypical numerical (and spatial) processing in the parietal area resulted in reduced parietal volume in the adult? Only a developmental approach can resolve such questions.

Although the vast majority of studies focus on the adult brain, one study by Boddaert and collaborators (2006) did find reduced grey matter in the parieto-occipital regions of children and adolescents with WS aged 5-15 years. However, by that age the WS brain has already engaged in a great deal of spatial and numerical processing, so until studies of the neonate brain are undertaken in a longitudinal design, our neuroconstructivist questions remain. Indeed, at present we lack sufficient information about the full course of development of the WS brain (and even of the TD brain) to answer these questions, but they highlight the need for future approaches to the WS brain to focus on the dynamics of brain atypicalities over developmental time (Karmiloff-Smith, 2010), using either longitudinal or cross-sectional developmental trajectory approaches. It is clear that adult neuropsychological models of the brain are not appropriate for understanding the dynamics of change in disorders of a developmental nature (Karmiloff-Smith, 1997, 1998). The WS brain should not be considered as a normal brain with parts intact and parts impaired, as some approaches to neurodevelopmental disorders hold, that is, that 'WS can be explained in terms of selective deficits to an otherwise normal modular system' (Clahsen & Temple, 2003) or in terms of static dichotomies such as 'sparing and breakdown' of function (Landau et al., 2005). Rather, as we shall see in the rest of this chapter, the anatomy, biochemistry, intraregional functional relations and inter-regional connectivity are all atypical in WS, indicating that the WS brain develops along a somewhat different developmental trajectory from the outset.

One particular advantage in studying brain activity in atypically developing individuals is that it can allow scientist to identify abnormalities in underlying neural activity despite the presence of seemingly intact behaviour. For instance, behavioural studies showed that individuals with WS have highly proficient face recognition abilities and seemingly intact point-light motion perception. Yet, when the brains of such individuals were studied while they were processing faces, their neural activity turned out to look different from that of matched controls (Karmiloff-Smith et al., 2004). The brain can reveal that what seems intact at the behavioural level is not intact after all (Karmiloff-Smith et al., 1997).

A developmental perspective is always essential when studying the atypically (and typically) developing brain. Indeed, if we are to understand the atypical brain, we need to take into account what happens very early in ontogeny and not merely focus on the adult end state. In this chapter, however, we will be obliged to concentrate almost exclusively on what is known about the adult brain in WS, although a few studies do now exist that offer snapshots of the WS infant and child brain (Boddaert et al., 2006; Jones et al., 2002). In any case, we shall also see that it is always crucial to exercise caution both methodologically and theoretically in interpreting differences between individuals with WS—or any other neurodevelopmental disorder—and controls if the comparison is based on templates derived from the normal brain.

Methods for measuring the atypical brain

There now exist numerous techniques for measuring the structure, intraregional function and inter-regional connectivity of the human brain as well as its biochemistry. These techniques are already providing exciting insights into the atypical brain. Before proceeding with an account of what we currently know about the WS brain and how it compares to brains in other neurodevelopmental disorders, it is worth briefly examining the advantages and limitations of various methodologies for studying the atypical brain (Johnson et al., 2002; Karmiloff-Smith, 2010). These include: post-mortem studies of brain tissue, structural magnetic resonance imaging (MRI), magnetic resonance spectroscopy (MRS), functional MRI (fMRI), diffusion tensor imaging (DTI), magnetoencephalography (MEG), electro-encephalography (EEG) together with event-related potentials (ERP), and functional near-infrared spectroscopy (fNIRS). Other more invasive systems also exist (e.g. positron emission tomography [PET], transcranial magnetic stimulation), which, for ethical reasons, are less suitable for use with individuals with neurodevelopmental disorders, although they are sometimes employed.

Of note, future approaches to studying the atypical brain will need to use a combination of these methods to achieve simultaneous data acquisition—as has been done, for instance, in comparing fNIRS and fMRI results across multiple cognitive tasks for healthy young adults (Cui et al., 2011)—in order to yield complementary, converging data about changes in the time course, spatial location and connectivity of neural activity in both the typical and the atypical brain (Casey et al., 2010; for multimodality approaches, see also Huppert et al., 2008, and Steinbrink et al., 2006).

Post-mortem studies

This method has, of course, a very long history and was one of the main approaches to understanding the human brain prior to the invention of modern technologies. Cytoarchitectonic evaluation of autopsy specimens is obviously limited by the availability of post-mortem brains, giving rise to ethical problems with respect to decisions to approach families at the moment of death. Moreover, in the atypical case, it can some-times be difficult to ascertain whether the actual cause of death altered brain morphology beyond the brain features typical of the targeted syndrome.

Structural magnetic resonance imaging

Structural MRI is noninvasive and uses magnetic fields and radio waves to produce two- and three-dimensional images of brain anatomy that are of very high quality. The participant's reclined body is moved into a large cylindrical magnet, which can cause claustrophobia. Also, individuals with neurodevelopmental disorders tend to be more disturbed by sounds/noise from equipment, although these can be significantly attenu-ated by training and desensitisation prior to the experiment. Both surface and deep brain structures can be imaged with high degrees of anatomical detail, including subtle differ-ences in regional boundaries and in the depths of sulci and gyri. The resulting images can be analysed in a variety of ways for comparison with TD brains or those from individuals with other neurodevelopmental disorders.

Structural or anatomical MRI only gives a static image of brain structure, more like a snapshot, but other methods exist to analyse the brain as it functions in real time, more like a film.

Functional magnetic resonance imaging

Scientists now have at their disposal powerful methods to examine brain activity in real time. One of these methods is fMRI. It relies on the magnetic properties of blood and detects changes in blood oxygenation and blood flow in response to neural activity while the participant views or listens to various stimuli. These changes are referred to as the blood-oxygen-level dependence (BOLD) signal. fMRI allows the researcher to determine with spatial precision which brain regions become active, how strong the activity is, whether several regions become active simultaneously or sequentially and for how long they remain active, although temporal resolution is relatively poor in fMRI. Deoxygenated haemoglobin attenuates the magnetic resonance signal, so that the vascular response leads to a signal increase that is related to the neural activity. This technology yields images that can potentially distinguish structures less than 1 mm apart. Indeed, one of the major advantages of fMRI, be it for developmental or adult neuroimaging, is its very fine spatial resolution.

Although there are many advantages to fMRI, interpretation of the BOLD signal remains somewhat unclear as do the effects on the signal of differences in vascular physiology in clinical populations (Church et al., 2010). Furthermore, because of the slow data acquisition (several seconds, compared with milliseconds in ERP and fNIRS), the fMRI signal can only distinguish anticipatory processing from stimulus-generated activity by inference from carefully designed event-related experiments, whereas this distinction can be detected more directly using ERP or fNIRS. In other words, if one aims to identify, for instance, the extent to which a group shows a shift from data-driven to top-down neural processing, this is more difficult to infer from fMRI data although not impossible. Moreover, when comparing atypical brains with TD ones, the BOLD signal cannot distinguish between moderate activation of a greater number of neurons versus increased activation within the same number of neurons (Karmiloff-Smith, 2010). Such contrasts could turn out to be relevant to neural differences between typical and atypical brains, with animal models providing illumination on this question (Bandettini & Ungerleider, 2001; Logothetis et al., 2001).

Diffusion tensor imaging

DTI allows the scientist to measure macro- and microstructural aspects of white-matter integrity. DTI has been the focus of recent research in TD children (Paus, 2010; Konrad & Eickhoff, 2010; Blakemore et al., 2010), but is still relatively rarely used in studies of atypical brains. This is an important method, however, because the two primary types of data available from longitudinal DTI studies (apparent diffusion coefficient of water and diffusion anisotropy measures) can reveal significant developmental changes in white matter over time, again highlighting the limitations of concentrating solely on the WS adult brain.

Positron emission tomography

Unlike the methods described already, PET is invasive because it involves a radiotracer, that is, the injection into the bloodstream of radioactively labelled chemicals that are carried to the brain, producing three-dimensional images of how these chemicals are accumulated and distributed throughout different neural regions. Using different compounds, PET can measure the amount of blood flow, oxygen consumption, glucose metabolism and specific receptor density/occupancy in different tissues of the active brain. The sensors in the PET scanner detect the radioactivity as the compounds accumulate in different brain areas. However, because of its invasive nature and the fact that it involves needles, it is rarely used with individuals with neurodevelopmental disorders.

Magnetic resonance spectroscopy

MRS is a noninvasive method that enables the scientist to characterise the ratios of various biochemicals in different regions of the brain (Marenco & Radulescu, 2010). Whereas MRI uses the signal from hydrogen protons to form anatomic images, as mentioned earlier, proton MRS uses this information to determine the concentration of specific brain metabolites in brain tissues, such as *N*-acetylaspartate (NAA, a chemical associated with the myelin sheaths of nerve cell fibres and a marker of neuronal integrity and synaptic abundance), choline (Cho, a chemical used to create cell membranes) and creatine (Cr, a chemical involved in the metabolism of energy). The neurons in our brains communicate by passing signals through the release and capture of neurotransmitter and neuromodulator chemicals. Although research into deficiencies in these neurochemicals has been very active in acquired disorders such as Parkinson disease, Alzheimer disease, depression, cancer and the like, such biochemical deficiencies have only rarely been studied with respect to neurodevelopmental disorders. However, as we shall see, three such MRS studies have been carried out on individuals with WS.

Magnetoencephalography

MEG is a technique for mapping brain activity by recording magnetic fields produced by electrical currents occurring naturally in the brain. It uses time-resolved methods to access deep brain tissue (as opposed to the surface tissue accessed by ERP and fNIRS, as discussed later). Although MEG and EEG signals originate from similar neurophysiological processes, there are some crucial differences. Magnetic fields are less distorted by the skull and the scalp than electrical fields, so brain activity measured with MEG can be localised with much greater accuracy. Furthermore, scalp EEG is sensitive to extracellular volume currents produced by postsynaptic potentials, whereas MEG primarily detects intracellular currents associated with these synaptic potentials.

MEG is also one of the preferred systems for studying cognitive processes in the TD fetus. Therefore, as genetic identification of fetuses developing atypically becomes increasingly sophisticated, this method might be used to investigate the extent to which there is already structural atypicality prior to birth.

Event-related potentials and high-density event-related potentials

Rather than measuring the magnetic field as is done in MEG, EEG measures patterns of electrical activity emanating from the brain. It is completely noninvasive and simply records the brain's activity; no electrical currents are sent into the brain. Within individual neurons, signals are formed by electrochemical pulses. This electrical activity can be detected on the surface of the scalp. So, unlike MEG and the magnetic resonance techniques described earlier, EEG measurements are restricted to the brain surface. The electrical signal can be time-locked to visual or auditory stimuli, creating an ERP. This technique is used to assess the temporal waveforms involved in the brain's processing of incoming input. From the waveforms, scientists can measure activity in the alpha band (e.g. while individuals are sleeping) through to the gamma band (e.g. thought to be an indication of active integration/binding of features when viewing/listening to a stimulus). In other words, by tracking differences in both amplitude and latency of the electrical activity tied to an auditory or visual stimulus, scientists can determine the simultaneous and sequential time course of patterns of activity across the brain, that is, the temporal brain signature tied to the processing of a particular kind of stimulus and how such brain signatures might differ between the typical and atypical brain.

ERP provides an excellent recording of the temporal processes of neural activity. Initially, it was limited by the small number of channels on the original electrode caps, but with the advent of the Geodesic Sensor Net (Electrical Geodesics Inc, Eugene, Oregon, USA), the scalp can now be fitted with some 260 channels in the adult net (128 channels in the infant net) covering the entire scalp, enabling the recording of high-density ERPs (HD-ERP). This has now become one of the methods of choice for understanding the temporal patterns of brain activity. Alas, as mentioned, WS studies have mainly concentrated on adults only, although this easily tolerated method would be very suitable for atypically developing infants.

Although HD-ERP yields relatively fine-grained scalp maps, the spatial location data are not as good as those provided by fMRI, MEG or fNIRS, so source reconstruction continues to pose a problem, particularly when the cognitive processes are complex and depend on large functional networks. Interestingly, though, the temporal patterns of ERP can be used to distinguish predictive responses directly from data-driven responses (Southgate et al., 2009), which may turn out to be very relevant for differentiating the processes underlying similar overt behaviours in typical and atypical populations. For example, in the case of so-called 'intact' face processing in WS, ERP studies have revealed differences between TD and WS individuals at the neural level (Grice et al., 2001, 2003; Karmiloff-Smith, 2009; Karmiloff-Smith et al., 2004).

Functional near-infrared spectroscopy

fNIRS is unique among the imaging methods in that it measures both oxygenated and deoxygenated haemoglobin signals (Cui et al., 2011). fNIRS also offers a number of advantages over fMRI because it is relatively inexpensive in comparison and is portable (Atsumori et al., 2009). Moreover, whereas fMRI requires participants to remain completely still, fNIRS can tolerate a degree of movement, which is critical when testing individuals with neurodevelopmental disorders who experience difficulty in inhibiting movement. fNIRS is even more suitable for infants than for older children and adults because the optical geometry of the infant head renders biological tissue more transparent to light in the near-infrared part of the spectrum (particularly in those with no hair). Moreover, fNIRS can acquire data at a rapid temporal rate (Huppert et al., 2006, 2008), overcoming some of the intrinsic limitations of fMRI mentioned above. fNIRS currently surpasses EEG in providing a better spatial resolution, thereby allowing more accurate localisation of brain responses to specific cortical regions (for an excellent review of fNIRS, see Lloyd-Fox et al., 2010). Another advantage is that fNIRS can potentially distinguish between anticipatory and reactive neural processes (Csibra et al., 2001). fNIRS can also be used for paradigms unsuitable for an MRI scanner such as face-to-face communication (Suda et al., 2010).

Although fNIRS produces better spatial resolution than EEG and better temporal resolution than fMRI, its temporal resolution is lower than that of EEG and its spatial resolution is not as good as that of fMRI because it is restricted to the cortical surface and therefore must be inferred. Moreover, the signal-to-noise ratio is low in fNIRS. Currently, fNIRS sits between the two methods in terms of its advantages and limitations, but that also constitutes its major strength. Unlike MRI, near-infrared spectroscopy does not lend itself to the measurement of brain structures (Minagawa-Kawai et al., 2007, 2009), so debates continue as to how to locate the origin of the haemodynamic response from the scalp measurements (Meek, 2002; Aslin & Mehler, 2005), although newer fNIRS devices are now allowing for three-dimensional marking of skull landmarks that can be calibrated with the same landmarks as those used for anatomical MRI (Cui et al., 2011).

Hitherto, there seem to have been no studies using fNIRS with individuals with neurodevelopmental disorders, but in my view the method has significant practical and theoretical potential for such an approach in future studies of the brains of children with neurodevelopmental disorders.

Structural and functional atypicalities in the WS brain

Approximately 22 of the 28 genes within the WS critical region are thought to be expressed in the brain (see Chapter 3), so their haploinsufficiency may well affect brain development in WS. However, as mentioned before, there are very few studies of the WS brain during the process of brain development over time, which will oblige us mainly to focus on the adult brain, although a couple of studies of the WS child brain at specific time points have been carried out (Boddaert et al., 2006; Jones et al., 2002). Moreover, the unique brain shape and size in individuals with WS obviously affects comparisons with TD controls, because considerable warping is necessary to normalise the WS brain image to a standard template, making it unclear whether the same brain regions are being compared in the two cases. Some studies have surmounted this by using individual regions of interest. However, comparisons between WS and TD brains always need to be treated with caution. For example, Meyer-Lindenberg and collaborators (2004) found reduced grey matter in the orbitofrontal cortex, whereas Reiss and collaborators (2004) reported the opposite finding, that is, increased grey matter in this same region. Such differences are likely to be attributable to brain image transformation procedures (Eckert et al., 2006). Moreover, as we shall see towards the end of the chapter, many of the atypicalities characteristic of the WS brain are also evident in the brains of individuals with other neurodevelopmental disorders. This means that particular regional differences are not syndrome-specific, although, as we will conclude, the overall pattern of atypicalities in the WS brain may indeed be unique.

Most children with WS present with reduced head circumference (Boddaert et al., 2006; Eisenberg et al., 2010; Schmitt et al., 2001), and indeed by adulthood, WS brains only reach about 80% of the TD brain volume (Chiang et al., 2007; Jernigan & Bellugi, 1994). Figure 2.1 illustrates volumetric maps of the WS brain (Chiang et al., 2007). The overall brain curvature in WS is reduced compared with TD brains (Schmitt et al., 2001a, 2001b)

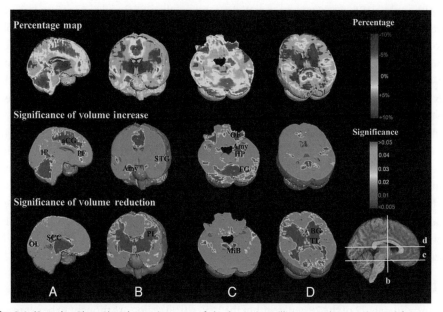

Fig. 2.1 (See also Plate 3) Volumetric maps of the brain in Williams syndrome, derived from magnetic resonance imaging. WS and control brain volumes were compared in the ICBM space to adjust for individual differences in total brain volumes. The ratio of the mean JICBM space in WS to the mean JICBM in control subjects was computed voxel-wise to map the three-dimensional profile of brain volume increases (colour-coded as red) or reductions (colour-coded as blue) (first row). Panels (A) to (D) show relative preservation of the volume (which is shown as increase in the volume percentage maps) in prefrontal and orbitofrontal areas, anterior cingulate gyrus, inferior parietal regions at the parieto-occipital junction, superior temporal gyrus, amygdala and part of hippocampus (especially on the right side), fusiform gyrus, and cerebellum. Occipital areas, parietal lobes close to temporo-parietal junction, splenium and posterior body of the corpus callosum, thalamus and the basal ganglia (including globus pallidus, putamen, and caudate nucleus), and midbrain are disproportionally reduced. The Mann–Whitney U test was used to obtain the significance maps for the volume increase (second row) or reduction (third row). Abbreviations: aCG = anterior cingulate gyrus; Amy = amygdala; BG = basal ganglia; FG = fusiform gyrus; HP = hippocampus; IP = inferior parietal region; JICBM = Jacobian determinant in the ICBM space; MiB = midbrain; OF = orbitofrontal area; OL = occipital lobe; PF = prefrontal area; PL = parietal lobe; SCC = splenium of the corpus callosum; STG = superior temporal gyrus; TL = thalamus. Reprinted from *NeuroImage*, **36** (4), Ming-Chang Chiang, Allan L. Reiss, Agatha D. Lee, Ursula Bellugi, Albert M. Galaburda, Julie R. Korenberg, et al, 3D pattern of brain abnormalities in Williams syndrome visualized using tensor-based morphometry, pp. 1096–1109, Copyright (2007), with permission from Elsevier.

and the cortical thickness is increased (Thompson, et al., 2005). Structural analyses also reveal increased gyral complexity, particularly in parieto-occipital regions, compared with TD brains (Eisenberg et al., 2010; Meyer-Lindenberg et al., 2006; Schmitt et al., 2001a, 2001b; Thompson et al., 2005), indicating abnormal cortical maturation in WS. Post-mortem studies have identified cytoarchitectonic anomalies in the occipital region of the WS brain (Gallaburda et al., 2002). Moreover, in several other regions of the cortex the WS brain has atypical neuronal density with abnormal neuronal layering, particularly in the primary visual cortex. Cells in some layers of the left peripheral visual cortex have been found to be densely packed and significantly smaller in size than those in TD brains (Gallaburda et al., 2002). By contrast, larger neurons and a greater cell-packing density were found in the primary auditory cortex (Holinger et al., 2005). These visual–auditory cortical differences would seem to reflect the differences in the visual and verbal modalities in the cognitive phenotype, but such inferences from brain region to cognition are often premature and the situation tends to turn out to be far more complex when connectivity analyses are undertaken.

Although an early study indicated a normal corpus callosum morphology in WS (Wang et al., 1992), subsequent research has identified several abnormalities (Chiang et al., 2007). Indeed, the corpus callosum—normally a wide, flat bundle of neural fibres beneath the cortex connecting the left and right cerebral hemispheres—turns out to have both an abnormal shape and an abnormal thickness in WS brains, with a less concave shape in midsaggital sections and overall a more flattened morphology compared with TD controls (Luders et al., 2007; Sampaio et al., 2010; Schmitt et al., 2001a, 2001b; Tomaiuolo et al., 2002). The abnormal corpus callosum morphology could impact on interhemispheric communication in the WS brain. Interestingly, corpus callosum abnormality has been linked to problems with shifting attention between visual fields (Hines et al., 2002), which could well contribute to some of the clear-cut visual problems evidenced in the WS cognitive phenotype. Although the corpus callosum is shorter in WS brains than in TD brains, one study found increased relative thickness in all callosal sections in the WS brain. Whether this relates to differences in intelligence as found in the TD population (Luders et al., 2007) remains to be investigated in the WS population.

After adjustment for total reduced brain volume, the frontal lobes, anterior cingulate, superior temporal gyrus, amygdala, fusiform gyrus and cerebellum in WS adult brains are all relatively preserved. By contrast, the parietal and occipital lobes, the thalamus, the basal ganglia and the midbrain are disproportionally small in volume. Interestingly, the amygdala and the cerebellum are proportionally somewhat larger than the rest of the WS brain, and in one of the rare developmental studies the atypicality of cerebellum size was shown to be present from early on (Jones et al., 2002). Indeed, a study by Jones and collaborators (2002) of nine infants and toddlers between the ages of 7 and 43 months revealed an atypically large cerebellum in proportion to other brain areas, suggesting an early structural abnormality in the WS brain. Moreover, the study also indicated that the magnitude of the cerebellar abnormalities did not vary as a function of age in this albeit small WS group. Of course, given the small sample size, such conclusions are very preliminary prior to replication on a larger group of young children.

Voxel-based morphometry has made it possible to examine specific brain regions for differences in grey-matter volume in WS brains compared with healthy controls. In WS, grey matter is reduced in several brain regions, namely the right fusiform gyrus, the left parieto-occipital regions, the intraparietal sulcus and the orbitofrontal regions (Eckert et al., 2006; Menghini et al., 2011). This obtains both for WS adults with intelligence scores in the normal range (Meyer-Lindenberg et al., 2004) and for the more typical WS adults with mild-to-moderate intellectual disability (Reiss et al., 2004). Some of this research has been carried out on children (5-12 years old: Boddaert et al., 2006; 11-15 years old: Campbell et al., 2009a), resulting in the identification of grey-matter reductions in right parieto-occipital regions, the right posterior cingulate gyrus and the basal ganglia. By contrast, significant grey-matter increases were found in the frontal lobes, the anterior cingulate gyrus and the left temporal lobe, together with increases in white matter bilaterally in the anterior cingulate (Campbell et al., 2009a).

An fMRI study by Golarai and collaborators (2010) defined the portion of the fusiform gyrus that is devoted to face processing (in contrast to the processing of houses) and found that the fusiform face area (FFA) in WS adults was twice the size of that in TD controls, in both absolute and relative terms, despite a reduced grey-matter volume of the anatomical region of the fusiform gyrus. This was a notable study because, instead of spatially normalising the WS brains to the TD brain, the functional analyses were based on individually defined regions of interest (Golarai et al., 2010).

These different studies raise the question of whether the lifelong fascination with faces that is so notable in this syndrome (see Chapter 14) is attributable to an early enlarged FFA in the neonate or whether the constant processing of faces has resulted in structural alterations in this region. It is even possible that the WS infants' fascination with faces stems from a combination of rather different factors: that they were fascinated with sound that they had already heard during the last 3 months in their mother's uterus, that the familiar sound of the mother's voice attracted them to her face at birth, that their problems with planning eye movements (Brown et al., 2003) kept them visually fixated on her face, that this drove the subsequent treatment of the face as a privileged input and that this ultimately resulted in the increasing size of the FFA (Karmiloff-Smith, 2009). Only a developmentally sensitive study can address such important questions.

Despite the small participant numbers and varied methods of analysis, remarkably consistent findings have emerged with respect to grey-matter reduction in posterior parietal areas (Eckert et al., 2006; Kippenhan et al., 2005; Menghini et al., 2011; Meyer-Lindenberg et al., 2004; Reiss et al., 2004; Schmitt et al., 2001a, 2001b; Thompson et al., 2005) as shown in Figures 2.1 and 2.2. In particular, studies have identified anomalies in the intraparietal sulcus, consisting of bilaterally reduced grey-matter volume (Meyer-Lindenberg et al., 2004; Reiss et al., 2004; Boddaert et al., 2006; Eckert et al., 2006) and bilateral reductions in sulcal depths in the intraparietal/occipitoparietal regions of individuals with WS (Eisenberg et al., 2010; Kippenhan et al., 2005; Van Essen et al., 2006). Interestingly, the structural finding of reduced parietal grey matter in the intraparietal sulcus turned out to be associated with hypoactivity in directly adjacent parietal regions during spatial localisation and visuospatial construction, with path analysis revealing reduced information flow

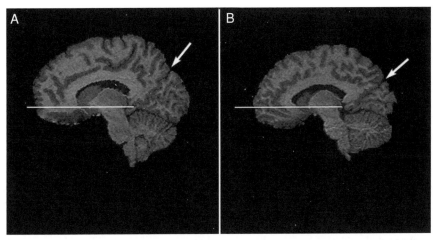

Fig. 2.2 Representative parasagittal magnetic resonance images (at the same anatomic location) from a young adult control participant (A) and an age- and gender-matched participant with Williams syndrome (B). The horizontal line on each image shows the location of the plane defined by the anterior and posterior commissures. Arrows point to the location of parieto-occipital fissure. Note the relatively greater amount of ventral prefrontal tissue inferior to the plane between the anterior and posterior commissures and the disproportionately small occipital lobe (posterior and inferior to the parieto-occipital fissure) in the participant with Williams syndrome. Figure reprinted with permission from *Journal of Neuroscience, 24*, 5009–5015.

from the intraparietal sulcus to these later dorsal-stream regions (Meyer-Lindenberg et al., 2004). Abnormal functional connectivity has also been identified between the parahippoc-ampal gyrus and the parietal cortex and between the fusiform gyrus and a network of brain regions including the amygdala and parts of the prefrontal cortex (Eisenberg et al., 2010; Sarpal et al., 2008), highlighting the importance of thinking in terms of connectivity rather than merely in terms of regional differences in attempting to understand the atypical brain. Other studies indicate that the intraparietal sulcus also presents with abnormal white-matter integrity (Meyer-Lindenberg et al., 2006). In fact, one consistent finding from DTI of white-matter integrity in the dorsal and ventral streams has been of higher fractional anisotropy (a measure of microstructural integrity) in the right superior longitudinal fasciculus in WS brains compared with the brains both of TD controls and of another group of developmentally delayed individuals (Hoeft et al., 2007; Marenco et al., 2007), again underlining the anomalous inter-regional network connectivity in the WS brain.

In a study initially indicating relatively normal activation of ventral streams (Sarpal et al., 2008), subsequent functional connectivity analyses revealed abnormalities in the interactions of the ventral visual areas with other systems known to by atypical in WS, such as the intraparietal sulcus. This abnormal connectivity in the WS brain is likely to contribute to the visuospatial problems characteristic of the syndrome (see Chapters 12 and 13). Moreover, whereas in TD brains there is a tight functional coupling between areas involved in face processing (intraparietal sulcus) and those involved in object processing (parahippocampal place area), in WS this coupling is significantly decreased.

For example, both the FFA, an area related to face processing (ventral stream), and the parahippocampal place area, an area that is crucial for spatial navigation, showed reduced connections to the intraparietal sulcus, which is part of the dorsal visual stream. Interestingly, Sarpal et al. (2008) also showed areas of increased connectivity in WS, which they hypothesise relates to compensatory functional reorganisation during development. The authors suggest that increased connectivity between the parahippocampal place area and the superior temporal cortex, an area that integrates information from dorsal and ventral streams and is involved in motion processing, might explain why not all motion-processing tasks elicit impaired performance in WS.

In contrast to the decreased grey matter in WS parieto-occipital regions, increased grey matter was identified in the amygdala circuit (Reiss et al., 2004). It is also the case that individuals with WS fail to recruit frontostriatal circuits (Mobbs et al., 2007) and display aberrant connectivity between the orbitofrontal cortex and the amygdala (Meyer-Lindenberg et al., 2006), which has been linked to their problems with inhibitory control and attention (see Chapters 6 and 9). Indeed, amygdala reactivity to threatening socially relevant stimuli has been shown to be significantly diminished in WS, whereas amygdala activation to nonsocial stimuli is abnormally increased (Meyer-Lindenberg et al., 2006). Rather than being a local dysfunction of the amygdala, the lack of interaction between the amygdala and the orbitofrontal cortex may well be a major contributor to the unusually uninhibited social phenotype in WS (Meyer-Lindenberg et al., 2006; see Chapter 15). The problems with inhibitory control in the WS social phenotype may be underpinned by more general problems with attention and inhibitory control outside the social domain (Menghini et al., 2011; Mobbs et al., 2007; Rhodes et al., 2010; see Chapter 9).

As already alluded to, Boddaert and collaborators (2006) reported that many of the significant anatomical abnormalities found in adult WS brains were not present in their paediatric group. Although they worked with a very small number of participants, these child data are interesting, and it may turn out that the adult abnormalities in the cerebellar, orbitofrontal and thalamic regions (Meyer-Lindenberg et al., 2004; Reiss et al., 2004) not found in children are the outcome in adults of atypical processing over developmental time. Of course, most of the studies on the WS brain have very small population sizes, so may suffer from insufficient statistical power. Nonetheless, it is worth noting that in the TD brain, grey matter develops earlier in the parietal cortex than in other cerebral regions (Giedd et al., 1999), suggesting that the parietal anomaly in the WS child brain may be a very basic developmental feature of the syndrome's brain. As stated earlier, studies of the WS neonate brain, and not just the child brain, are crucial for understanding the developmental roots of the atypicalities in the WS adult brain. In other words, we still need to document the full time course of WS brain growth from the earliest points in development.

In summary, accumulating evidence is available pointing to gross morphological alterations in WS such as reduced brain size, reduced overall curvature and increased gyral complexity, in conjunction with reductions in parietal and limbic regional volumes, all of which seem to coexist with the functional atypicalities found in WS neural processing (Eisenberg et al., 2010). In particular, parieto-occipital abnormality is evidenced in both structural and functional studies of the WS brain, together with atypical connectivity of the amygdala, the orbitofrontal cortex and related limbic pathways.

The biochemistry of the Williams syndrome brain

The cerebellum and hippocampus have been the main focus of interest in studies of the biochemistry of the WS brain, with research revealing normal ratios of Cho to Cr but particularly abnormal ratios of both Cho to NAA and Cr to NAA (Rae et al., 1998). Of particular interest is the fact that the atypical NAA:Cho and NAA:Cr ratios in the WS cerebellum correlate strongly with individual differences in various cognitive tasks, but most strongly with what is known as inspection time, that is, how long one needs to see stimuli to make a decision about them (e.g. which is larger) before they are masked. The particularly strong correlation between NAA concentration and inspection time indicates that the biochemical abnormalities may have a domain-general effect on cognitive outcome. NAA biochemical abnormalities were replicated in a later study by Meyer-Lindenberg and collaborators (2005), who identified a reduced NAA:Cr ratio in the left hippocampal formation. Interestingly, these regions do not show a relative volume reduction, pointing to functional impairment of neurons rather than volume loss. These biochemical findings indicate an overall depression of energy metabolism and synaptic activity in the cerebellum and hippocampus of the WS brain, which may contribute to the visuo-motor control problems they experience when negotiating stairs (Cowie et al., in press).

The electrophysiology of the Williams syndrome brain

ERP studies have suggested possible developmental arrest compared with the TD brain. Indeed, in several areas of cognition, for example face and language processing, the TD brain will initially process incoming input bilaterally, but with development a progressive specialisation and localisation of brain function occurs giving rise to a shift to increasingly specialised unilateral processing (predominantly right hemisphere for faces, predominantly left hemisphere for the morphosyntax of language). Several studies have now shown that the WS brain tends to continue processing faces and language bilaterally, even in adulthood (Grice et al., 2001, 2003; Neville et al., 1994; Mills et al., 2000). In other words, whereas in the TD brain we witness a gradual specialisation and hemispheric localisation of function over time, this does not seem to occur in the same way in the development of the WS brain (Karmiloff-Smith, 2009). Moreover, the brain signature for faces becomes increasingly specific over developmental time in TD brains, whereas WS brains tend to process faces, cars and other objects with the same temporal signature (Grice et al., 2001; Karmiloff-Smith, 2009; see also Golarai et al., 2010, for similar differences between TD and WS in fMRI studies).

Cross-syndrome comparisons of the atypical brain

There are few studies that directly compare brain anatomy, brain biochemistry and brain functional connectivity across syndromes. Yet, it is crucial to understand whether the observed atypicalities in the WS brain are merely the nonspecific results of having a genetic disorder or whether they are specific to WS. Moreover, it is quite often the case that authors claim a causal relationship between, say, increased volume in a cortical area and atypical cognitive processing with respect to one syndrome, and yet associate similar atypical cognition with decreased volume in the same area in another syndrome. As with the cognitive phenotype, it is crucial to ask whether the abnormalities in the WS brain are syndrome-specific or also found in other neurodevelopmental disorders, and whether similar brain abnormalities give rise to similar cognitive atypicalities across syndromes. In other words, how syndrome-specific are the brain abnormalities identified in WS?

Take the abnormalities identified in the corpus callosum morphology of the WS brain. Are these specific to WS? Studies of the brains of individuals with other syndromes—for example autism (Vidal et al., 2006), schizophrenia (Frumin et al., 2002; Innocenti et al., 2003) and Tourette syndrome (Plessen et al., 2006)—have also revealed corpus callosum atypicalities compared with TD controls. So, corpus callosum atypicality is not in and of itself unique to WS, but the type of abnormality and how it contributes to cognitive outcome may well be. Further longitudinal, more in-depth cross-syndrome comparisons of the corpus callosum are required to establish this.

The consistent finding of anomalies in the posterior parietal lobe in WS also turns out to be characteristic of other syndromes. For example, it is found in severe dyscalculia (Butterworth, 1999), Turner syndrome (Molko et al., 2003) and 22q syndrome (Campbell et al., 2009b). Moreover, reduced parietal grey matter has been identified in adolescents born prematurely but with no frank brain damage (Isaacs et al., 2001), with the grey-matter volume correlating with problems in numerical cognition in these adolescents. Frontostriatal circuitry abnormalities identified in WS have also been associated with attention deficit hyperactivity disorder (Castellanos et al., 2002), obsessive compulsive disorder (van den Heuvel et al., 2005) and fragile X syndrome (Menon et al., 2004). In other words, there is little about the WS brain's regional structural and functional abnormalities that seem entirely specific to WS, except perhaps the very enlarged FFA. Again, a longitudinal study of the time course of FFA development is critical to understanding how this increase originated and what it means in terms of reorganisation of functional connectivity as the WS brain develops.

There exist two studies that set out to directly compare the WS brain with another neurodevelopmental disorder involving a hemizygous microdeletion, namely 22q syndrome, otherwise known as velocardiofacial syndrome or DiGeorge syndrome (Campbell et al., 2009b; Eisenberg et al., 2010). Both WS and 22q syndrome are associated with mild-to-moderate intellectual disability, but they differ with respect to their social phenotypes: individuals with 22q syndrome show poor social skills and have a high prevalence of psychosis, whereas individuals with WS display strong albeit atypical social skills and no psychosis. Unlike autism and dyslexia, which are found predominantly in males, WS and 22q have no gender bias, so affected individuals can be matched on chronological age, full-scale IQ and gender. However, there are key similarities and differences in their cognition and neuroanatomy. In particular, cognitively they differ in the distribution of verbal and nonverbal skills. Individuals with 22q are significantly stronger than those with WS on nonverbal tasks, whereas those with WS perform better on verbal, social and facial tasks. Individuals with either syndrome experience sensitive hearing, anxiety, overactivity and problems with peer relations and attention.

In the Campbell et al. (2009b) cross-syndrome comparative study using identical MRI methodologies with WS and 22q, there were 12 matched participants between 6 and 16 years of age for each syndrome. Similarities and differences across the two syndromes emerged in brain anatomy despite overall similarities in brain volume. Manual tracing was used to determine volumetric differences. Midline anomalies were more common in the 22q group, as were regional differences such as increased striatal volumes and reduced cerebellar volumes. By contrast, as we have seen, the size of the cerebellum was relatively increased in WS. Both syndromes revealed reduced grey-matter volume in parieto-occipital regions. By contrast, whereas the amygdala was reduced in 22q syndrome, its volume was increased in WS. Compared with TD control brains, the basal ganglia region was larger in individuals with 22q, whereas it was volumetrically smaller in those with WS. Campbell and colleagues (2009b) identified structural alterations of the cerebellum and the fusiform gyrus in 22q, whereas these regions were closer to TD brains in WS, albeit with atypical connectivity. Grey and white striatal matter was increased in the 22q group compared with the WS group. By contrast, the 22q group displayed decreased grey matter in the cerebellum, cingulate gyrus and parietal lobes compared with WS. Furthermore, greater white-matter reductions were observed in 22q posterior regions compared with WS. The greater problems with white-matter integrity in 22q may contribute to their vulnerability to psychotic symptoms (Simon et al., 2005).

Possibly linked to their differing social profiles, with WS individuals being hypersocial and 22q individuals being shy and withdrawn, is evidence of a distinct difference in midline cerebellar structures, notably the vermis, which displays reductions in 22q syndrome (Eliez et al., 2001) and fragile X syndrome, but has an increased size in WS (Schmitt et al., 2001a, 2001b). The Campbell et al. (2009b) study confirmed this striking cross-syndrome anatomical difference, but determining the extent to which it explains the differing social phenotypes requires deeper analysis.

In terms of cross-syndrome comparisons of temporal aspects of the brain, one study (Grice et al., 2001) looked at gamma-band activity in WS and autism in response to face stimuli, because gamma-band bursts are thought to relate to the binding of features and both WS and autism are characterised by a focus on features at the expense of the configural whole. The findings yielded very significant differences between individuals with autism and those with WS. The brains of the former displayed regular gamma bursts, although, unlike in TD controls, these bursts were not as tightly tied to stimulus onset and showed no difference in response to upright versus inverted faces. By contrast, what characterised the WS brains was an almost complete lack of gamma-band activity in response to the face stimuli irrespective of their upright or inverted orientation, a pattern usually only seen in very young infants.

Cross-syndrome comparisons highlight the importance of trying to characterise the atypical brain in terms of a set of functionally connected atypicalities, rather than by comparing isolated brain regions. The linking of brain anatomy to cognitive outcome is not straightforward, even with respect to the TD brain, because the cognitive outcome is the result of much lower-level processes that impact on basic brain architecture, such as differences in neurons, axons, dendrites, bursts of growth followed by periods of synaptic consolidation when unused connections are pruned, and so forth. So brain networks are constantly changing and there are no neat direct mappings between brain and cognition.

Concluding thoughts

It is clear that the WS brain develops atypically at multiple levels—anatomy, biochemistry and functional connectivity—with different spatial and temporal patterns compared with TD brains. It is also clear that the WS brain is not unique in each of its atypicalities in particular brain regions. On the other hand, if we look at the *overall pattern* of brain abnormalities, then the WS brain is indeed unique in its phenotypic outcome. As Allan Reiss pointed out in an email on 13 January 2011: 'I can spot a WS brain just by walking past a computer with the anatomy on the screen—a gestalt that I have picked up from seeing hundreds of these anatomic MRIs of the WS brain.' This unique pattern includes a reduced grey-matter volume in the parieto-occipital lobe, a greater 'bending' of the corpus callosum and cerebrum and prominence of the orbitofrontal cortex relative to the plane between the anterior and posterior commissures (AC–PC plane) (see figure 3 in Reiss et al., 2004). In other words, the WS brain seems to be uniquely characterised by the relatively greater amount of ventral prefrontal tissue inferior to the AC–PC plane and the disproportionately small occipital lobe (posterior and inferior to the parieto-occipital fissure).

What remains to be identified is whether this typical pattern of WS brain atypicalities also holds true for those with WS who have more unusual sociocognitive profiles than the majority with WS. So, the importance of individual differences at the cognitive and neural levels will probably be a critical area of future research. We know that there are enormous interindividual differences not only across syndromes but also within syndromes, attributable in part to genetic backgrounds but also to the influence of dynamic environmental forces (Haas et al., 2010). However, even subtle initial differences can alter the velocity of brain development and the density of neurons, cause delays in myelination, result in volumetric differences and disrupt the integrity of regional connectivity. Moreover, brains are not static; they change over developmental time, and plasticity holds for both the typical and atypical brains. A developing brain such as that of individuals with WS is highly unlikely, in my view, to result in a normal brain with parts intact and parts impaired, as some like to characterise it. Rather, it is a brain that develops in subtly different ways throughout its trajectory, resulting in some small and some more serious brain, cognitive and behavioural atypicalities in the phenotypic outcome.

Editor commentary (Emily K. Farran & Annette Karmiloff-Smith)

This chapter explored the impact of genetic mutations and atypical environmental experiences on brain development from a neuroconstructivist stance. The chapter clearly illustrated, using multilevel analysis, why we should not consider the brain of an individual with a developmental disorder in terms of 'parts intact' and 'parts impaired'. Examples were given of seemingly typical overt behaviour that is actually driven by atypical neural activation, and of areas of the brain that show largely typical structure and function but atypical neural connections and evidence for increased functional connectivity, all of which may be indicative of compensatory functional reorganisation in the atypical brain. Among many other considerations, the chapter also discussed the likelihood that brain development can be altered by environmental input, using the example that the large FFA in WS adults may be the outcome of increased attention to faces in infancy. Such considerations are widely applicable across neurodevelopmental syndromes. For example, Sahyoun et al. (2010) report that in autism, although performance on a visual task seemed typical, neural activation in frontal and temporal regions showed reduced activation relative to typical development, which is indicative of a dissociation in task completion strategies.

Multilevel analysis has also been beneficial to determine the environmental impact of intervention. For example, Shaywitz et al. (2003) report that in dyslexia, the neural circuits activated when reading are atypical, suggestive of functional reorganisation. Interestingly, activation becomes more typical after intervention, demonstrating the plasticity of the brain and potential effects of environmental input.

In summary, while knowledge of the adult brain at the gross level of structural brain anatomy is useful, it is vital that we take a multidisciplinary approach to consider how genetic and environmental factors affect the organisation of the cortex. Future research should also explore the development of the functions and structures of the typical and typical brain from infancy onwards.

References

Aslin, R., & Mehler, J. (2005). Near-infrared spectroscopy for functional studies of brain activity in human infants: promises, prospects and challenges. *Journal of Biomedical Optics*, 10, 11009.

Atsumori, H., Kiguchi, M., Obata, A., Sato, H., Katura, T., Funane, T., et al. (2009). Development of wearable optical topography system for mapping the prefrontal cortex activation. *Review of Scientific Instrumuments*, 80, 043704.

Bandettini, P.A., & Ungerleider, L.G. (2001). From neuron to BOLD: new connections. *Nature Neuroscience*, 4, 864–67.

Blakemore, S.-J., Burnett, S., & Dahl, R.E. (2010). The role of puberty in the developing brain. *Human Brain Mapping*, 31, 926–33.

Boddaert, N., Mochel, F., Meresse, I., Seidenwurm, D., Cachia, A., Brunelle, F., et al. (2006). Parieto-occipital grey matter abnormalities in children with Williams syndrome. *NeuroImage*, 30, 721–25.

Brown, J.H., Johnson, M.H, Paterson, S.J., Gilmore, R., Longhi, E., & Karmiloff-Smith, A. (2003). Spatial representation and attention in toddlers with Williams syndrome and Down syndrome. *Neuropsychologia*, 41, 10371046.

Butterworth, B. (1999). *The Mathematical Brain*. Macmillan, London.

Clahsen, H., & Temple, C. (2003). Words and rules in children with Williams syndrome. In Y. Levy & J.C. Schaeffer (Eds), *Language Competency Across Populations: Towards a Definition of Specific Language Impairment* (pp. 323–52). Hillsdale, NJ: Lawrence Erlbaum.

Campbell, L.E., Daly, E., Toal, F., Stevens, A, Azuma, R., Karmiloff-Smith, A., et al. (2009a). Brain structural differences associated with the behavioural phenotype in children with Williams syndrome. *Brain Research*, 1258, 96–107.

Campbell, L.E., Stevens, A., Daly, E., Toal, F., Azuma, R., Karmiloff-Smith, A., et al. (2009b). A comparative study of cognition and brain anatomy between two neurodevelopmental disorders: 22q11.2 deletion syndrome and Williams syndrome. *Neuropsychologia*, **47**, 1034–44.

Casey, B., Soliman, F., Bath, K.G., & Glatt, C.E. (2010). Imaging genetics and development: challenges and promises. *Human Brain Mapping*, **31**, 838–51.

Castellanos, F.X., Lee, P.P., Sharp, W., Jeffries, N.O., Greenstein, D.K., Clasen, L.S., Blumenthal, et al. (2002). Developmental trajectories of brain volume abnormalities in children and adolescents with attention-deficit/hyperactivity disorder. *Journal of the American Medical Association*, **288**, 1740–48.

Chiang, M.-C., Reiss, A.L., Lee. A., Bellugi, U., Galaburda, A., Kroenberg, J., et al. (2007). 3D pattern of brain abnormalities in Williams syndrome visualized using tensor-based morphometry. *NeuroImage*, **36**, 1096–1109.

Church, J.A., Peterson, S.E., & Schlaggar, B.L. (2010). The 'Task B problem' and other considerations in developmental functional neuroimaging. *Human Brain Mapping*, **31**, 852–62.

Cowie, D., Braddick, O., & Atkinson, J. (in press). Visually guided locomotion in children with Williams syndrome. *Developmental Science*.

Csibra, G., Tucker, L., & Johnson, M.H. (2001). Differential frontal cortex activation before anticipatory and reactive saccades in infants. *Infancy*, **2**, 159–74.

Cui, X., Bray, S., Bryant, DM, Glover, GH., & Reiss, A. m. (2011). A quantitative comparisobn of NIRS and fMRI across multiple cognitive tasks. *NeuroImage*, **54**, 2808–21.

Eckert, M.A., Galaburda, A.M., Mills, D.L., Bellugi, U., Korenberg, J.R., & Reiss, A.L. (2006). The neurobiology of Williams syndrome: cascading influences of visual system impairment? *Cellular and Molecular Life Sciences*, **63**, 1867–75.

Eisenberg, D.P., Jabbi, M., & Berman, K.F. (2010). Bridging the gene behaviour divide through neuroimaging deletion syndromes: velocardiofacial (22q11.2 deletion) and Williams (7q11.23 deletion) syndromes. *NeuroImage*, **53**, 857–69.

Eliez, S., Blasey, C.M., Schmitt, E.J., White, C.D., Hu, D., & Reiss, A.L. (2001). Velocardiofacial syndrome: are structural changes in the temporal and mesial temporal regions related to schizophrenia? The *American Journal of Psychiatry*, **158**, 447–53.

Frumin, M., Golland, P., Kikinis, R., Hiravasu, Y., Salisbury, D.F., Hennen, J., et al. (2002). Shape differences in the corpus callosum in first-episode schizophrenia and first-episode psychotic affective disorder. *The American Journal of Psychiatry*, **159**, 866–68.

Gallaburda, A., Holinger, D., Bellugi, U., & Shermanm, G. (2002). Williams syndrome: neuronal size and neuronal-packing density in primary visual cortex. *Archives of Neurology*, **59**, 1461–67.

Giedd, J.N., Blumenthal, J., Jeffries, N.O., Castellanos, F.X., Liu, H., Zijdenbos, A., et al. (1999). Brain development during childhood and adolescence: a longitudinal MRI study. *Nature Neuroscience*, **2**, 861–63.

Golarai, G., Hong, S., Haas, B., Galaburda, A., Mills, D., Bellugi, U., et al. (2010). The fusiform face area is enlarged in Williams syndrome. *The Journal of Neuroscience*, **30**, 6700–6712.

Grice, S.J., de Haan, M., Halit, H., Johnson, M.H., Csibra, G., Grant, J., et al. (2003). ERP abnormalities of visual perception in Williams syndrome. *NeuroReport*, **14**, 1773–77.

Grice, S., Spratling, M.W., Karmiloff-Smith, A., Halit, H., Csibra, G., de Haan, M., et al. (2001). Disordered visual processing and oscillatory brain activity in autism and Williams syndrome. *NeuroReport*, **12**, 2697–2700.

Haas, B.W., Hoeft, F., Searcy, Y.M., Mills, D., Bellugi, U., & Reiss, A. (2010). Individual differences in social behaviour predict amygdala response to fearful facial expressions in Williams syndrome. *Neuropsychologia*, **48**, 1283–88.

Hines, R.J., Paul, L.K., & Brown, W.S. (2002). Spatial attention in agenesis of the corpus callosum: shifting attention between visual fields. *Neuropsychologia*, **40**, 1804–1814.

Hoeft, F., Barnea-Goraly, N., Hass, B.W., Golarai, G., Ng, D., Mills, D., et al. (2007). More is not always better: increased fasciculus associated with poor visuospatial abilities in Williams syndrome. *The Journal of Neuroscience*, **27**, 11960–65.

Holinger, D.P., Bellugi, U., Mills, D.L., Korenberg, J.R., Reiss, A.L., Sherman, G.F., et al. (2005). Relative sparing of primary auditory cortex in Williams syndrome. *Brain Research*, **1037**, 35–42.

Huppert, T.J., Diamond, S.G., & Boas, D.A. (2008). Direct estimation of evoked haemoglobin changes by multimodality fusion imaging. *Journal of Biomedical Optics*, **13**, 054031.

Huppert, T.J., Hoge, R.D., Diamond, S.G., Franceschini, M.A., & Boas, D.A. (2006). A temporal comparison of BOLD, ASl and NIRS haemodynamic responses to motor stimuli in adult humans. *NeuroImage*, **29**, 368–82.

Huttenlocher, P.R. (2002). *Neural Plasticity: The Effects of the Environment on the Development of the Cerebral Cortex*. Cambridge, MA: Harvard University Press.

Innocenti, G.M., Ansermet, F., & Parnas, J. (2003). Schizophrenia, neurodevelopment and corpus callosum. *Molecular Psychiatry*, **8**, 261–74.

Isaacs, E.B., Edmonds, C.J., Lucas, A., & Gadian, D.G. (2001). Calculation difficulties in children of very low birthweight. *Brain*, **124**, 1701–1707.

Jernigan, T.L., & Bellugi, U. (1994). Neuroanatomical distinctions between Willisms and Down syndromes. In S. Broman & J. Grafnab (Eds), *Atuypical Cognitive Deficits in Developmental Disorders: Implications in Brain Function* (pp. 57–66). Hillsdale, NJ: Lawrence Erlbaum.

Johnson, M.H. (2001). Functional brain development in humans. *Nature Reviews Neuroscience*, **2**, 475–83.

Johnson, M.J., Halit, H., Grice, S.J., & Karmiloff-Smith, A. (2002). Neuroimaging of typical and atypical development: a perspective from multiple levels of analysis. *Development and Psychopathology*, **14**, 521–36.

Jones, W., Hesselink, J.R., Courchesne, E., Duncan, T., Matsuda, K., & Bellugi, U. (2002). Cerebellar abnormalities in infants and toddlers with Williams syndrome. *Developmental Medicine and Child Neurology*, **44**, 688–94.

Karmiloff-Smith, A. (1997). Crucial differences between developmental cognitive neuroscience and adult neuropsychology. *Developmental Neuropsychology*, **13**, 513–24.

Karmiloff-Smith, A. (1998). Development itself is the key to understanding developmental disorders. *Trends in Cognitive Sciences,* **2**, 389–98.

Karmiloff-Smith, A. (2009). Nativism versus neuroconstructivism: rethinking the study of developmental disorders. special issue on the interplay of biology and environment. *Developmental Psychology*, **45**, 56–63.

Karmiloff-Smith, A. (2010). Neuroimaging of the developing brain: taking "developing" seriously. *Human Brain Mapping*, **31**, 934–41.

Karmiloff-Smith, A., Grant, J., Berthoud, I., Davies, M., Howlin, P., & Udwin, O. (1997). Language and Williams syndrome: how intact is "intact"? *Child Development*, **68**, 246–62.

Karmiloff-Smith, A., Grant, J., Ewing. S., Carette, M.J., Metcalfe, K., Donnai, D., et al. (2003). Using case study comparisons to explore genotype-phenotype correlations in Williams Beuren syndrome. *Journal of Medical Genetics*, **40**, 136–40.

Karmiloff-Smith, A., Thomas, M., Annaz, D., Humphreys, K., Ewing, S., Brace, N., et al. (2004). Exploring the Williams syndrome face-processing debate: the importance of building developmental trajectories. *Journal of Child Psychology and Psychiatry*, **45**, 1258–74

Kippenhan, J., Olsen, R., Mervis, C., Morris, C., Kohn, P., Meyer-Lindenberg, A., et al. (2005). Genetic contributions to human gyrification: sulcal morphometry in Williams syndrome. *Journal of Neuroscience*, **25**, 7840–46.

Konrad, K., & Eickhoff, S.B. (2010). Is the ADHD brain wired differently? A review on structural and functional connectivity in attention deficit hyperactivity disorder. *Human Brain Mapping*, **31**, 904–916.

Landau, B., Hoffman, J.E., & Kurz, N. (2005). Object definition with severe spatial deficits in Williams syndrome: sparing and breakdown. *Cognition*, **100**, 483–510.

Lloyd-Fox, S., Blasi, A., & Elwell, C.E. (2010). Illuminating the developing brain: the past, present and future of functional near infrared spectroscopy. *Neuroscience and Biobehavioural Reviews*, **34**, 269–84.

Logothetis, N.K., Pauls, J., Augath, M., Trinath, T., & Oeltermann, A. (2001). Neurophysiological investigation of the basis of the fMRI signal. *Nature*, **412**, 150–57.

Luders, E., Narr, K.L., Bilder, R.M., Thompson, P.M., Szeszko, P.R., Hamilton, L., et al. (2007). Positive correlations between corpus callosum thickness and intelligence. *NeuroImage*, **37**, 1457–64.

Marenco, S., & Radulescu, E. (2010). Imaging genetics of structural brain connectivity and neural integrity markers. *NeuroImage*, **53**, 848–56.

Marenco, S., Siuta, M., Kippenhan, J., Grodofsky, S., Chang, W.-L., Kohn, P., et al. (2007). Genetic contributions to white matter architecture revealed by diffusion tensor imaging in Williams syndrome. *Proceedings of the National Academy of Sciences of the USA*, **104**, 155117–22.

Martens, M.A., Wilson, S.J., & Reutens, D.C. (2008). Williams syndrome: a critical review of the cognitive, behavioural, and neuroanatomical phenotype. *The Journal of Child Psychology and Psychiatry*, **49**, 576–608.

Meek, J. (2002). Basic principles of optical imaging and application to the study of infant development. *Developmental Science*, **5**, 371–80.

Menghini, D., Di Paola, M., Federico, F., Vicari, S., Petrosini, L., Caltagirone, C., et al. (2011). Relationship between brain abnormalities and cognitive profile in Williams syndrome. *Behavioural Genetics*, **41**, 394–402.

Menon, V., Leroux, J., White, C.D., & Reiss A.L. (2004). Frontostriatal deficits in fragile x syndrome: relation to FMR1 gene expression. *Proceedings of the National Academy of Sciences of the USA*, **101**, 3615–20.

Meyer-Lindenberg, A., Kohn, P., Mwervis, C.B., Jippenhan, J.S., Olsen, R.K., Morris, C.A., et al. (2004). Neural basis of genetically determined visuospatial construction deficit in Williams syndrome. *Neuron*, **43**, 623–31.

Meyer-Lindenberg, A., Mervis, C.B., & Berman, K.F. (2006). Neural mechanisms in Williams syndrome: a unique window to genetic influences on cognition and behaviour. *Nature Reviews Neuroscience*, **7**, 380–93.

Meyer-Lindenberg, A., Mervis, C.B., Sarpal, D., Koch, P., Steele, S., Kohn, P., et al. (2005). Functional, structural, and metabolic abnormalities of the hippocampal formation in Williams syndrome. *Journal of Clinical Investigation*, **115**, 1888–95.

Mills, D.L., Alvarez, T.D., St. George, M., Appelbaum, L.G., Bellugi, U., & Neville, H. (2000). Electrophysiological studies of face processing in Williams syndrome. *Journal of Cognitive Neuroscience*, **12**, 47–64.

Minagawa-Kawai, Y., Mori, K., Naoi, N., & Kojima, S. (2007). Neural attunement processes in infants during the acquisition of a language-specific phonemic contrast. *Journal of Neuroscience*, **27**, 315–21.

Minagawa-Kawai, Y., Naoi, N., Naoko, K., Yamamoto, J.-I., Nakamura, K., & Kojima, S. (2009). Cerebral laterality for phonemic and prosodic cue decoding in children with autism. *NeuroReport*, **20**, 1219–24.

Mobbs, D., Eckert, M.A., Mills, D., Korenberg, J., Bellugi, U., Galaburda, A.M., et al. (2007). Frontostriatal dysfunction during response inhibition in Williams syndrome. *Biological Psychiatry*, **62**, 256–61.

Molko, N., Cachia, A., Riviere, D., Mangin, J.-F., Bruandet, M., Le Bihan, D., et al. (2003). Functional and structural alterations of the intraparietal sulcus in a developmental dyscalculia of genetic origin. *Neuron*, **40**, 847–58.

Neville, H.J., Mills, D.L., & Bellugi, U. (1994). Effects of altered auditory sensitivity and age of language acquisition on the development of language-relevant neural systems: preliminary studies of Williams syndrome. In S. Broman & J. Grafman (Eds), *Atypical Cognitive Deficits in Developmental Disorders: Implications for Brain Function* (pp. 67–83). Hillsdale, NJ: Lawrence Erlbaum.

Paus, T. (2010). Growth of white matter in the adolescent brain: myelin or axon? *Brain and Cognition*, 72, 26–35.

Plessen, K.J., Gruner, R., Lundervold, A., Hirsch, J.G., Xu, D., Bansal, R., et al. (2006). Reduced white matter connectivity in the corpus callosum of children with Tourette syndrome. *The Journal of Child Psychology and Psychiatry*, 47, 1013–22.

Rae, C., Karmiloff-Smith, A., Lee, M.A., Dixon, R.M., Grant, J., Blamire, A.M., et al. (1998). Brain biochemistry in Williams syndrome: evidence for a role of the cerebellum in cognition? *Neurology*, 51, 33–40.

Reiss, A.L., Eckert, M.A., Rose, F.E., Karcheminskiy, A., Kesler, S., Reynolds, M.F., et al. (2004). An experiment of nature: brain anatomy parallels cognitition and behaviour in Williams syndrome. *Journal of Neuroscience*, 24, 5009–5015.

Rhodes, S.M., Riby, D.M., Park, J., Fraser, E., & Campbell, L.E. (2010). Executive neuropsychological functioning in individuals with Williams syndrome. *Neuropsychologia*, 48, 1216–26.

Sahyoun, C.P., Belliveau, J.W., Soulières, I., Schwartz, S., & Mody, M. (2010). Neuroimaging of the functional and structural networks underlying visuospatial vs. linguistic reasoning in high-functioning autism. *Neuropsychologia*, 48, 86–95.

Sampaio, A., Bouix, S., Sousa, N., Prieto, M., & Vasconcelos, C. (2010). Morphometry and connectivity of corpus callosum: indices of neural development in Williams syndrome. *International Journal of Developmental Neuroscience*, 28, 716.

Sarpal, D., Buchsbaum, B.R., Kohn, P.D., Kippenhan, J.S., Mervis, C.B., Morris, C.A, et al. (2008). A genetic model for understanding higher order visual processing: functional interactions of the ventral visual stream in Williams syndrome. *Cerebral Cortex*, 18, 24022409.

Schmitt, J.E., Eliez, S., Bellugi, U., & Reiss, A. (2001). Analysis of cerebral shape in Williams syndrome. *Archives of Neurology*, 58, 283–87.

Schmitt, J.E., Eliez, S., Warsofsky, I.S., Bellugi, U., & Reiss, A. (2001a). Corpus callosum morphology of Williams syndrome: relation to genetics and behaviour. *Developmental Medicine Child Neurology*, 43, 155–59.

Schmitt, J.E., Eliez, S., Warsofsky, I.S., Bellugi, U., & Reiss.A.L. (2001b). Enlarged cerebellar vermis in Williams syndrome. *Journal of Psychiatric Research*, 35, 225–29.

Shaywitz, S.E., Shaywitz, B.A., Fulbright, R.K., Skudlarski, P., Mencl, W.E., Constable, R.T., et al. (2003). Neural systems for compensation and persistence: young adult outcome of childhood reading disability. *Biological Psychiatry*, 54, 25–33.

Simon, T.J., Bish, J.P., Bearden, C.E., Ding, L., Ferrante, S., Nguyen, V., et al. (2005). A multilevel analysis of cognitive dysfunction and psychopathology associated with chromosome 22q11.2 deletion syndrome in children. *Developmental psycholpathology*, 17, 753–84.

Southgate, V., Johnson, M.H., Osborne, T., & Csibra, G. (2009). Predictive motor activation during action observation in human infants. *Biology Letters*, 5, 769–72.

Steinbrink, J., Villringer, A., Kempf, F., Haux, D., Boden, S., & Obrig, H. (2006). Illuminating the BOLD signal: combined fMRI-fNIRS studies. *Magnetic Resonance Imaging*, 24, 495–505.

Suda, M., Takei, Y. Aoyama, Y., Narita, K., Sato, T., Fukuda, M., et al. (2010). Frontopolar activation during face-to-face conversation: an in situ study using near-infrared spectroscopy. *Neuropsychologia*, 48, 441–47.

Thompson, P.M., Lee, A.D., Dutton, R.A., Geaga, J.A., Hayashi, K.M., Eckert, M.A., et al. A.L. (2005). Abnormal cortical complexity and thickness profiles mapped in Williams syndrome. *The Journal of Neuroscience*, 25, 4146–58.

Tomaiuolo, F., Di Paola, M., Caravale, B., Vicari, S., Petrides, M., & Caltagirone, C. (2002). Morphology and morphometry of the corpus callosum in Williams syndrome: a T1-weighted MRI study. *NeuroReport*, 13, 2281–84.

Van den Heuvel, O.A., Veltman, D.J., Groenewegen, H.J., Cath, D.C., van Balkom, A.J.L.M., van

Hartskamp, J., et al. (2005). Frontal-striatal dysfunction during planning in obsessive-compulsive disoder. *Archives of General Psychiatry*, **62**, 301–309.

Van Essen, D.C., Dierker, D., Snyder, A.Z., Raichle, M.E., Reiss, A.L., & Korenberg, J. (2006). Symmetry of cortical folding abnormalities in Williams syndrome revealed by surface-based analyses. *The Journal of Neuroscience*, **26**, 5470–83.

Vidal, C.N., Nicolson, R., DeVito, T.J., Hayashi, K.M., Geaga, J.A., Drost, D.J., et al. (2006). Mapping corpus callosum deficits in autism: an index of aberrant cortical connectivity. *Biological Psychiatry*, **60**, 218–25.

Wang, P.P., Doherty, S., Hesselink, J.R., & Bellugi, U. (1992). Callosal morphology concurs with neurobehavioural and neuropathological findings in two neurodevelopmental disorders. *Archives of Neurology*, **42**, 1999–2002.

Chapter 3

Genes: The gene expression approach

Lucy R. Osborne

Introduction

Williams syndrome (WS) is caused by the hemizygous deletion (deletion of one of the two copies) of more than 25 genes on the long arm of human chromosome 7 (Table 3.1; Figure 3.1). The deletion occurs during meiosis, the swapping of genetic material between chromosomes as the egg or sperm cells are generated, so it can arise in either parent even though they show no symptoms of WS. The presence of large blocks of almost identical DNA sequences flanking the WS chromosome region leads to incorrect alignment of the two chromosomes as they swap genetic material and can result in either deletion or duplication of the intervening region (Osborne & Mervis, 2007). This mechanism leads to a common deletion size, with only rare cases of shorter deletions that can help link specific genes with aspects of the complex phenotype (C.A. Morris, 2010). The gene encoding elastin (*ELN*) is still the only gene that has been unequivocally linked with any aspect of WS; haploinsufficiency for *ELN* causes cardiovascular disease, hypertension and soft-tissue changes (Pober, 2010). However, evidence from individuals with atypical deletions and from mouse models points to particular genes—*LIMK1*, *CLIP2*, *GTF2I* and *GTF2IRD1*—within the WS region that are likely to play a significant role in the many other phenotypic features of this disorder (C.A. Morris, 2010).

To fully understand how the complex clinical, cognitive and behavioural phenotype of WS develops and why it can vary so much between individuals, it is crucial to determine the role of each of the deleted genes throughout development and adulthood and to map the effects of other genetic and environmental factors. WS is a developmental disorder that affects many different body systems. Since reduced expression of multiple genes is responsible for the varied phenotypic consequences, knowledge of their expression throughout pre- and postnatal development is important if we are to understand the molecular basis for these symptoms or generate effective therapies. When trying to understand the impact of altered gene expression in WS, we must examine the precise spatial and temporal expression of the genes that contribute to the WS phenotype.

The majority of mammalian genes have changing patterns of expression during development, depending on their role at any given time, and this is also true of genes from the WS region. Since WS is a dominant disorder, we must also consider the effects of altered gene dosage rather than complete loss of gene function, and how this impacts on specific tissues or developmental stages. Some of the genes deleted in WS are general transcription factors

Table 3.1 Expression of genes from the Williams syndrome region

Gene[a]	Expression in the developing brain	Expression in the adult brain	Splice variants[1]
NOP2/Sun domain family, member 5			
Nsun5	n/a	Yes[2]; low in reticular nucleus, olfactory bulb, thalamus, cortex, hippocampus, Purkinje cells[3]	No
NSUN5	n/a	Yes[4]	Yes
Tripartite motif containing 50			
Trim50	n/a	No[2,3,5]	Yes
TRIM50	n/a	No[2]	Yes
FK506 binding protein 6			
Fkbp6	n/a	No[2,6]; entire cortex, medulla, amygdala, Purkinje cells, molecular layer of cerebellum[3]	Yes
FKBP6	Yes[7]	Yes[4,7]	Yes
Frizzled homologue 9			
Fzd9	E11.5 ventricular zone of cortex, E14.5 cortical plate, E12.5 hippocampus, P8 Purkinje cells[8,9]	Yes[2]; no[3]; Cortex layer II/III, CA region, dentate gyrus of hippocampus[8]	No
FZD9	n/a	Yes[4]	No
Bromodomain adjacent to zinc finger domain, 1B			
Baz1b	E8.5 presumptive hindbrain, headfolds[10]; E13.5 midbrain and hindbrain[11]	Yes[2,12]; Entire brain, higher in hippocampus, granular layer of cerebellum[3]	No
BAZ1B	Gestational weeks 19-23[12]	Yes[4,12]	No
B-cell chronic lymphocytic leukaemia/lymphoma 7B			
Bcl7b	n/a	Yes[2]; low in cortex, medulla, hippocampus, Purkinje cells[3]	Yes
BCL7B	Fetal brain[13]	Yes[4,13]; no[14]	Yes
Transducin (beta)-like 2			
Tbl2	n/a	Yes[2]; weak expression[15]; no[3]	Yes
TBL2	Fetal brain[13]	Yes[4]; weak expression[13,15]	Yes
MLX interacting protein-like			
Mlxipl	Yes[16]	No[2,3,17]	Yes
MLXIPL	No[13]	Yes[4,15]; no[12,17,18]	Yes
Vacuolar protein sorting 37 homolog D			
Vps37d	n/a	Yes[2,5]; entire brain, high in cortex layer II/III, granular layer of cerebellum, hippocampus[3]	Yes
VPS37D	n/a	Yes[4]	Yes

(Continued)

Table 3.1 (Cont'd)

Gene[a]	Expression in the developing brain	Expression in the adult brain	Splice variants[1]
DnaJ (heat shock protein 40) homolog, subfamily C, member 30			
Dnajc30	n/a	Yes[2]	Yes
DNAJC30	n/a	Yes[4,19]	No
Williams–Beuren syndrome chromosome region 22			
Wbscr22	n/a	Yes[2]; low throughout brain, higher in cortex, hippocampus, Purkinje cells[3]	Yes
WBSCR22	n/a	Yes[4]; low level[19]	Yes
Syntaxin 1A			
Stx1a	n/a	Yes[2]; high exclusively in cerebral cortex, hippocampus[3]	Yes
STX1A	Gestational weeks 5.3-10 in spinal cord and dorsal root ganglia[20]	Yes[4]; molecular layer of the cortex, amygdala, hippocampus, cerebellum[20]	Yes
Abhydrolase domain containing 11			
Abhd11	n/a	Yes[2]; low throughout brain[3]	Yes
ABHD11	n/a	Yes[4,19]	Yes
Claudin 3			
Cldn3	n/a	No[2]	Yes
CLDN3	n/a	No[4]	No
Claudin 4			
Cldn4	n/a	No[2,3,21]	No
CLDN4	No[21]	Very few expressed sequence tags[4]; no[20]	No
Williams–Beuren syndrome chromosome region 27			
Wbscr27	n/a	No[2,3,5]	Yes
WBSCR27	n/a	No[4]	Yes
Williams–Beuren syndrome chromosome region 28			
Wbscr28	n/a	No[2,5]	No
WBSCR28	n/a	No[4]	Yes
Elastin			
Eln	E10.5 neuroepithelia[22]	Yes[2]; in blood vessels[3]	No
ELN	n/a	Yes[4]	Yes
LIM domain kinase 1			
LIMK1	Diffuse expression throughout CNS; Purkinje cells, hippocampus, cortex layer II/III[23]	Yes[2,3]; cortex (layers III, V, VI), thalamus, Purkinje cell layer, deep nuclei of cerebellum[23]	Yes
LIMK1	n/a	Yes[4]	Yes

(Continued)

Table 3.1 (Cont'd)

Gene[a]	Expression in the developing brain	Expression in the adult brain	Splice variants[1]
\multicolumn{4}{l}{Eukaryotic translation initiation factor 4H}			
Eif4h	n/a	Yes[2]; high throughout brain especially hippocampus, cortex layer II/III, granular layer of cerebellum[3]	Yes
EIF4H	n/a	Yes[4]	Yes
\multicolumn{4}{l}{microRNA 590}			
miR-590	n/a	No[24]	No
MIR590	n/a	No[24]	No
\multicolumn{4}{l}{Linker for activation of T-cells family, member 2}			
Lat2	n/a	Yes[2,25]; no[3]	Yes
LAT2	n/a	Yes[4,25,26]	Yes
\multicolumn{4}{l}{Replication factor C subunit 2}			
Rfc2	n/a	Yes[2]; low in hippocampus[3]	No
RFC2	n/a	Yes[4]	Yes
\multicolumn{4}{l}{Cytoplasmic linker 2 (CAP-GLY domain containing linker protein 2)}			
Clip2	n/a	Yes[2]; high in pyramidal cells of CA1 and CA3 in hippocampus, lower in cortex, Purkinje cells[3,27]	Yes
CLIP2	n/a	Yes[4]	Yes
\multicolumn{4}{l}{General transcription factor II-I repeat domain containing 1}			
Gtf2ird1	E13.5 - E18.5 diffuse throughout brain, except telecephalon/cortex[28]	Yes[2]; low throughout brain, high in Purkinje cells, olfactory bulb, cortex layer V[3,28–30]; granular cells of cerebellum[31]	Yes
GTF2IRD1	n/a	Yes[4]	Yes
\multicolumn{4}{l}{General transcription factor II-I}			
Gtf2i	E8.0 neural ectoderm, E9.0 neural tube[32]; E18.5 uniform expression, but becomes restricted by P7[31]	Yes[2]; low throughout brain, high in hippocampus, Purkinje cells[3,31,32]; cortex layer II/III, granule layer of hippocampus and dentate gyrus[28]	Yes
GTF2I	n/a	Yes[4]	Yes
\multicolumn{4}{l}{Neutrophil cytosolic factor 1}			
Ncf1	n/a	Yes[2]	Yes
NCF1	n/a	Yes[4]	Yes

(Continued)

Table 3.1 (Cont'd)

Gene[a]	Expression in the developing brain	Expression in the adult brain	Splice variants[1]
General transcription factor II-I repeat domain containing 2			
Gtf2ird2	n/a	Yes[2]; widely expressed, high in hippocampus, Purkinje cells, olfactory bulb, cortex layer II/II[3]	Yes
GTF2IRD2	n/a	Yes[4]	Yes

Abbreviations: CNS = central nervous system; E = embryonic day; n/a = data not available; P = postnatal day.
[a] Lower-case gene names refer to genes from mouse and upper-case gene names refer to genes from human.
Sources: [1] Based on the presence of alternative transcripts present in Ensembl (European Bioinformatics Institute & Wellcome Trust Sanger Institute, 2000); [2] Based on the presence of mouse expressed sequence tags generated from brain libraries (National Center for Biotechnology Information, n.d.); [3] Based on expression data in the *Allen Mouse Brain Atlas* (Allen Institute for Brain Science, 2009); [4] Based on the presence of human expressed sequence tags generated from brain libraries (National Center for Biotechnology Information, n.d.); [5] Micale et al., 2009; [6] Crackower et al., 2003; [7] Meng et al., 1998b; [8] Zhou et al., 2010; [9] Wang et al., 1999; [10] Ashe et al., 2008; [11] Gray et al., 2004; [12] Peoples et al., 1998; [13] Meng et al., 1998b; [14] Jadayel et al., 1998; [15] Pérez-Jurado et al., 1999; [16] Cairo et al., 2001; [17] de Luis et al., 2000; [18] Iizuka et al., 2004; [19] Merla et al., 2002; [20] Botta et al., 1999; [21] Paperna et al., 1998; [22] Lakkakorpi et al. 1999; [23] Mori et al., 1997; [24] Computational Biology Center at Memorial Sloan-Kettering Cancer Center (n.d.); [25] Martindale et al., 2000; [26] Doyle et al., 2000; [27] Hoogenraad et al., 2002; [28] Palmer et al., 2007; [29] Young, 2010; [30] Proulx et al., 2010; [31] Danoff et al., 2004; [32] Fijalkowska et al., 2010.

that control the expression of many other genes, so the downstream effects of their altered expression may be broad. Other genes from the region have a paralogue (paralogues are pairs of genes derived from the same ancestral gene) that may compensate for the reduced expression in some tissues, but not in others. Moreover, some of the WS genes are members of parallel pathways that converge on the same biological process, so compounding the effects of altered expression of each individual gene. Although not firmly established, there may also be an epigenetic component to WS, where the parent of origin of the deletion

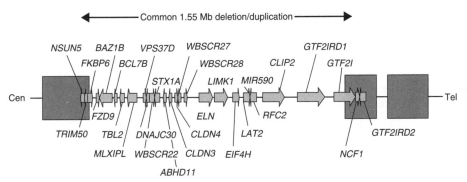

Fig. 3.1 The Williams syndrome region on chromosome 7q11.23. Genes within the 1.55-Mb commonly deleted/duplicate region at 7q11.23 are represented by shaded arrows indicating the direction of transcription. The flanking low-copy repeats that mediate deletion or duplication of the region are represented by dark shaded boxes. Abbreviations: Cen = centromeric region; Tel = telomeric region; for full versions of the gene names see Table 3.1. With kind permission from Springer Science+Business Media: Genomic Disorders: The Genomic Basis of Disease, Williams-Beuren syndrome, 2006, pp. 221–236, Scherer, S.W., & Osborne, L.R.

impacts on the severity of some phenotypic features (epigenetic changes refer to heritable changes in gene activity that are not caused by alteration of the genetic code). Finally, it is essential to understand the role of gene expression in adulthood versus development to determine the origin of the phenotypic features of WS. Many characteristic symptoms of WS are evident at birth, but it is not known whether these are reversible during postnatal life or even in adulthood. Recent therapeutic treatments have been at least partially successful in mouse models of neurodevelopmental disorders such as fragile X syndrome and Rett syndrome, and newly developed mouse models of WS will be invaluable in establishing therapeutics for cardiovascular and neurological symptoms of WS.

Central nervous system development

In vertebrates, most organ and tissue development occurs during the prenatal stages of embryogenesis, with postnatal changes primarily concerned with growth. However, this is not the case in the central nervous system, where a significant amount of morphological development, cell differentiation and acquisition of function takes place during postnatal development (Noback et al., 2005). Complex but structured molecular mechanisms are involved, and characterising these genetic programs and multigene pathways is one of the most challenging aspects of modern biology.

The adult brain consists of approximately 100 billion neurons that between them make trillions of synaptic connections. The control and coordination that are necessary for the development of this complex living system come from a combination of genetic programming and interaction with the environment. Brain changes and adaptation occur throughout the lifetime, but the most dramatic and probably most important periods are the earliest. In early gestation, neurons are forming at the fantastic rate of thousands per minute and this continues throughout prenatal development and into early postnatal development, with a maximum number reached at around 2 years of age (Noback et al., 2005). Cortical development also continues postnatally into late adolescence following the trajectory of neural proliferation, migration and differentiation, followed by axonal and dendritic growth, synaptogenesis, myelination and, finally, neuronal death through sculpting and pruning (Noback et al., 2005). This process is subject to modifications driven by stimulation and experience, but a proportion is predetermined by a precise genetic program. For example, the blueprint for the body plan in different animal species, including the plan for hindbrain development, is determined by the same set of transcription factor genes (homeobox genes) (Tümpel et al., 2009). In mice, synaptogenesis is initiated by the coordinated expression of many synapse protein genes before activity-dependent gene expression and morphological changes occur (Valor et al., 2007). Neurons themselves are among the most transcriptionally active cells in the body, with complex transcription programs that allow them to become highly specialised with individual electrophysiological signatures (Nelson et al., 2006). The advent of microarray technology has provided a way of analysing gene expression on a genome-wide scale and the ability to differentiate and sort specific cell types will allow in-depth characterisation of neuronal subtypes (Díaz, 2009).

Expression of genes from the WS region

Although the complex genetic programming of human brain development remains poorly understood, it is possible to examine the expression of the specific genes deleted in WS to help understand their potential roles. Of the 28 transcripts that lie within the WS deletion region, 22 are expressed in the brain (Table 3.1), although the temporal and spatial dynamics and the cell types in which they are expressed have not yet been well-studied in most cases. Preliminary data on expression are available in mice for some genes, where either messenger RNA (mRNA) or protein expression can be analysed through RNA *in situ* hybridisation or the use of a *LacZ* reporter gene. Insertion of a *LacZ* reporter into a gene locus results in the expression of a fusion protein under the control of the endogenous promoter, so allowing the analysis of spatial and temporal protein expression (Mountford et al., 1994). For example, Hoogenraad et al., (2002) used a LacZ marker to identify tissues where cytoplasmic linker 2 (Clip2) was expressed in the adult mouse brain and found robust expression in the hippocampus, amygdala, cerebral cortex and cerebellum. Syntaxin 1A (STX1A) was found to be widely expressed throughout the developing and adult brain, probably because of its essential role in neurotransmission, where it facilitates the fusion of neurotransmitter-containing vesicles at the presynaptic membrane (Allen Institute for Brain Science, 2009; Bennett et al., 1992; Botta et al., 1999).

LIM domain kinase 1

LIM domain kinase 1 (LIMK1), which is encoded near the centre of the common WS deletion, controls actin dynamics via the phosphorylation and inactivation of cofilin (Arber et al., 1998). The rapid turnover of actin required for dynamic processes such as growth cone motility and neurite outgrowth is achieved through cofilin, which depolymerises the actin filaments, allowing them to be reassembled in a different position. Interfering with this process by changing the activity of cofilin through the increase or decrease of the amount of LIMK1 can have dramatic effects on the morphology and growth of neurites both in culture and in the mammalian brain (Endo et al., 2003; Endo et al., 2007; Meng et al., 2002). LIMK1 is expressed in the developing human midbrain, cerebellum, spinal cord and peripheral nervous system (Frangiskakis et al., 1996). Pröschel et al. (1995) found mRNA expression in the adult spinal cord, cortex, cerebellum and placenta of the mouse, and expressed sequence tag evidence indicates that it is expressed in many adult tissues (National Center for Biotechnology Information, n.d.). Rather than being expressed throughout the developing brain, however, LIMK1 is restricted to the ependymal layer, where neurons are generated, which is consistent with its important role in growth cone motility and with an essential function in neurogenesis (Frangiskakis et al., 1996; Pröschel et al., 1995).

   Although disruption of *Limk1* in a mouse model caused abnormal neuronal spine morphology, altered synaptic function and some mild cognitive abnormalities, complete lack of LIMK1—somewhat unexpectedly considering its function—produced viable animals (Meng et al., 2002). This was hypothesised to be attributable to functional redundancy by a paralogue, LIMK2, which shares approximately 50% amino acid identity with LIMK1 and can also phosphorylate cofilin (Sumi et al., 1999). Both genes seem to be expressed in the central nervous system during development, but differential expression was seen in specific regions such as the cerebellum and cortex, where LIMK1 expression was predominant (Mori et al., 1997). However, mice lacking both LIMK1 and LIMK2 were still viable and showed no gross abnormalities of the central nervous system and normal home cage behaviour (Meng et al., 2004). The mice showed similar changes in synaptic function to the *Limk1* knockout mice, but were even less efficient at phosphorylating cofilin (Meng et al., 2004).

In addition to developmental control of *Limk1* expression, hormonal control of LIMK1 activity has been shown during the oestrus cycle of mice. Activation of LIMK1 in the hippocampus, but not the cortex, was found to be highest when circulating steroid hormone levels were at their highest level and lowest when these hormones were at their lowest circulating levels (Spencer et al., 2008). This study raises the possibility that actin remodelling in the hippocampus is affected by fluctuations in endogenous oestradiols in females during the oestrus cycle, although it remains to be seen whether there is a real physiological effect on behaviour or cognition (see Chapter 12 for discussion of a possible role for *LIMK1* in visuospatial cognition).

General transcription factor II-I genes

The three general transcription factor II-I genes *GTF2I*, *GTF2IRD1* and *GTF2IRD2* code for TFII-I, TFII-IRD1 and TFII-IRD2, the sole members of a family of proteins that contain helix-loop-helix domains and are able to dimerise (two protein molecules joining together) and bind DNA (Hinsley et al., 2004). The genes are thought to have evolved from a single ancestral locus, probably *GTF2IRD1* because this gene is most similar to the only *GTF2I*-like gene present in zebrafish and frogs (Makeyev et al., 2004). The TFII-I proteins are proposed to act as transcriptional activators and/or repressors and therefore may have wide-ranging effects on the expression of other genes during development. These proteins are expressed in regions of the brain implicated in the pathophysiology of WS and show a dynamic pattern of spatial and temporal expression. All three genes are expressed more widely and abundantly during development than in adulthood, particularly in the brain (Danoff et al., 2004; Fijalkowska et al., 2010; Allen Institute for Brain Science, 2009), and TFII-I and TFII-IRD1 seem to be expressed throughout pre- and postimplantation embryogenesis (Bayarsaihan et al., 2003; Enkhmandakh et al., 2004) (see Chapters 12 and 15 for discussion of WS phenotypic characteristics that might be associated with deletion of the *GTF2I* genes).

The reports of *Gtf2i* and TFII-I expression in the mouse are quite consistent, with data derived from mRNA *in situ* hybridisation, immunohistochemistry with specific antibodies and knock-in LacZ reporter proteins (Danoff et al., 2004; Enkhmandakh et al., 2004; Fijalkowska et al., 2010; Palmer et al., 2007). Reported temporal and spatial expression of *Gtf2ird1* and TFII-IRD1, however, differs between publications, depending on the method by which the data were generated. Bayarsaihan et al. (2003) used a

TFII-IRD1 antibody for immunohistochemistry on sections from the developing mouse, but Western blot analysis detected multiple bands, indicating that this antibody may not be specific for TFII-IRD1. Palmer et al. (2007) used a knock-in *LacZ* reporter to assay TFII-IRD1 protein expression and although there was some overlap with the antibody data, overall the correlation was poor. A subsequent *LacZ* reporter mouse showed expression consistent with Palmer et al. (2007), but no developmental time points were assayed (Proulx et al., 2010).

TFII-I and TFII-IRD1 expression during mouse embryogenesis

In the postimplantation mouse embryo, TFII-I is expressed in the neural ectoderm and neural tube between embryonic day (E) 8.0 and E9.0 (mouse gestation is 19 days), and becomes uniformly expressed in the brain during the second half of gestation (Danoff et al., 2004; Fijalkowska et al., 2010). By postnatal day 7, expression has become more restricted and resembles the distribution seen in the adult brain (Danoff et al., 2004). Isoform-specific antibodies have also detected differences in immunoreactivity between cell types within the developing brain, indicating that different sets of genes may be altered in a complex temporal and spatial manner (Danoff et al., 2004). Immunohistochemistry with a TFII-IRD1 antibody showed immunoreactivity throughout the developing mouse brain up until E15.5, when expression was no longer detected (Bayarsaihan et al., 2003). Analysis of mice expressing a TFII-IRD1 knock-in LacZ protein showed expression throughout the midbrain and hindbrain during the second half of gestation (E13.5-E18.5) with highest levels in the pituitary, the thalamic and hypothalamic tissues, the roof of the midbrain and the ventral hindbrain (Palmer et al., 2007). This study also found high expression in specific tissues (e.g. brown adipose tissue) that did not show immunoreactivity in the study by Bayarsaihan et al. (2003).

TFII-I and TFII-IRD1 expression in the adult mouse brain

In the adult mouse, TFII-I shows highest levels of protein expression in the Purkinje cells of the cerebellum, the pyramidal and interneurons of the hippocampus and dentate gyrus and the large neurons of the cortex (Danoff et al., 2004; Young, 2010). TFII-IRD1 also shows a restricted expression in the adult brain, predominantly in the cerebellum and regions of the cortex (piriform cortex, superior colliculus, raphe nucleus) (Palmer et al., 2007; Proulx et al., 2010). Although these evolutionarily related proteins are expressed in the same brain region, their patterns of expression can be quite distinct. For example, in the cortex, TFII-I is expressed predominantly in layer II/III, whereas TFII-IRD1 is expressed in the large pyramidal neurons of layer V (Figure 3.2; Proulx et al., 2010; Young, 2010). In the cerebellum, both TFII-I and TFII-IRD1 have been shown to be present predominantly in the Purkinje cells (Danoff et al., 2004; Fijalkowska, et al., 2010; Palmer et al., 2007; Young, 2010), although one study reported TFII-IRD1 only in the granular cells (Danoff et al., 2004). There is certainly some overlap in expression between these two proteins, and specific target genes have been shown to be coordinately regulated by TFII-I and TFII-IRD1, with one protein promoting and the other repressing transcription (Jackson et al., 2005; Ku et al., 2005).

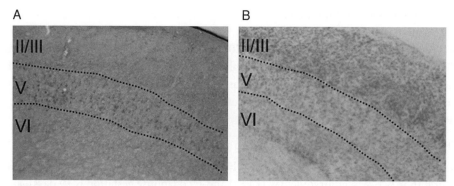

Fig. 3.2 (See also Plate 4) Patterns of TFII-IRD1 and TFII-I expression. (A) Coronal sections (50 µm) from the medial prefrontal cortex from *Gtf2ird1*$^{Gt(XS0608)Wtsi}$ adult mice. (B) Coronal sections (50 µm) from the medial prefrontal cortex from *Gtf2i*$^{Gt(YTA365)Byg}$ adult mice. Expression of the LacZ fusion protein in sections from each mouse line was visualised by X-gal staining. The Roman numerals indicate layers of the cortex.

Cellular localisation of TFII-I and TFII-IRD1

Although TFII-I and TFII-IRD1 are regarded as transcription factors, both proteins have been localised not only to the nucleus, where they would be expected to reside, but also to the cell cytoplasm. Danoff et al. (2004) saw TFII-I immunoreactivity in both the nucleus and the cell body of Purkinje cells and hippocampal neurons in the adult mouse, and Fijalkowska et al. (2010) saw differences in TFII-I cellular localisation at specific developmental stages. At E8.0, they found cytoplasmic expression in the neural ectoderm, whereas 1 day later they saw localisation to both nucleus and cytoplasm in the brain. An alternative cellular function for TFII-I was identified in B-cells, where it was shown to negatively regulate agonist-induced calcium entry into the cell (Caraveo et al., 2006). It is possible that TFII-I could have a similar cellular function in neurons, where intracellular calcium ion concentration plays a vital role in regulating fundamental cellular processes as well as neuronal excitability and synaptic plasticity (Selvaraj et al., 2010). Bayarsaihan et al. (2003) noted cytoplasmic localisation of TFII-IRD1 during early gastrulation in the mouse embryo between E3.5 and E6.5, indicating that it too may have a second, as yet undetermined, role within the cell. It has also been suggested that the levels of expression of TFII-I and TFII-IRD1 may affect the cellular localisation of the respective other protein when the proteins are co-expressed, although these studies have been carried out *in vitro* and there is no evidence for an *in vivo* effect (Ku et al., 2005; Tussié-Luna et al., 2001).

A role for epigenetics in WS

Epigenetics refers to heritable modifications to DNA other than alterations to the primary DNA sequence. Epigenetic mechanisms play key roles in the development of the mammalian nervous system and the disruption of epigenetically regulated genes or pathways can have severe consequences. Several neurodevelopmental disorders have been linked to the dysregulation of epigenetic marks or epigenetic mechanisms, including Rett syndrome, Prader–Willi syndrome, Angelman syndrome, Beckwith–Wiedemann syndrome,

Rubinstein–Taybi syndrome, fragile X syndrome, ATRX syndrome and autism spectrum disorders (Gräff & Mansuy, 2009; De Sario, 2009; Grafodatskaya et al., 2010). These disorders are characterised by alterations to DNA methylation or histone modification that affect gene expression without changing the DNA sequence. Given the number of disorders involving intellectual disability where epigenetic mechanisms are implicated, it is worth considering whether the WS deletion impacts epigenetic control and whether any symptoms of WS may be related to changes in epigenetically regulated genes.

Although there is currently no strong evidence for imprinted genes (genes with differential expression depending on which parent they were inherited from) within the WS region, there is some indication that epigenetic factors may contribute to the phenotypic variation. Three studies have looked at the effect of the parent of origin of the WS deletion on the phenotypic characteristics of individuals with WS. One small study reported significant parent-of-origin effects for head circumference, height and weight, with maternal origin of the deletion related to worse outcomes (Pérez-Jurado et al., 1996). However, only the head circumference finding was replicated in a larger sample of 66 individuals (Del Campo et al., 2006). In the third study, which looked at parent-of-origin effects on intellectual ability, *GTF2I* expression was reported to be lower in individuals with a deletion of maternal origin (Collette et al., 2009). In all three reports, the results should be interpreted with caution because the sample sizes were small, making statistical analyses problematic; however, they are suggestive of the need for further investigation using a large cohort with balanced participant parent-of-origin and gender numbers.

Three genes (*GTF2I*, *GTF2IRD1* and *BAZ1B*) from the WS critical region are known to be involved in epigenetic processes, indicating that deletion of the WS interval may result in generalised alterations in DNA methylation or histone modification. TFII-I (the protein product of *GTF2I*) has been copurified with histone deacetylase 3 (HDAC3) (Wen et al., 2003), and both TFII-I and TFII-IRD1 (the protein product of *GTF2IRD1*) have been shown to functionally interact with HDAC3 *in vitro* (Tussié-Luna et al., 2002). HDAC3 is a class I histone deacetylase that commonly resides in the nucleus and helps regulate histone acetylation in combination with other histone acetylases and histone acetyltransferases (Fischer et al., 2010). As well as having a role in histone modification, HDAC3 is known to have wide-ranging effects on gene expression through multiprotein complexes with co-repressors (Karagianni & Wong, 2007). Although the exact nature of the interplay between the TFII-I proteins and HDAC3 is not clear, it is hypothesised that HDAC3 may help to repress the transcriptional activity of TFII-I- or TFII-IRD1-regulated promoters (Wen et al., 2003).

BAZ1B, which lies towards the centromeric end of the common WS deletion, codes for a major subunit that is shared by two different ATP-dependent chromatin remodelling complexes, WINAC (mediates transcriptional control) and WICH (essential for DNA repair) (Kitagawa et al., 2011; Yoshimura et al., 2009). In the WINAC complex, BAZ1B interacts directly with acetylated histones through its bromodomain. In addition, it interacts with the vitamin D receptor to mediate the transrepression of 1-alpha-hydroxylase, a key enzyme in vitamin D biosynthesis (Fujiki et al., 2005). When contained within the WICH complex, BAZ1B binds to replication foci, where it is hypothesised to maintain chromatin accessibility for other factors that are needed to maintain the epigenetic state of newly synthesised DNA (Poot et al., 2005). If BAZ1B is depleted, heterochromatin is formed leading to an overall decrease in transcriptional activity (Poot et al., 2004).

Genotypic and phenotypic variation

Variation in the genome

The phenotypic presentation of WS has common core elements that result from the deletion of genes from the critical region, but there is significant variation in the expression of genes throughout the genome that can have a considerable effect on the severity and penetrance of clinical features. As with all developmental disorders, there is a natural variation across the entire spectrum of symptoms in WS, including cognitive function and behaviour (Martens et al., 2008).

General cognitive ability is known to have a strong genetic component. Over the entire range of learning abilities, Haworth & Plomin (2010) found that heritability estimates were approximately 50%, meaning that approximately half of the variance in learning abilities could be attributed to genetic differences and half to nongenetic factors. These genetics differences could be qualitative, meaning that specific genes contain nucleotide changes that alter the amino acid sequence, and therefore the function, of the translated protein. They could also be quantitative, where specific genes are expressed at different levels because of changes to their regulatory elements.

The expression of each individual gene is governed by the binding of specific proteins that orchestrate its spatial and temporal expression pattern through binding to regulatory elements. These tissue- or time-specific protein interactions occur near the start of the gene, often within the promoter region, and allow the pre-initiation complex to start the process of transcription (Lee & Young, 2000). A recent analysis of the expression of 49 genes in three inbred and four wild-derived inbred mouse strains revealed that over 50% of genes showed interstrain expression variation, with differences concentrated in higher-order brain regions such as the cortex and hippocampus (J.A. Morris et al., 2010). In addition, the variability in gene expression patterns reflected the genetic similarity between strains. There is strong evidence of the effect of genetic variation from mouse studies, where researchers use strains that have been selectively inbred to generate a homogenous genetic background. Behavioural phenotypes can be dramatically different depending upon the strain, presumably because of differences in gene expression (Spencer et al., 2011; Zambello et al., 2010).

Single-copy genes

The remaining single-copy genes within the WS deletion region might be expected to contribute significantly to phenotypic variation in WS because any polymorphic variation that produces even a small functional effect on the protein would be amplified owing to the absence of the other gene copy. Association studies of single nucleotide polymorphisms (SNPs) in genes from the WS region have been carried out in other clinical populations with varying results. Individual SNPs and haplotypes across *ELN* have been associated with susceptibility to intracranial aneurysms (Akagawa et al., 2006). These are not commonly seen in WS and because these associated SNPs are presumably present in the WS population, it would be interesting to see whether they modify the phenotypic features of WS. SNPs of *STX1A* have been associated with migraine in two studies of Spanish and Portuguese populations (Corominas et al., 2009; Lemos et al., 2010). An initial study also found an association with schizophrenia (Wong et al., 2004), but a subsequent attempt to replicate this finding in a different population was unsuccessful (Kawashima et al., 2008). Perhaps the most intriguing finding was that of elevated levels of *STX1A* expression in white blood cells from individuals with high-functioning autism (Nakamura et al., 2008), although the significance of this finding awaits further investigation, particularly because a follow-up study by the same group found lower levels of STX1A mRNA in post-mortem brain (Nakamura et al., 2011).

Copy number variation

A survey of a large cohort of individuals with severe developmental delay revealed a 520-kb deletion of chromosome 16p12.1 that was found not only in some of the cases but also in their unaffected parents (Girirajan et al., 2010). Further investigation showed that in a quarter of the individuals with developmental delay, the deletion co-occurred with a second, larger deletion or duplication elsewhere in the genome (a 'second hit'). In most cases, the clinical features resembled those associated with the larger copy number variant but were consistently more severe with additional phenotypes present, indicating that their phenotype was being modified by the 16p12.1 deletion (the 'first hit'). There have been previous case reports of the co-occurrence of different genomic disorders (Okamoto et al., 2010; South et al., 2008), but the study by Girirajan et al. introduces the concept that the second hit may be relatively benign on its own, yet still modify the syndromic phenotype either additively or epistatically by impacting on a pathway that is shared with one or several genes found on 16p12.1. A small study of individuals with WS, also reported by Girirajan et al. (2010), did not reveal an elevated proportion with a second copy-number-variant hit. However, the phenotypic spectrum of these individuals was not described and future studies would probably focus on individuals with severe or unusual clinical features.

Environmental response

Environmental factors can play important roles in the modulation of gene expression, not only during early development but also during later stages of childhood and adulthood. The regulation of gene expression in response to environmental stimuli is one of the major mechanisms of neural plasticity, and activation of the autonomic nervous system and the hypothalamo-pituitary-adrenal axis enables us to respond to acute stress and to adapt the stress response for future situations. Chronic stress, however, can produce prolonged periods of elevation of the stress response and is well known to induce changes in the morphology or function of neurons in the mammalian brain (McEwen, 2007). The hippocampus is one of the most sensitive areas of the brain and many studies have demonstrated chronic stress-associated changes in dendritic morphology along with accompanying alterations in synaptic transmission and plasticity in rodents (Sandi et al., 2003).

Recently, investigations have turned towards understanding the molecular changes that underlie these alterations in brain function and several microarray analyses have surveyed the changes in gene transcription in response to chronic stress (Andrus et al., 2010; Datson et al., 2010; Lisowski et al., 2011). Not surprisingly, genes involved in neurogenesis and neuron differentiation were differentially expressed in the hippocampus of chronically mildly stressed animals, but genes involved in programmed cell death and chromatin remodelling (shifting of nucleosome cores along the DNA molecule to alter binding of regulatory proteins) were also altered (Lisowski et al., 2011). Further evidence of an epigenetic component to stress-induced gene expression comes from the finding that changes in the transcription of brain-derived neurotrophic factor in the rat hippocampus in response to stressful stimuli are, at least in part, regulated by the histone acetylation status (Fuchikami et al., 2010).

In considering the effects of the environment on gene expression and, subsequently, on the symptoms of WS, it is important to bear in mind that the prevalence of chronic stress and anxiety in this population could be a contributing factor. Individuals with WS exhibit high levels of anxiety, which can be manifest as generalised anxiety disorder or, most often, as specific phobias (Leyfer et al., 2009; Chapter 5). As with many neurodevelopmental disorders, sleep disturbance is also common in WS (Goldman et al., 2009; Annaz et al., 2011) (see Chapter 7). Short-term sleep deprivation, although less studied, is known to affect cognitive function and behaviour, and long-term sleep disturbances are postulated to lead to neuronal damage, probably through cellular stress in susceptible structures such as the hippocampus (Jan et al., 2010).

The ageing brain
Genetic changes associated with ageing

As our bodies age, different systems and tissues age at different rates. The brain experiences a gradual decrease in volume, loss of synapses and cognitive decline, but these processes are probably driven, at least in part, by changes in gene expression. Studies of post-mortem human brain tissue have found that changes in gene expression appear in the absence of demonstrable neuronal loss or decrease in synapse numbers, suggesting that they precede histological changes (Burger, 2010; Loerch et al., 2008). Gene expression in the brain during ageing seems to have a distinct pattern in primates compared with mice (Loerch et al., 2008; Zahn et al., 2007). There are genes that show age-related changes in both primates and mice (e.g. apolipoprotein D, which is neuroprotective and is upregulated with age, and calcium/calmodulin-dependent kinase IV, a synaptic signalling gene that is downregulated with age), but overall a dramatic downregulation of neuronal genes seems to occur during ageing in primates (Erraji-Benchekroun et al., 2005; Loerch et al., 2008). This transcriptional repression may have evolved only in the longer-lived primates, but further studies of other species will be necessary to confirm this. Somel et al. (2010) proposed that many of these changes are not actually features of ageing but merely an extension of a lifelong expression pattern. In a study of prefrontal cortex in humans and macaques, Somel et al. (2010) found that many mRNA transcripts, microRNAs and even proteins that seemed to decline in later life in fact started their repressive pattern in childhood.

Gene expression is also affected by epigenetic changes and these are well known to occur throughout the life of an organism. Hernandez et al. (2011) recently used genome-wide methylation arrays to examine the effect of age on the DNA methylation status in the human brain. They reported a strong correlation between DNA methylation and age and also found that these methylated sites usually lay within CpG islands (regions containing a high frequency of adjacent cytosine and guanine nucleotides) that were associated with genes involved in transcriptional regulation. They therefore hypothesise that age-related DNA methylation has a broad impact on gene expression in the brain.

The advancement of tissue preservation and of microarray and sequencing technologies will enable more in-depth studies of gene expression in a wide array of tissues and species and provide a better understanding of the dynamic expression of genes over the human lifespan.

Ageing in WS

In addition to the normal processes associated with ageing, mild accelerated ageing might occur in individuals with WS, and this could lead to a deterioration in intellectual function and cognitive skills at earlier ages than in the general population (Devenny et al., 2004; Cherniske et al., 2004; Pober, 2010). Physical findings, such as premature greying of the hair and earlier onset of cataracts and hearing loss, support the theory of accelerated ageing. However, there has not yet been a longitudinal study to look at the physical features of WS over the lifespan (see Chapter 5 for discussion of longitudinal cognitive and social outcomes).

Physical findings in people with WS may also have additive effects over and above those seen in the general population. Hypertension and poorly controlled hyperglycaemia have both been shown to cause microangiopathies in the brains of the elderly, leading to vascular dementia (Cherubini et al., 2010). Hypertension and glucose intolerance are both common features in adults with WS and may therefore impact negatively on cognitive function if not treated appropriately (Cherniske et al., 2004; Pober, 2010).

Therapeutic advances in treating neurodevelopmental disorders

Neurodevelopmental disorders have traditionally been regarded as unlikely targets for therapeutic intervention because it was assumed that the presence of the causative genetic defect during pre- and postnatal development would result in irreversible impacts on brain structure and function. In the past few years, however, there has been considerable progress towards the development of therapeutic strategies for the reversal of deficits caused by neurodevelopmental disorders such as fragile X, Rett, Rubinstein–Taybi, tuberous sclerosis and Down syndrome (Ehninger et al., 2008; Wetmore & Garner, 2010).

The strategy for pharmacological intervention has been to target well-studied pathways that have been shown to be compromised with drugs that are already in use, thus bypassing the usual arduous process for regulatory approval and rapidly accelerating the route to human clinical trials. Perhaps the most progress has been made in the treatment of fragile X syndrome, the most common genetic cause of comorbid autism, where a triplet repeat expansion in the 5' untranslated region of the fragile X mental retardation 1 (*FMR1*) gene leads to a protein deficiency that affects the translation of multiple other proteins important for synaptic development and plasticity (Hagerman et al., 2010). Abnormalities in metabotropic glutamate receptor 5 (GRM5) signalling and gamma-aminobutyric acid (GABA)ergic inhibition have been identified in fragile X syndrome, and human clinical trials of GRM5 antagonists and $GABA_A$ agonists as well as minocycline, an inhibitor of matrix metalloproteinase 9, are currently underway after encouraging results in animal studies (Berry-Kravis et al., 2009; Bilousova et al., 2009; de Vrij et al., 2008; Hagerman et al., 2010; Krueger & Bear, 2010; Paribello et al., 2010; Yan et al., 2005).

Similar approaches in WS await demonstration of the dysfunction of a specific biochemical pathway where existing, approved pharmacological agents can be used. At the current time, no such pathways are known and pharmacological intervention for WS, although possible, is not yet feasible. However, the presence of common mechanisms of dysfunction in neurodevelopmental disorders with different phenotypic presentations suggests that WS too may be linked to imbalance among neurotransmitter systems or the disruption of local protein translation in neurons (Meyer-Lindenberg et al., 2005; Rae et al., 1998). If so, the initiation of treatment trials for cognitive and behavioural features of this syndrome may come sooner rather than later.

Editor commentary (Emily K. Farran & Annette Karmiloff-Smith)

As exciting as it is to discover which particular genes are mutated in a neurodevelopmental syndrome, the really crucial questions for fully understanding the phenotypic outcome— and the focus taken in this chapter—are when and where genes are expressed, how gene expression changes during prenatal development, postnatal development and ageing, and how epigenetic, genetic and environmental factors interact to influence the phenotype. However, this neuroconstructivist stance is no simple endeavour. As the chapter showed, methodological problems abound in both animal and human models and there are thus differing findings with respect to the temporal and spatial expression of some of the WS genes. Currently, the only clear-cut genotype/phenotype correlation identified is between *ELN* and connective-tissue problems affecting the heart and other organs. However, it now seems to be clear that the four telomeric genes (*GTF2I*, *GTF2IRD1*, *LIMK1* and *CLIP2*) in the WS critical region are the most likely candidates for critically contributing to the full WS phenotype. Patients with only a partial deletion of the critical region who have retained both copies of those four genes tend not to show the full classic phenotype. The precise details of how these genes contribute to the specific cognitive features that we discuss in the rest of the book and to individual differences in such expression–outcome correlations remain to be identified. Indeed, there is significant variation in the expression of genes throughout the genome and those in the WS critical region are no exception to this. Therefore, allelic variation in the expression of each of the remaining genes on the nondeleted chromosome may well help to explain individual variation in the cognitive outcome. As difficult as this endeavour may seem, rapid technological advances in genetics leave us with much hope, so the more we understand about gene expression over developmental time, the more likely is the initiation of treatment trials for cognitive and behavioural features of neurodevelopmental syndromes.

References

Akagawa, H., Tajima, A., Sakamoto, Y., Krischek, B., Yoneyama, T., Kasuya, H., et al. (2006). A haplotype spanning two genes, ELN and LIMK1, decreases their transcripts and confers susceptibility to intracranial aneurysms. *Human Molecular Genetics*, 15, 1722–34.

Allen Institute for Brain Science. (2009). *Allen Brain Atlas Resources* [online database] <http://www.brain-map.org> accessed 28 June 2011.

Andrus, B.M., Blizinsky, K., Vedell, P.T., Dennis, K., Shukla, P.K., Schaffer, D.J., Radulovic, J., et al. (2010). Gene expression patterns in the hippocampus and amygdala of endogenous depression and chronic stress models. *Molecular Psychiatry*. [Epub ahead of print 16 November 2010].

Annaz, D., Hill, C.M., Ashworth, A., Holley, S., & Karmiloff-Smith, A. (2011). Characterisation of sleep problems in children with Williams syndrome. *Research in Developmental Disabilities*, 32, 164–69.

Arber, S., Barbayannis, F.A., Hanser, H., Schneider, C., Stanyon, C.A., Bernard, O., et al. (1998). Regulation of actin dynamics through phosphorylation of cofilin by LIM- kinase. *Nature*, 393, 805–809.

Ashe, A., Morgan, D.K., Whitelaw, N.C., Bruxner, T.J., Vickaryous, N.K., Cox, L.L., et al. (2008). A genome-wide screen for modifiers of transgene variegation identifies genes with critical roles in development. *Genome Biology*, 9, R182.

Bayarsaihan, D., Bitchevaia, N., Enkhmandakh, B., Tussié-Luna, M.I., Leckman, J.F., Roy, A., et al. (2003). Expression of BEN, a member of TFII-I family of transcription factors, during mouse pre- and postimplantation development. *Gene Expression Patterns*, 3, 579–89.

Bennett, M.K., Calakos, N., & Scheller, R.H. (1992). Syntaxin: a synaptic protein implicated in docking of synaptic vesicles at presynaptic active zones. *Science*, 257, 255–59.

Berry-Kravis, E., Hessl, D., Coffey, S., Hervey, C., Schneider, A., Yuhas, J., et al. (2009). A pilot open label, single dose trial of fenobam in adults with fragile X syndrome. *Journal of Medical Genetics*, 46, 266–71.

Bilousova, T.V., Dansie, L., Ngo, M., Aye, J., Charles, J.R., Ethell, D.W., et al. (2009). Minocycline promotes dendritic spine maturation and improves behavioural performance in the fragile X mouse model. *Journal of Medical Genetics*, 46, 94–102.

Botta, A., Sangiuolo, F., Calza, L., Giardino, L., Potenza, S., Novelli, G., et al. (1999). Expression analysis and protein localization of the human HPC-1/syntaxin 1A, a gene deleted in Williams syndrome. *Genomics*, 62, 525–28.

Burger, C. (2010). Region-specific genetic alterations in the aging hippocampus: implications for cognitive aging. *Frontiers in Aging Neuroscience*, 2, 140.

Cairo, S., Merla, G., Urbinati, F., Ballabio, A., & Reymond, A. (2001). WBSCR14, a gene mapping to the Williams–Beuren syndrome deleted region, is a new member of the Mlx transcription factor network. *Human Molecular Genetics*, 10, 617–27.

Caraveo, G., van Rossum, D.B., Patterson, R.L., Snyder, S.H., & Desiderio, S. (2006). Action of TFII-I outside the nucleus as an inhibitor of agonist-induced calcium entry. *Science*, 314, 122–25.

Cherniske, E.M., Carpenter, T.O., Klaiman, C., Young, E., Bregman, J., Insogna, K., Schultz, R.T., et al. (2004). Multisystem study of 20 older adults with Williams syndrome. *American Journal of Medical Genetics Part A*, 131A, 255–64.

Cherubini, A., Lowenthal, D.T., Paran, E., Mecocci, P., Williams, L.S., & Senin, U. (2010). Hypertension and cognitive function in the elderly. *Disease-a-Month*, 56, 106–47.

Collette, J.C., Chen, X.N., Mills, D.L., Galaburda, A.M., Reiss, A.L., Bellugi, U., et al. (2009). William's syndrome: gene expression is related to parental origin and regional coordinate control. *Journal of Human Genetics*, 54, 193–98.

Computational Biology Center at Memorial Sloan-Kettering Cancer Center. (n.d.). *microRNA Target Predictions and Expression Profiles* [online database] (August 2010 release) <http://www.microRNA.org> accessed 28 June 2011.

Corominas, R., Ribasés, M., Cuenca-León, E., Narberhaus, B., Serra, S.A., del Toro, M., et al. (2009). Contribution of syntaxin 1A to the genetic susceptibility to migraine: a case-control association study in the Spanish population. *Neuroscience Letters*, 455, 105–109.

Crackower, M.A., Kolas, N.K., Noguchi, J., Sarao, R., Kikuchi, K., Kaneko, H., et al. (2003). Essential role of Fkbp6 in male fertility and homologous chromosome pairing in meiosis. *Science*, 300, 1291–95.

Danoff, S.K., Taylor, H.E., Blackshaw, S., & Desiderio, S. (2004). TFII-I, a candidate gene for Williams syndrome cognitive profile: parallels between regional expression in mouse brain and human phenotype. *Neuroscience*, 123, 931–38.

Datson, N.A., Speksnijder, N., Mayer, J.L., Steenbergen, P.J., Korobko, O., Goeman, J., et al. (2010). The transcriptional response to chronic stress and glucocorticoid receptor blockade in the hippocampal dentate gyrus. *Hippocampus*. [Epub ahead of print 23 December 2010].

Del Campo, M., Antonell, A., Magano, L., Muñoz, F., Flores, R., Bayés, M., et al. (2006). Hemizygosity at the NCF1 gene in Williams Beuren syndrome patients decreases their risk of hypertension. *American Journal of Human Genetics*, 78, 533–42.

De Sario, A. (2009). Clinical and molecular overview of inherited disorders resulting from epigenomic dysregulation. *European Journal of Medical Genetics*, 52, 363–72.

Devenny, D.A., Krinsky-McHale, S.J., Kittler, P.M., Flory, M., Jenkins, E., & Brown, W.T. (2004). Age-associated memory changes in adults with Williams syndrome. *Developmental Neuropsychology*, 26, 691–706.

Díaz, E. (2009). One decade later: what has gene expression profiling told us about neuronal cell types, brain function and disease? *Current Genomics*, 10, 318–25.

Doyle, J.L, DeSilva, U., Miller, W., & Green, E.D. (2000). Divergent human and mouse orthologs of a novel gene (WBSCR15/Wbscr15) reside within the genomic interval commonly deleted in Williams syndrome. *Cytogenetics and Cell Genetics*, 90, 285–90.

Ehninger, D., Li, W., Fox, K., Stryker, M.P., & Silva, A.J. (2008). Reversing neurodevelopmental disorders in adults. *Neuron*, 60, 950–60.

Endo, M., Ohashi, K., & Mizuno, K. (2007). LIM kinase and slingshot are critical for neurite extension. *Journal of Biological Chemistry*, 282, 13692–13702.

Endo, M., Ohashi, K., Sasaki, Y., Goshima, Y., Niwa, R., Uemura, T., & Mizuno, K. (2003). Control of growth cone motility and morphology by LIM kinase and Slingshot via phosphorylation and dephosphorylation of cofilin. *Journal of Neuroscience*, 23, 2527–37.

Enkhmandakh, B., Bitchevaia, N., Ruddle, F., & Bayarsaihan, D. (2004). The early embryonic expression of TFII-I during mouse preimplantation development. *Gene Expression Patterns*, 4, 25–28.

Erraji-Benchekroun, L., Underwood, M.D., Arango, V., Galfalvy, H., Pavlidis, P., Smyrniotopoulos, P., et al. (2005). Molecular aging in human prefrontal cortex is selective and continuous throughout adult life. *Biological Psychiatry*, 57, 549–58.

European Bioinformatics Institute & Wellcome Trust Sanger Institute. (2000). *Ensembl Genome Browser* [online database] (updated April 2011) <http://uswest.ensembl.org/index.html> accessed 28 June 2011.

Fijalkowska, I., Sharma, D., Bult, C.J., & Danoff, S.K. (2010). Expression of the transcription factor, TFII-I, during post-implantation mouse embryonic development. *BMC Research Notes*, 3, 203.

Fischer, A., Sananbenesi, F., Mungenast, A., & Tsai, L.H. (2010). Targeting the correct HDAC(s) to treat cognitive disorders. *Trends in Pharmacological Science*, 31, 605–617.

Frangiskakis, J.M., Ewart, A.K., Morris, C.A., Mervis, C.B., Bertrand, J., Robinson, B.F., et al. (1996). LIM-kinase1 hemizygosity implicated in impaired visuospatial constructive cognition. *Cell* 86, 59–69.

Fuchikami, M., Yamamoto, S., Morinobu, S., Takei, S., & Yamawaki, S. (2010). Epigenetic regulation of BDNF gene in response to stress. *Psychiatry Investigation*, 7, 251–56.

Fujiki, R., Kim, M.S., Sasaki, Y., Yoshimura, K., Kitagawa, H., & Kato, S. (2005). Ligand-induced transrepression by VDR through association of WSTF with acetylated histones. *EMBO Journal*, **24**, 3881–94.

Girirajan, S., Rosenfeld, J.A., Cooper, G.M., Antonacci, F., Siswara, P., Itsara, A., et al. (2010). A recurrent 16p12.1 microdeletion supports a two-hit model for severe developmental delay. *Nature Genetics*, **42**, 203–209.

Goldman, S.E., Malow, B.A., Newman, K.D., Roof, E., & Dykens, E.M. (2009). Sleep patterns and daytime sleepiness in adolescents and young adults with Williams syndrome. *Journal of Intellectual Disability Research*, **53**, 182–88.

Grafodatskaya, D., Chung, B., Szatmari, P., & Weksberg, R. (2010). Autism spectrum disorders and epigenetics. *Journal of the American Academy of Child and Adolescent Psychiatry*, **49**, 794–809.

Gräff, J., & Mansuy, I.M. (2009). Epigenetic dysregulation in cognitive disorders. *European Journal of Neuroscience*, **30**, 1–8.

Gray, P.A., Fu, H., Luo, P., Zhao, Q., Yu, J., Ferrari, A., et al. (2004). Mouse brain organization revealed through direct genome-scale TF expression analysis. *Science*, **306**, 2255–57.

Hagerman, R., Hoem, G., & Hagerman, P. (2010). Fragile X and autism: intertwined at the molecular level leading to targeted treatments. *Molecular Autism*, **1**, 12.

Haworth, C.M., & Plomin, R. (2010). Quantitative genetics in the era of molecular genetics: learning abilities and disabilities as an example. *Journal of the American Academy of Child and Adolescent Psychiatry*, **49**, 783–93.

Hernandez, D.G., Nalls, M.A., Gibbs, J.R., Arepalli, S., van der Brug, M., Chong, S., et al. (2011). Distinct DNA methylation changes highly correlated with chronological age in the human brain. *Human Molecular Genetics*, **20**, 1164–72.

Hinsley, T.A., Cunliffe, P., Tipney, H.J., Brass, A., & Tassabehji, M. (2004). Comparison of TFII-I gene family members deleted in Williams-Beuren syndrome. *Protein Science*, **13**, 2588–99.

Hoogenraad, C.C., Koekkoek, B., Akhmanova, A., Krugers, H., Dortland, B., Miedema, M., et al. (2002). Targeted mutation of Cyln2 in the Williams syndrome critical region links CLIP-115 haplo-insufficiency to neurodevelopmental abnormalities in mice. *Nature Genetics*, **32**, 116–27.

Iizuka, K., Bruick, R.K., Liang, G., Horton, J.D., & Uyeda, K. (2004). Deficiency of carbohydrate response element-binding protein (ChREBP) reduces lipogenesis as well as glycolysis. *Proceedings of the National Academy of Sciences of the USA*, **101**, 7281–86.

Jackson, T.A., Taylor, H.E., Sharma, D., Desiderio, S., & Danoff, S.K. (2005). Vascular endothelial growth factor receptor-2: counter-regulation by the transcription factors, TFII-I and TFII-IRD1. *Journal of Biological Chemistry*, **280**, 29856–63.

Jadayel, D.M., Osborne, L.R., Coignet, L.J., Zani, V.J., Tsui, L.C., Scherer, S.W., et al. (1998). The BCL7 gene family: deletion of BCL7B in Williams syndrome. *Gene*, **224**, 35–44.

Jan, J.E., Reiter, R.J., Bax, M.C., Ribary, U., Freeman, R.D., & Wasdell, M.B. (2010). Long-term sleep disturbances in children: a cause of neuronal loss. *European Journal of Paediatric Neurology*, **14**, 380–90.

Karagianni, P., & Wong, J. (2007). HDAC3: taking the SMRT-N-CoRrect road to repression. *Oncogene*, **26**, 5439–49.

Kawashima, K., Kishi, T., Ikeda, M., Kitajima, T., Yamanouchi, Y., Kinoshita, Y., et al. (2008). No association between tagging SNPs of SNARE complex genes (STX1A, VAMP2 and SNAP25) and schizophrenia in a Japanese population. *American Journal of Medical Genetics Part B: Neuropsychiatric Genetics*, **147B**, 1327–31.

Kitagawa, H., Fujiki, R., Yoshimura, K., Oya, H., & Kato, S. (2011). Williams syndrome is an epigenome-regulator disease. *Endocrine Journal*, **58**, 77–85.

Krueger, D.D., & Bear, M.F. (2010). Toward Fulfilling the promise of molecular medicine in fragile X syndrome. *Annual Review of Medicine*, **62**, 411–29.

Ku, M., Sokol, S.Y., Wu, J., Tussie-Luna, M.I., Roy, A.L., & Hata, A. (2005). Positive and negative regulation of the transforming growth factor beta/activin target gene goosecoid by the TFII-I family of transcription factors. *Molecular and Cellular Biology*, **25**, 7144–57.

Lakkakorpi, J., Li, K., Decker, S., Korkeela, E., Piddington, R., Abrams, W., et al. (1999). Expression of the elastin promoter in novel tissue sites in transgenic mouse embryos. *Connective Tissue Research*, **40**, 155–62.

Lee, T.I., & Young, R.A. (2000). Transcription of eukaryotic protein-coding genes. *Annual Review of Genetics*, **34**, 77–137.

Lemos, C., Pereira-Monteiro, J., Mendonça, D., Ramos, E.M., Barros, J., Sequeiros, J., et al. (2010). Evidence of syntaxin 1A involvement in migraine susceptibility: a Portuguese study. *Archives in Neurology*, **67**, 422–27.

Leyfer, O., Woodruff-Borden, J., & Mervis, C.B. (2009). Anxiety disorders in children with Williams syndrome, their mothers, and their siblings: implications for the etiology of anxiety disorders. *Journal of Neurodevelopmental Disorders*, **1**, 4–14.

Lisowski, P., Juszczak, G.R., Goscik, J., Wieczorek, M., Zwierzchowski, L, & Swiergiel, A.H. (2011). Effect of chronic mild stress on hippocampal transcriptome in mice selected for high and low stress-induced analgesia and displaying different emotional behaviors. *European Neuropsychopharmacology*, **21**, 45–62.

Loerch, P.M., Lu, T., Dakin, K.A., Vann, J.M., Isaacs, A., Geula, C., Wang, et al. (2008). Evolution of the aging brain transcriptome and synaptic regulation. *PLoS One*, **3**, e3329.

de Luis, O., Valero, M.C., & Jurado, L.A. (2000). WBSCR14, a putative transcription factor gene deleted in Williams-Beuren syndrome: complete characterisation of the human gene and the mouse ortholog. *European Journal of Human Genetics*, **8**, 215–22.

Makeyev, A.V., Erdenechimeg, L., Mungunsukh, O., Roth, J.J., Enkhmandakh, B., Ruddle, F.H., et al. (2004). GTF2IRD2 is located in the Williams–Beuren syndrome critical region 7q11.23 and encodes a protein with two TFII-I-like helix–loop–helix repeats. *Proceedings of the National Academy of Sciences of the USA*, **101**, 11052–57.

Martens, M.A., Wilson, S.J., & Reutens, D.C. (2008). Williams syndrome: a critical review of the cognitive, behavioral, and neuroanatomical phenotype. *Journal of Child Psychology and Psychiatry*, **49**, 576–608.

Martindale, D.W., Wilson, M.D., Wang, D., Burke, R.D., Chen, X., Duronio, V., et al. (2000). Comparative genomic sequence analysis of the Williams syndrome region (LIMK1-RFC2) of human chromosome 7q11.23. *Mammalian Genome*, **11**, 890–98.

McEwen, B.S. (2007). Physiology and neurobiology of stress and adaptation: central role of the brain. *Physiology Reviews*, **87**, 873–904.

Meng, X., Lu, X., Li, Z., Green, E.D., Massa, H., Trask, B.J., et al. (1998b). Complete physical map of the common deletion region in Williams syndrome and identification and characterization of three novel genes. *Human Genetics*, **103**, 590–99.

Meng, X., Lu, X., Morris, C.A., & Keating, M.T. (1998a). A novel human gene FKBP6 is deleted in Williams syndrome. *Genomics*, **52**, 130–37.

Meng, Y., Takahashi, H., Meng, J., Zhang, Y., Lu, G., Asrar, S., Nakamura, T., et al. (2004). Regulation of ADF/cofilin phosphorylation and synaptic function by LIM-kinase. *Neuropharmacology*, **47**, 746–54.

Meng, Y., Zhang, Y., Tregoubov, V., Janus, C., Cruz, L., Jackson, M., et al. (2002). Abnormal spine morphology and enhanced LTP in LIMK-1 knockout mice. *Neuron*, **35**, 121–33.

Merla, G., Ucla, C., Guipponi, M., & Reymond, A. (2002). Identification of additional transcripts in the Williams-Beuren syndrome critical region. *Human Genetics*, **110**, 429–38.

Meyer-Lindenberg, A., Mervis, C.B., Sarpal, D., Koch, P., Steele, S., Kohn, P., et al. (2005). Functional, structural, and metabolic abnormalities of the hippocampal formation in Williams syndrome. *Journal of Clinical Investigation*, **115**, 1888–95.

Micale, L., Fusco, C., Augello, B., Napolitano, L.M., Dermitzakis, E.T., Meroni, G., et al. (2008). Williams-Beuren syndrome TRIM50 encodes an E3 ubiquitin ligase. *European Journal of Human Genetics*, **16**, 1038–1049.

Mori, T., Okano, I., Mizuno, K., Tohyama, M., & Wanaka, A. (1997). Comparison of tissue distribution of two novel serine/threonine kinase genes containing the LIM motif (LIMK-1 and LIMK-2) in the developing rat. *Molecular Brain Research*, **45**, 247–54.

Morris, C.A. (2010). Introduction: Williams syndrome. *American Journal of Medical Genetics Part C: Seminars in Medical Genetics*, **154C**, 203–208.

Morris, J.A., Royall, J.J., Bertagnolli, D., Boe, A.F., Burnell, J.J., Byrnes, E.J., et al. (2010). Divergent and nonuniform gene expression patterns in mouse brain. *Proceedings of the National Academy of Sciences of the USA*, **107**, 19049–54.

Mountford, P., Zevnik, B., Düwel, A., Nichols, J., Li, M., Dani, C., et al. (1994). Dicistronic targeting constructs: reporters and modifiers of mammalian gene expression. *Proceedings of the National Academy of Sciences of the USA*, **91**, 4303–4307.

Nakamura, K., Anitha, A., Yamada, K., Tsujii, M., Iwayama, Y., Hattori, E., et al. (2008). Genetic and expression analyses reveal elevated expression of syntaxin 1A (STX1A) in high functioning autism. *International Journal of Neuropsychopharmacology*, **11**, 1073–84.

Nakamura, K., Iwata, Y., Anitha, A., Miyachi, T., Toyota, T., Yamada, S., et al. (2011). Replication study of Japanese cohorts supports the role of STX1A in autism susceptibility. *Progress in Neuro-Psychopharmacology and Biological Psychiatry*, **35**, 454–58.

National Center for Biotechnology Information. (n.d.) UniGene [online database] <http://www.ncbi.nlm.nih.gov/unigene> accessed 28 June 2011.

Nelson, S.B., Hempel, C., & Sugino, K. (2006). Probing the transcriptome of neuronal cell types. *Current Opinions in Neurobiology*, **16**, 571–76.

Noback, C.R., Ruggerio, D.A., Demarest, R.J., & Strominger, N.L. (Eds), (2005). *The Human Nervous System*. Totowa NJ: Humana Press.

Okamoto, N., Akimaru, N., Matsuda, K., Suzuki, Y., Shimojima, K., & Yamamoto, T. (2010). Co-occurrence of Prader-Willi and Sotos syndromes. *American Journal of Medical Genetics Part A*, **152A**, 2103–2109.

Osborne, L.R., & Mervis, C.B. (2007). Rearrangements of the Williams-Beuren syndrome locus: molecular basis and implications for speech and language development. *Expert Reviews in Molecular Medicine*, **9**, 1–16.

Palmer, S.J., Tay, E.S., Santucci, N., Cuc Bach, T.T., Hook, J., Lemckert, F.A., et al. (2007). Expression of Gtf2ird1, the Williams syndrome-associated gene, during mouse development. *Gene Expression Patterns*, **7**, 396–404.

Paperna, T., Peoples, R., Wang, Y.K., Kaplan, P., & Francke, U. (1998). Genes for the CPE receptor (CPETR1) and the human homolog of RVP1 (CPETR2) are localized within the Williams-Beuren syndrome deletion. *Genomics*, **54**, 453–59.

Paribello, C., Tao, L., Folino, A., Berry-Kravis, E., Tranfaglia, M., Ethell, I.M., et al. (2010). Open-label add-on treatment trial of minocycline in fragile X syndrome. *BMC Neurology*, **10**, 91.

Peoples, R.J., Cisco, M.J., Kaplan, P., & Francke, U. (1998). Identification of the WBSCR9 gene, encoding a novel transcriptional regulator, in the Williams-Beuren syndrome deletion at 7q11.23. *Cytogenetics and Cell Genetics*, **82**, 238–46.

Pérez-Jurado, L.A., Peoples, R., Kaplan, P., Hamel, B.C., & Francke, U. (1996). Molecular definition of the chromosome 7 deletion in Williams syndrome and parent-of-origin effects on growth. *American Journal of Human Genetics*, **59**, 781–92.

Pérez-Jurado, L.A., Wang, Y.-K., Francke, U., & Cruces, J. (1999). TBL2, a novel transducin family member in the WBS deletion: characterization of the complete sequence, genomic structure, transcriptional variants and the mouse ortholog. *Cytogenetics and Cell Genetics*, **86**, 277–84.

Pober, B.R. (2010). Williams-Beuren syndrome. *New England Journal of Medicine*, **362**, 239–52.

Poot, R.A., Bozhenok, L., van den Berg, D.L., Hawkes, N., & Varga-Weisz, P.D. (2005). Chromatin remodeling by WSTF-ISWI at the replication site: opening a window of opportunity for epigenetic inheritance? *Cell Cycle*, **4**, 543–46.

Poot, R.A., Bozhenok, L., van den Berg, D.L., Steffensen, S., Ferreira, F., Grimaldi, M., et al. (2004). The Williams syndrome transcription factor interacts with PCNA to target chromatin remodelling by ISWI to replication foci. *Nature Cell Biology*, **6**, 1236–44.

Pröschel, C., Blouin, M.J., Gutowski, N.J., Ludwig, R., & Noble, M. (1995). Limk1 is predominantly expressed in neural tissues and phosphorylates serine, threonine and tyrosine residues in vitro. *Oncogene*, **11**, 1271–81.

Proulx, E., Young, E.J., Osborne, L.R., & Lambe, E.K. (2010). Enhanced prefrontal serotonin 5-HT(1A) currents in a mouse model of Williams-Beuren syndrome with low innate anxiety. *Journal of Neurodevelopmental Disorders*, **2**, 99–108.

Rae, C., Karmiloff-Smith, A., Lee, M.A., Dixon, R.M., Grant, J., Blamire, A.M., et al. (1998). Brain biochemistry in Williams syndrome: evidence for a role of the cerebellum in cognition? *Neurology*, **51**, 33–40.

Sandi, C., Davies, H.A., Cordero, M.I., Rodriguez, J.J., Popov, V.I., & Stewart, M.G. (2003). Rapid reversal of stress induced loss of synapses in CA3 of rat hippocampus following water maze training. *European Journal of Neuroscience*, **17**, 2447–56.

Scherer, S.W., & Osborne, L.R. (2006). Williams-Beuren syndrome, In P.T. Stankiewicz & J.R. Lupski (Eds) *Genomic Disorders: The Genomic Basis of Disease* (pp. 221–36). Totowa, NJ: Humana Press.

Selvaraj, S., Sun, Y., & Singh, B.B. (2010). TRPC channels and their implications for neurological diseases. *CNS and Neurological Disorders - Drug Targets*, **9**, 94–104.

Somel, M, Guo, S., Fu, N., Yan, Z, Hu, H.Y., Xu, Y., et al. (2010). MicroRNA, mRNA, and protein expression link development and aging in human and macaque brain. *Genome Research*, **20**, 1207–1218.

South, S.T., Whitby, H., Maxwell, T., Aston, E., Brothman, A.R., & Carey, J.C. (2008). Co-occurrence of 4p16.3 deletions with both paternal and maternal duplications of 11p15: modification of the Wolf-Hirschhorn syndrome phenotype by genetic alterations predicted to result in either a Beckwith-Wiedemann or Russell-Silver phenotype. *American Journal of Medical Genetics Part A*, **146A**, 2691–97.

Spencer, C.M., Alekseyenko, O., Hamilton, S.M., Thomas, A.M., Serysheva, E., Yuva-Paylor, L.A., et al. (2011). Modifying behavioral phenotypes in Fmr1KO mice: genetic background differences reveal autistic-like responses. *Autism Research*, **4**, 40–56.

Spencer, J.L., Waters, E.M., Milner, T.A., & McEwen, B.S. (2008). Estrous cycle regulates activation of hippocampal Akt, LIM kinase, and neurotrophin receptors in C57BL/6 mice. *Neuroscience*, **155**, 1106–1119.

Sumi, T., Matsumoto, K., Takai, Y., & Nakamura, T. (1999). Cofilin phosphorylation and actin cytoskeletal dynamics regulated by rho- and Cdc42-activated LIM-kinase 2. *Journal of Cell Biology*, **147**, 1519–32.

Tümpel, S., Wiedemann, L.M., & Krumlauf, R. (2009). Hox genes and segmentation of the vertebrate hindbrain. *Current Topics in Developmental Biology*, **88**, 103–37.

Tussié-Luna, M.I., Bayarsaihan, D., Ruddle, F.H., & Roy, A.L. (2001). Repression of TFII-I-dependent transcription by nuclear exclusion. *Proceedings of the National Academy of Sciences of the USA*, **98**, 7789–94.

Tussié-Luna, M.I., Bayarsaihan, D., Seto, E., Ruddle, F.H., & Roy, A.L. (2002). Physical and functional interactions of histone deacetylase 3 with TFII-I family proteins and PIASxbeta. *Proceedings of the National Academy of Sciences of the USA*, **99**, 12807–12.

Valor, L.M., Charlesworth, P., Humphreys, L., Anderson, C.N., & Grant, S.G. (2007). Network activity-independent coordinated gene expression program for synapse assembly. *Proceedings of the National Academy of Sciences of the USA*, **104**, 4658–63.

de Vrij, F.M., Levenga, J., van der Linde, H.C., Koekkoek, S.K., De Zeeuw, C.I., Nelson, D.L., et al. (2008). Rescue of behavioral phenotype and neuronal protrusion morphology in Fmr1 KO mice. *Neurobiology of Disease*, **31**, 127–32.

Wang, Y.K., Sporle, R., Paperna, T., Schughart, K., & Francke, U. (1999). Characterization and expression pattern of the frizzled gene Fzd9, the mouse homolog of FZD9 which Is deleted in Williams–Beuren syndrome. *Genomics*, **57**, 235–48.

Wen, Y.D., Cress, W.D., Roy, A.L., & Seto, E. (2003). Histone deacetylase 3 binds to and regulates the multifunctional transcription factor TFII-I. *Journal of Biological Chemistry*, **278**, 1841–47.

Wetmore, D.Z., & Garner, C.C. (2010). Emerging pharmacotherapies for neurodevelopmental disorders. *Journal of Developmental & Behavioral Pediatrics*, **31**, 564–82.

Wong, A.H., Trakalo, J., Likhodi, O., Yusuf, M., Macedo, A., Azevedo, M.H., et al. (2004). Association between schizophrenia and the syntaxin 1A gene. *Biological Psychiatry*, **56**, 24–29.

Yan, Q.J., Rammal, M., Tranfaglia, M., & Bauchwitz, R.P. (2005). Suppression of two major fragile X syndrome mouse model phenotypes by the mGluR5 antagonist MPEP. *Neuropharmacology*, **49**, 1053–66.

Yoshimura, K., Kitagawa, H., Fujiki, R., Tanabe, M., Takezawa, S., Takada, I., et al. (2009). Distinct function of 2 chromatin remodeling complexes that share a common subunit, Williams syndrome transcription factor (WSTF). *Proceedings of the National Academy of Sciences of the USA*, **106**, 9280–85.

Young, E.J. (2010). Genomic rearrangements in human and mouse and their contribution to the Williams-Beuren syndrome phenotype. (Doctoral dissertation). University of Toronto, Toronto, ON, Canada.

Zahn, J.M., Poosala, S., Owen, A.B., Ingram, D.K., Lustig, A., Carter, A., et al. (2007). AGEMAP: a gene expression database for aging in mice. *PLoS Genetics*, **3**, e201.

Zambello, E., Zanetti, L., Hédou, G.F., Angelici, O., Arban, R., Tasan, R.O., et al. (2010). Neuropeptide Y-Y2 receptor knockout mice: influence of genetic background on anxiety-related behaviors. *Neuroscience*, **176**, 420–30.

Zhou, W., Zhang, Y., Li, Y., Wei, Y.S., Liu, G., Liu, D.P., et al. (2010). A transgenic Cre mouse line for the study of cortical and hippocampal development. *Genesis*, **48**, 343–50.

Part 2

Clinical and Practical Outcomes

Chapter 4

Clinical profile: Diagnosis and prognosis

Kay Metcalfe

Introduction

Williams syndrome (WS) is a multisystem neurodevelopmental disorder with a prevalence of between 1 in 7500 and 1 in 20 000 live births (Morris et al., 1988; Stromme et al., 2002). It is caused by a contiguous gene deletion on chromosome 7q11.23 that arises in meiosis owing to nonallelic homologous recombination between blocks of low-copy repeat DNA with high sequence homology. The nonallelic homologous recombination is interchromosomal in two-thirds and intrachromosomal in one-third of cases (Baumer et al., 1998; Dutly & Schinzel, 1996; Thomas et al., 2006).

In 'classic' WS, depending on which low-copy repeat blocks are involved, the resultant deletion is usually 1.55 Mb containing 26 genes (95%) or 1.8 Mb containing 28 genes (5%) (Bayes et al., 2003). Rarer larger or smaller deletions are typically associated with a more or less severe phenotype, respectively (Botta et al., 1999; Dai et al., 2009; Frangiskakis et al., 1996; Gagliardi et al., 2003; Heller et al., 2003; Hirota et al., 2003; Howald et al., 2006; Karmiloff-Smith et al., 2003; Korenberg et al., 2000; Morris et al., 2003; Tassabehji et al., 1999). An inversion polymorphism estimated to be present in around 6% in the general population is enriched to approximately 25% in the transmitting parent of the deleted chromosome in WS (Bayes et al., 2003; Osborne et al., 2001). Hobart et al. (2010) have calculated that the chance to have a child with WS is approximately 1 in 750 for a parent carrying one copy of the inversion polymorphism compared with a 1 in 9500 chance for a parent without the inversion.

WS is associated with a characteristic physical, behavioural and neurodevelopmental phenotype. While haploinsufficiency for the elastin gene (*ELN*) probably explains the cardiovascular abnormalities, herniae, hoarse voice, lax joints and bladder and bowel diverticulae often associated with WS (Tassabehji et al., 1999), the mechanism by which deletion of other genes contributes to the phenotype is not fully ascertained (see Chapter 3). WS can act as a useful model for the dissection of genotype–phenotype correlations in chromosomal microdeletion disorders.

The diagnosis of 'classic' WS can be made by an experienced clinician on the basis of the dysmorphic features, medical problems and behavioural phenotype. However, the diagnosis is usually confirmed by genetic testing. Routine chromosome analysis is typically normal, but the deletion can be confirmed by a variety of molecular cytogenetic methods including fluorescence *in situ* hybridisation (FISH), analysis of microsatellite markers, multiplex ligation-dependent probe amplification, quantitative polymerase chain reaction and microarray analysis. FISH using a DNA probe targeted to the *ELN* gene has been used most commonly, the deletion being confirmed by presence of a signal from only one rather than both chromosome 7 homologues. Rarely, *ELN* can be deleted in isolated autosomal dominant supravalvular aortic stenosis (Fryssira et al., 1997) and is conversely not deleted in a small minority of patients with WS who have atypical deletions (Edelmann et al., 2007; Tassabehji et al., 1999). Microarray analysis, although currently more expensive, has the advantage of delineating precisely which genes are involved in the deletion and so may be particularly useful in atypical WS and for research purposes.

It is clearly important to try to characterise a disorder from as many areas as possible. How should a syndrome such as WS be defined in the light of expanding knowledge about genotypes and phenotypes? Should this be by physical appearance, by combinations of phenotypic features including cognitive data, by molecular genetic data or a combination of all of these? Although in a research context we are interested in both an expanded phenotype and the mildest end of the spectrum, should a child without physical features but with a typical cognitive profile and a small deletion or point mutation within a single gene be said to have WS? The definition is important for families wishing to seek support from other affected families or for those seeking prognostic information.

The presence or severity of individual or combined clinical phenotypic features in WS by and large does not correlate with cognitive outcomes, although for example the severity of cardiovascular features or hypercalcaemia may correlate with morbidity and mortality.

As for many other chromosomal disorders, there is wide phenotypic variability even in those with an identical sized deletion. Presumably, this relates in part to the effects of environmental factors and to the importance of genetic background, modifying genes or polymorphisms (see Chapter 3).

Physical appearance

Individuals with WS have characteristic facial dysmorphology that tends to be more obvious in the early childhood years. In childhood, the forehead is broad with bitemporal narrowing. The nose is very characteristic being upturned with a depressed nasal bridge, bulbous tip and anteverted nares (nostrils). The cheeks are full and droopy, with flattening of the malar regions (area over the cheekbones) and the chin is small. The mouth is wide and the lips, particularly the lower lips, are full. A variety of dental abnormalities are described and the primary teeth are small and widely spaced. The philtrum (the area between nose and mouth) may appear subjectively long. The ears have prominent lobes. Periorbital fullness (puffiness around the eyes) and epicanthic folds (folds of skin at the inner corner of the eye) are most apparent in infancy and tend to be lost with age. Convergent strabismus is common. The hair is typically dark and curly and the irises most commonly blue and with a stellate (star-like) pattern representing stromal hypoplasia.

In adulthood, the face may appear 'scrawnier' with loss of subcutaneous fat and, combined with early greying of the hair, this gives a somewhat prematurely aged appearance.

Compared with the younger face, the nasal root is narrower and the bridge less depressed although the tip remains bulbous. The supraorbital ridges are more prominent. The chin remains small and the permanent dentition has a tendency to be crowded and maloccluded.

The shoulders are narrow and sloping, and the neck appears longer with prominence of the hyoid (horseshoe-shaped bone in the midline of the neck between the chin and thyroid cartilage). There is a characteristic standing posture with rounding of the shoulders, forward thrust of the neck and flexion at the hips and knees (Joseph & Parrott, 1958; Metcalfe, 2001; Williams et al., 1961).

Within a research setting, techniques such as three-dimensional facial imaging can be a helpful tool in drawing out the more subtle nuances of facial appearance in the context of a given syndrome (Hammond et al., 2004; see Conclusion, this volume).

Cardiac problems

Cardiovascular abnormalities in WS are related to elastin haploinsufficiency (see Chapter 3). Thickening of the vascular media owing to smooth muscle cell proliferation occurs predominantly in the large and medium-sized elastic arteries. Vascular stenoses (narrowing of blood vessels) are particularly likely to occur at sites of arterial origin and can be discreet or diffuse. Studies with different ascertainment methods have given rather variable figures for the occurrence of individual heart defects, although the overall rate of cardiovascular abnormality has been generally around 75% (Bruno et al., 2003; Collins et al., 2010; Eronen et al., 2002; Hallidie-Smith & Karas, 1988; Morris et al., 1988; Perez-Jurado et al., 1996; Wang et al., 2007). The hallmark cardiac defect is supravalvular aortic stenosis, which is a narrowing of the aortic artery, present in around 32-76%; it can be progressive, particularly in the first few years, and requires intervention in 40-60% of cases, the majority in infancy (Bruno et al., 2003; Collins et al., 2010; Eronen et al., 2002; Wessel et al., 2004). Restenosis (further narrowing of the aorta after a corrective procedure) at graft site appears to be more common in patients with aortic hypoplasia (underdevelopment of the aorta) (Wang et al., 2007; Wessel et al., 1994). Peripheral pulmonary artery stenosis (narrowing of the arteries to the lungs) occurs in around 3-35% and, by contrast, often improves over time without treatment (Giddins et al., 1989; Wang et al., 2007; Wessel et al., 1994). Renal artery stenosis and narrowing of other peripheral vessels including carotid, innominate, subclavian, coeliac and mesenteric vessels are also reported.

A range of other abnormalities have been reported including aortic coarctation (narrowing of the aorta, often discrete) or diffuse aortic hypoplasia (a small, underdeveloped aorta, not limited to a discrete segment), middle aortic syndrome (narrowing of a segment of the descending thoracic or abdominal aorta, often associated with a narrowing of the arteries to the kidneys and bowel with high blood pressure and abdominal pain), bicuspid aortic valve (an aortic valve with two cusps instead of the usual three), supravalvular or valvular pulmonary stenosis (narrowing either above or at the pulmonary valve), mitral valve prolapse (movement of a usually thickened mitral valve into the left atrium during heart contraction; reported in up to 20% of adults), atrial and ventricular septal defects (a hole connecting the right and left atria or the ventricles of the heart) and anomalous pulmonary venous return (a situation in which the blood vessels returning oxygenated blood from the lungs to the heart do not enter the left atrium normally). Hypertension is an important complication of WS and may occur in children and in around 50% of adults. Generalised arterial stiffening, renal artery stenosis and increased sympathetic activity (adrenaline response) may be contributory (Broder et al., 1999; Morris et al., 1988; Wessel et al., 1997).

Sudden death and myocardial infarction have also been reported. A number of these deaths occurred during cardiac catheterisation or surgery and those with severe biventricular outflow obstruction or coronary artery stenosis seem to be at most risk (Bird et al., 1996; Wessel et al., 2004).

There have been a number of reports of stroke in WS, secondary to cerebral arterial narrowing (Ardinger et al., 1994; Kaplan et al., 1995; Putman et al., 1995; Soper et al., 1995; Wollack et al., 1996), although overall this seems to be an infrequent complication. An increased carotid artery intima-media thickness was reported by Sadler et al. (1998), but Cherniske et al. (2004) reported only one in nine adults undergoing carotid artery Doppler (a technique used to look at blood flow in the carotid artery using ultrasound) having any narrowing.

Cardiovascular complications represent the major cause of death in WS. In an analysis of 293 patients with WS representing 5190 patient years of follow-up, Wessel et al. (2004) reported ten deaths, of which five were classed as sudden. This represented a risk 25-100 times that for controls. Ongoing monitoring of blood pressure and cardiac status is an important part of medical follow-up throughout life.

Hypercalcaemia

Although it was recognised early on that transient idiopathic infantile hypercalcaemia (a high blood level of calcium) is a feature of WS, documented evidence of hypercalcaemia is present in a minority. Between studies, the reported incidence varies from 5% to 50% with an overall figure of around 15%. Symptoms of hypercalcaemia usually present within the first year of life, peaking at 5-8 months of age. These commonly include food refusal, vomiting, constipation, colic, failure to thrive and irritability, although it should be noted that these symptoms seem common even in those with normal calcium levels. Hypercalcaemia is usually restricted to infancy and early childhood, but later hypercalcaemia has been occasionally described (Black & Bonham Carter, 1963; Morris et al., 1990). The precise underlying defect in hormonal control of calcium in WS remains unknown. Hypercalciuria (increased urine calcium) can accompany hypercalcaemia or can occur alone. Ultrasound studies indicate that nephrocalcinosis (excess calcium deposits in the kidneys) occurs in less than 5% (Pober et al., 1993; Pankau et al., 1996; Sforzini et al., 2002).

Orthopaedic and other connective-tissue problems

Joints are often lax in the younger child with around 5% having dislocation or subluxation (incomplete or partial dislocation of a joint) at the patella (kneecap). Some 10% have clinical evidence of radioulnar synostosis (bony or soft-tissue connection between the two bones of the forearm, radius and ulna; Dupont et al., 1970; Pagon et al., 1987; Morris & Carey, 1990). With age, there is stiffening and contracture of the joints, predominantly of the lower limbs, and tightening of the heel cords resulting in a stooped habit. Scoliosis of childhood or juvenile onset occurs in 12-17% (Morris et al., 1988; Metcalfe, 2001), but more common is increased lumbar lordosis, an exaggerated inward curve of the lower spine. Inflammatory arthritis has not been a feature.

Inguinal and umbilical herniae (herniae in the groin or belly button area), either singly or in combination, are common affecting around 38% of infants (Morris et al., 1988).

The voice is characteristically deep, gruff or 'brassy' even in infancy, presumably because of reduced elastin in the vocal cords (Vaux et al., 2003).

Growth and puberty

The majority (89%) of babies with WS are born at term, with an average birth weight of 2.76 kg and mean birth weight standard deviation score of −1.49 (Metcalfe, 2001). Problems with feeding and weight gain are commonly encountered in the first year, particularly in children with hypercalcaemia, and children tend to be of slim build with 62% being below the 10th centile (Metcalfe, 2001). However, obesity can be a problem in adulthood affecting one-half to one-third (Morris et al., 1988), with a particular propensity for females to have increased fat distribution around buttocks and thighs. More recently, Cherniske et al. (2004) have reported that approximately two-thirds of adults with WS are overweight or obese. Further, they indicate that this is consistent with the rates of obesity in the general population, so may not reflect a disposition towards weight problems in WS.

Most are short for their families (Morris et al., 1988; Partsch et al.,1999). The average adult height for British women with WS is 151.5 cm and that for British men with WS is 161 cm, equating to a height between the 0.4th and 2nd percentile on the standard UK growth charts. UK-derived WS-specific growth charts are available (Martin et al., 2007).

Head circumference tends to be below the 50th centile, but only around a quarter have microcephaly (small head size).

Puberty occurs around 2 years earlier than in the typical population for both males and females (Morris et al., 1988; Cherniske et al., 2004; Partsch et al., 1999; Pankau et al., 1992) and contributes to reduced adult height. True precocious puberty has been occasionally described (Scothorn & Butler, 1997).

There are limited data on fertility, but individuals with WS of both sexes have reproduced (Metcalfe et al., 2005; Morris et al., 1993; Sadler et al., 1993).

Genitourinary abnormalities

Structural urinary tract abnormalities occur with a much higher prevalence than in the general population (18% compared with 1.5%; Pober et al., 1993; Pankau et al., 1996; Sheih et al., 1989). Described abnormalities include renal agenesis (absent kidney), duplicated kidney, ectopic kidney (kidney in an abnormal position), renal dysplasia (a collection of conditions in which kidneys start to develop but development fails), renal cysts, vesicoureteric reflux (movement of the urine back up the ureters towards the kidneys) and nephrocalcinosis (calcification of the kidneys). Multiple bladder diverticulae (out-pouchings of the bladder wall) are present in around 45% on cystourethrogram, an X-ray that images the bladder and urethra while the bladder is full and passing urine (Babbitt et al., 1979; Sammour et al., 2006). Urinary tract infections and functional abnormalities including urinary frequency, urgency and nocturnal enuresis (incontinence) are common. Sammour et al. (2006) found that bladder capacity was reduced and detrusor instability (weakness or irritability of muscle in the bladder wall) present in 60%. Renal artery stenosis has been reported in up to 50% of individuals with hypertension undergoing arteriography (imaging of blood vessels) (Pober et al., 1993; Sforzini et al., 2002).

Hearing and vision

Hyperacusis, a subjective sensitivity to sound, and phonophobia, a reaction of distress in response to certain sounds, affects almost all individuals with WS, although over time there is often some modification of the behavioural response (Davies et al., 1997; Gothelf et al., 2006; Klein et al., 1990; Levitin et al., 2005; Metcalfe, 2001; Morris et al., 1988). The most problematic sounds are mechanical noises such as vacuum cleaners, food processors, drills, airbrakes and sudden unexpected sounds such as balloons popping, fireworks and dogs barking. Hyperacusis can lead to anxiety and phobias and can adversely affect the quality of life in WS. Individuals with WS report discomfort at sound intensities that are 20 dB lower than the respective threshold for controls (Gothelf et al.,2006), and in individuals with WS who have hyperacusis, hyperexcitability of the auditory efferent system and absence of acoustic reflexes have been found (Attias et al., 2008; Johnson et al., 2001).

High-frequency sensorineural hearing loss or mixed hearing loss in the mild-to-moderate range has been reported in 60-70% of school-aged children with WS (Marler et al., 2005, 2009; Gothelf et al., 2006) compared with 7% of the typical population at school age (Bess et al., 1998; Niskar et al.,1998). Mild-to-moderate high-frequency sensorineural hearing loss is reported in 75% of adults (Cherniske et al., 2004; Johnson et al., 2001).

Convergent squint and refractive error, mainly long-sightedness, affect around 50% of individuals with WS (Braddick & Atkinson,1995; Winter et al., 1996). Suboptimal binocular vision has been reported (Sadler et al., 1996) and individuals with WS often have difficulty in negotiating stairs and uneven surfaces (see Chapters 9 and 13).

Endocrine abnormalities

Although overt hypothyroidism (an underactive thyroid) is uncommon, around two-thirds of persons with WS have thyroid hypoplasia, an underdeveloped thyroid gland (Selicorni et al., 2006; Cambiaso et al., 2007; Stagi et al., 2005). There is a high rate of elevated thyroid-stimulating hormone with normal thyroid hormones (free thyroxine and free triiodothy-ronine) particularly in infancy, which tends to normalise with age.

A complication that has recently come to light is that of diabetes mellitus. Although earlier literature mentions a few cases of overt diabetes mellitus (Morris et al., 1988; Lopez-Rangel et al., 1992; Plissart et al., 1994; Imashuku et al., 2000; Nakaji et al., 2001), it is only more recent systematic studies that have shown that around 75% of adults with WS have prediabetes or type II diabetes on the basis of oral glucose tolerance tests (Pober et al., 2010; Cherniske et al., 2004). Of the adults over 35 years, only 1 in 17 had a normal glucose tolerance test. Impaired glucose tolerance and diabetes were, as expected, more common in individuals with a body mass index of more than 25 kg/m^2, but also occurred in approximately 60% of those with a body mass index of less than 25 kg/m^2. Larger systematic studies are required to confirm this high incidence and to help dissect out contributions from concurrent medication, obesity and lack of exercise. However, Pober et al. (2010) state that they have additional unpublished data showing an increased rate of prediabetes even in individuals with WS aged 10-17 years, prior to onset of obesity or medications, suggesting a true genetic predisposition.

Neurological problems

Hyperreflexia of knee jerks occurs in around 45% of individuals with WS (Metcalfe, 2001; Morris et al., 1988). A higher incidence of left-hand dominance is reported (Bellugi et al., 1990). Epilepsy is uncommon except in those with deletions greater than 1.8 Mb, in whom deletion of the gene *MAGI2* is proposed to lead to an increased risk for infantile spasms (Marshall et al., 2008). Individuals with WS are easily fatigued with a low tolerance for repetitive tasks.

Gastrointestinal problems

Feeding difficulties and poor weight gain in infancy feature strongly. Babies are often described as having poor sucking ability, being slow to feed, having persistent vomiting and being irritable/colicky (Martin et al., 1984; Morris et al., 1988; Metcalfe, 2001; Perez-Jurado et al., 1996). These problems can occur with or independently of hypercalcaemia. Oral sensitivity to textures may contribute to difficulties in weaning onto solids. Inguinal hernias occur in approximately 38% and affect both sexes (compared with a rate of approximately 4% in the general population and a 6:1 male-to-female ratio). Constipation can be severe and was associated with rectal prolapse in 11% in one study (Metcalfe, 2001). Ongoing constipation is a problem at all ages and should be treated aggressively. By contrast, however, 13% have ongoing diarrhoea, for reasons that are unclear but that may include irritable bowel syndrome, increased anxiety or coeliac disease. Giannotti et al. (2001) reported a consecutive series of 63 Italian patients with WS who were screened for coeliac disease by analysis of the dosage of antigliadin immunoglobulin A antibodies and antiendomisium antibodies, with small bowel biopsy in those with positive antibodies. The prevalence of coeliac disease in their series of patients with WS was 9.5% (6/63), compared with 0.54% (1/184) in a published series of Italian students (p<0.001), indicating that the prevalence of coeliac disease in WS is higher than in the general population and is comparable with that reported in Down syndrome and Turner syndrome.

A combination of constipation and reduced elastin in the bowel probably explains the increase in diverticular disease (outpouchings of the bowel wall) in adults with WS. For example, Cherniske et al. (2004) describe an incidence of diverticulosis/diverticulitits of 8 in

20 adults with WS. Bowel surgery was required in 6 of the 20 adults (4 had partial colonic resection for diverticular disease, 1 had a cholecystectomy and 1 had a haemorrhoidectomy).

Partsch et al.'s (2005) retrospective survey of 128 adults with WS reported an increased prevalence of sigmoid diverticulitis (inflamed outpouchings in the lower part of the colon) in adult patients with WS (8% versus 2% in the typical population in the age group below 40 years). Gastroesophageal reflux is reported in 25% of adults (Cherniske et al., 2004).

Development

Acquisition of early motor milestones and language development tend to be delayed in WS. Independent walking is achieved at a mean of 21-27 months but with a broad range (Metcalfe, 2001, Morris et al., 1988). Language development is initially delayed and the mechanisms of language acquisition may not follow the normal path (Karmiloff-Smith et al., 1997). Children with WS show surprising abilities on formal language tests assessing vocabulary, morphology and syntax for their overall IQ. However, language functions are not intact and they show weakness in relational language and pragmatics (see Chapters 10 and 11).

Full-scale IQ averages 50-60 in noninstitutionalised individuals, indicating mild-to-moderate intellectual impairment in most, but with a few having a normal IQ or severe impairment (Davies et al., 1997; Martens et al., 2008; Morris et al., 1988). However, the overall IQ hides an uneven profile of cognitive abilities, termed the WS cognitive profile (Howlin et al., 1998; Mervis et al., 2000). As discussed in Part 4, language, verbal short-term memory, facial processing and social cognition are relative strengths, with greater difficulties in spatial cognition, number, planning and problem solving (Bellugi et al., 1990; Bihrle et al., 1989; Udwin & Yule, 1991). Visuospatial processing in WS, when assessed by drawing tests and block construction tests, follows a local hierarchical pattern in contrast to Down syndrome, where it tends to follow a global processing pattern (Bihrle et al., 1989; see Chapter 12).

Reading skills of adults with WS are generally poor with around one-third of adults with WS lacking basic reading skills and those who can read having a mean reading age equivalent of 8-9 years (Howlin et al., 1998). Reading comprehension is typically poorer (see Chapter 17). Individuals with WS have difficulties with fine motor skills such as writing and drawing and problems with time-telling and mathematics (O'Hearn & Landau, 2007; Paterson et al., 2006; Udwin et al., 1996; see Chapter 16).

Personality and behaviour

Most individuals with WS are described as being of a happy, friendly, outgoing and affection-ate nature, as was recognised in Beuren's initial description of them having 'the same kind of friendly nature—they love everyone, are loved by everyone and are very charming' (Beuren et al., 1964; von Arnim & Engel, 1964). A propensity to regard faces is evident even from babyhood and there is a strong natural tendency to approach strangers and engage them in conversation, regarding everyone as their friend (see Chapters 14 and 15).

Their overfriendliness and poor social judgement leaves them vulnerable to inappropriate advances/abuse (Davies et al., 1997; Elison et al., 2010; see Chapter 5).

This lack of social anxiety contrasts with high levels of fears, phobias and anxiety with studies showing that approximately 50% have a specific phobia and 16-85% have an anxiety disorder (Dykens, 2003; Leyfer et al., 2006; Stinton et al., 2010). Specific phobias are often directed towards loud noises, blood tests or injections and persist over time (Woodruff-Borden et al., 2010). Particularly prominent is anticipatory anxiety, for example, for forthcoming events. Although individuals with WS display high levels of empathy and often anxiety about the health of others, social disinhibition means that they may make socially inappropriate comments. They can be emotionally labile being easily upset by criticism (Elison et al., 2010; Klein-Tasman & Mervis, 2003) (see Chapter 5).

Individuals with WS frequently exhibit preoccupations or obsessions with people, objects or activities such as weather phenomena, lawnmowers and car washes. These can be very pervasive and be to the detriment of normal conversations and daily activities. Some 2-12% of individuals with WS meet diagnostic criteria for obsessive compulsive disorder (Cherniske et al., 2004; Dykens, 2003; Stinton et al., 2010).

Young children display hyperactivity and attention deficit hyperactivity disorder (Arnold et al., 1985; Dilts et al., 1990; Greer et al., 1997; Kennedy et al., 2006; Leyfer et al., 2006). Although hyperactivity reduces, distractibility persists into adulthood (Davies et al., 1998).

Individuals with WS have often been described as having a 'cocktail-party manner', a term initially coined by Hadenius et al. (1962) in reference to hydrocephalic children and defined by Tew (1979) as having four of the following five characteristics: perseveration of response, either echoing the examiner or repeating an earlier statement made by the child; an excessive use of social phrases in conversation; an overfamiliarity in a manner not expected at that age; a habit of introducing personal experience into the conversation in irrelevant and inappropriate contexts; fluent and normally well-articulated speech.

Sleeping difficulties are particularly frequent in infancy and early childhood but can persist (see Chapter 7). Suggested mechanisms include anxiety, restless legs and being easily disturbed by noise (Annaz et al., 2011; Arens et al., 1998; Mason & Arens, 2006).

Individuals with WS tend to have a strong interest in music but, contrary to early reports, do not in most cases seem to have any special musical ability (Hopyan et al., 2001; Levitin et al., 2004).

Adaptive behaviour

People with WS have lower adaptive behavioural skills than expected for their measured IQ and rarely attain full independence (see also Chapter 5). Most adults live with carers or in some form of supervised/sheltered housing. Limited fine motor ability, lack of persistence and distractibility mean that most individuals with WS need prompting and supervision even for carrying out fairly simple tasks. Difficulties in numeracy and planning make budgeting and financial independence a challenge. WS characteristics of overfriendliness and social naivety may mean that carers are reluctant to give independence outside of the home (Davies et al., 1997; Elison et al., 2010; Mervis et al., 2001).

In Davies et al.'s (1997) study of 70 adults with WS, around a quarter of the subjects required some assistance when using the toilet and around half needed at least some assistance with washing and dressing. Some 80-94% were wholly dependent on others for preparation of food and domestic chores. Elison et al. (2010) report their findings on a cohort of 92 adults, 43 of whom were followed longitudinally. Overall 77% required no or minor assistance with self-care, 52% had little or no ability to undertake household chores, 49% were unable to undertake any independent travel and 49% had no ability to make their own purchases. However, Elison et al. noted that adults with WS continued to make slow but steady progress in skills of self-help, daily living and independence. Mervis and John (2010) reported adaptive behaviour performance for 122 children with WS aged 4-15 years, finding lowest scores in the domains of broad independence, community living skills and motor skills. Social skills training and applied behavioural analysis based interventions could help improve levels of independence in some areas.

Prognosis

Detailed studies in adults with WS are still lacking and understanding of the adult phenotype is still evolving. There are insufficient longitudinal data to determine the life expectancy, but this seems largely dependent on cardiovascular problems. The quality of life for adults with WS is strongly influenced by mental health problems, emotional well-being, personal opportunity and support for independence. There is a need for further research and for education of carers and physicians about potential complications in order to optimise preventative care and improve the life experiences of individuals with WS.

Editor commentary (Emily K. Farran & Annette Karmiloff-Smith)

Across the majority of this book, we focus on developmental interactions in relation to the cognitive and behavioural profile of WS. This chapter, by contrast, highlighted the phenotypic profile across a wide range of physical characteristics and their impact on an individual's life. The chapter pinpointed the huge interindividual variation within the WS population with respect to the presence or absence of clinical features and their severity, emphasising that even when individuals have the same genetic deletion, clinical outcome is the product of a highly interactive neuroconstructivist system.

Many clinical characteristics, such as hyperacusis, cardiac problems, reduced bladder capacity and delayed acquisition of motor milestones, place environmental and physical constraints on day-to-day functioning, with serious downstream effects on the course of development. To illustrate this, consider the following four examples. First, hyperacusis: it has been shown that the time taken for individuals with WS to grow out of hyperacusis can be reduced by increased exposure to noise from a young age (Marriage, 1996). This environmental influence might impact neural development and have a positive effect on later prognosis of anxieties and phobias. Second, cardiac problems: cardiac or other health problems can impact the quality of carer–child interactions and might yield behavioural constraints such as reduced active play during childhood. This, in turn, can influence both gene expression and neural development. Third, reduced bladder capacity: reduced bladder capacity can have an impact on the quality of sleep. As will be discussed in Chapter 7, poor sleep quality has cascading effects on brain maturation and the consolidation of learning. Finally, delayed acquisition of motor milestones: in typical development, infants generate sensory inputs by manipulating their environment (e.g. young infants' exploration of nearby objects by arm waving and kicking). This, in turn, leads to modifications of neural networks (e.g. Bertenthal et al., 1994). Impaired or delayed motor development in WS suggests that this cascading sequence of events might well be constrained.

In summary, the clinical profile described in this chapter represents an important piece in the jigsaw of our understanding of how atypical development proceeds in WS. Such considerations are applicable regardless of the neurodevelopmental disorder. For example the impact of hearing loss on phonological processing and later language development in Down syndrome, the effects of obesity on motor exploration in Prader–Willi syndrome, and the effects of digestive problems, a restricted or obsessive diet or sleep disturbance on attention in autism. In examining the cascading effects of seemingly small clinical problems, our neuroconstructivist approach is particularly relevant.

References

Annaz, D., Hill, C.M., Ashworth, A., Holley, S., & Karmiloff-Smith, A. (2011). Characterisation of sleep problems in children with Williams syndrome. *Research in Developmental Disabilities*, **32**, 164–69.

Ardinger, R.H., Jr., Goertz, K.K., & Mattioli, L.F. (1994). Cerebrovascular stenosis with cerebral infarction in a child with Williams syndrome. *American Journal of Medical Genetics*, **51**, 200–202.

von Arnim, G., & Engel, P. (1964). Mental retardation related to hypercalcaemia. *Developmental Medicine and Child Neurology*, **6**, 366–77.

Arnold, R., Yule, W., & Martin, N. (1985). The psychological characteristics of infantile hypercalcaemia: a preliminary investigation. *Developmental Medicine and Child Neurology*, **27**, 49–59.

Arens, R., Wright, B., Elliott, J., Zhao, H., Wang, P.P., Brown, C.W., et al. (1998). Periodic limb movement in sleep in children with Williams syndrome. *Journal of Pediatrics*, **133**, 670–74.

Attias, J., Raveh, E., Ben-Naftali, N.F., Zarchi, O., & Gothelf, D. (2008). Hyperactive auditory efferent systems and lack of acoustic reflexes in Williams syndrome. *Journal of Basic and Clinical Physiology and Pharmacology*, **19**, 193–207.

Babbitt, D.P., Dobbs, J., & Boedecker, R.A. (1979). Multiple bladder diverticula in Williams 'Elfin-Facies" syndrome. *Pediatric Radiology*, **8**, 29–31.

Baumer, A., Dutly, F., Balmer, D., Riegel, M., Tukel, T., Krajewska-Walasek, M., et al. (1998). High level of unequal meiotic crossovers at the origin of the 22q11.2 and 7q11.23 deletions. *Human Molecular Genetics*, **7**, 887–94.

Bayes, M., Magano, L.F., Rivera, N., Flores, R., & Perez Jurado, L.A. (2003). Mutational mechanisms of Williams-Beuren syndrome deletions. *American Journal of Human Genetics*, **73**, 131–51.

Bellugi,U., Bihrle,A., Jernigan,T., Trauner,D., & Doherty,S. (1990). Neuropsychological, neurological and neuroanatomical profile of Williams syndrome. *American Journal of Medical Genetics, Supplement*, **6**, 115–25.

Bertenthal, B.I., Campos, J.J., Kermoian, R. (1994). *Current Directions in Psychological Science*, **3**, 140–45.

Bess, F.H., Dodd-Murphy, J., & Parker, R.A. (1998). Children with minimal sensorineural hearing loss: prevalence, educational performance, and functional status. *Ear and Hearing*, **19**, 339–54.

Beuren, A., Schulze, C., Eberle, P., Harmjanz, D., & Apitz, J. (1964). The syndrome of supravalvular aortic stenosis, peripheral pulmonary stenosis, mental retardation and similar facial appearance. *The American Journal of Cardiology*, **13**, 471–83.

Bihrle, A.M., Bellugi, U., Delis, D., & Marks, S. (1989). Seeing either the forest or the trees: dissociation in visuospatial processing. *Brain and Cognition*, 11, 37–49.

Bird, L.M., Billman, G.F., Lacro, R.V., Spicer, R.L., Jariwala, L.K., Hoyme, H.E., et al. (1996). Sudden death in Williams syndrome:Report of ten cases. *Journal of Pediatrics*, 29, 926–31.

Black, J.A., & Bonham Carter, R.E. (1963). Association between aortic stenosis and facies of severe infantile hypercalcaemia. *The Lancet*, II, 745–49.

Botta, A., Novelli, G., Mari, A., Novelli, A., Sabani, M., Korenberg, J., et al. (1999). Detection of an atypical 7q11.23 deletion in Williams syndrome patients which does not include the STX1A and FZD3 genes. *Journal of Medical Genetics*, 36, 478–80.

Braddick, O.J., & Atkinson, J. (1995). Visual and visuospatial development in young Williams syndrome children. *Investigative Ophthalmology and Visual Science (Supplement)*, 36, S954.

Broder, K., Reinhardt, E., Ahern, J., Lifton, R., Tamborlane, W., & Pober, B. (1999). Elevated ambulatory blood pressure in 20 subjects with Williams syndrome. *American Journal of Medical Genetics*, 83, 356–60.

Bruno, E., Rossi, N., Thuer, O., Cordoba, R., & Alday, L.E. (2003). Cardiovascular findings and clinical course in patients with Williams syndrome. *Cardiology in the Young*, 13, 532–36.

Cambiaso, P., Orazi, C., Diglio, C., Loche, S., Capolino, R., Tozzi, A., et al. (2007). Thyroid morphology and subclinical hypothyroidism in children and adolescents with Williams syndrome. *Journal of Pediatrics*, 150, 62–65.

Cherniske, E.M., Carpenter, T.O., Klaiman, C., Young, E., Bregman, J., Insogna, K., et al. (2004). Multisystem study of 20 older adults with Williams syndrome. *American Journal of Medical Genetics*, 131, 255–64.

Collins, R.T., Kaplan, P., Somes, G.W., & Rome, J.J. (2010). Long-term outcomes of patients with cardiovascular abnormalities and Williams syndrome. *The American Journal of Cardiology*, 105, 874–78.

Dai, L., Bellugi, U., Chen, XN., Pulst-Korenberg, AM., Järvinen-Pasley, A., Tirosh-Wagner, T., et al. (2009). Is it Williams syndrome? GTF21RD1 implicated in visual-spatial construction and GTF21 in sociability revealed by high resolution arrays. *American Journal of Medical Genetics Part A*, 149A, 302–314.

Davies, M., Howlin, P., & Udwin, O. (1997). Independence and adaptive behaviour in adults with Williams syndrome. *American Journal of Medical Genetics*, 70, 188–95.

Davies, M., Udwin, O., & Howlin, P. (1998). Adults with Williams syndrome. Preliminary study of social, emotional and behavioural difficulties. *The British Journal of Psychiatry*, 172, 273–76.

Dilts, C.V., Morris, C.A., & Leonard, C.O. (1990). Hypothesis for development of a behavioural phenotype in Williams syndrome. *American Journal of Medical Genetics, Supplement*, 6, 126–31.

Dupont, B., Dupont, A., Bliddal, J., Holst, C., Melchior, K., & Ottesen, O.E. (1970). Idiopathic hypercalcaemia of infancy. The elfin face syndrome. *Danish Medical Bulletin*, 17, 33–46.

Dutly, F., & Schinzel, A. (1996). Unequal interchromosomal rearrangements may result in elastin gene deletions causing the Williams-Beuren syndrome. *Human Molecular Genetics*, 5, 1893–98.

Dykens, E.M. (2003). Anxiety, fears, and phobias in persons with Williams syndrome. *Developmental Neuropsychology*, 23, 291–316.

Edelmann, L., Prosnitz, A., Pardo, S., Bhatt, J., Cohen, N., Lauriat, T., et al. (2007). An atypical deletion of the Williams-Beuren syndrome interval implicates genes associated with defective visuospatial processing and autism. *Journal of Medical Genetics*, 44, 136–43.

Elison, S., Stinton, C., Howlin, P. (2010). Health and social outcomes in adults with Williams syndrome: findings from cross-sectional and longitudinal cohorts. *Research in Developmental Disabilities*, 31, 587–99.

Eronen, M., Peippo, M., Hiippala, A., Raatikka, M., Arvio, M., Johansson, R., et al. (2002). Cardiovascular manifestations in 75 patients with Williams syndrome. *Journal of Medical Genetics*, 39, 554–58.

Frangiskakis, J.M., Ewart, A.K., Morris, C.A., Mervis, C.B., Bertrand, J., Robinson, B.F., et al. (1996). LIM-kinase1 hemizygosity implicated in impaired visuospatial constructive cognition. *Cell*, **86**, 59–69.

Fryssira, H., Palmer, R., Hallidie-Smith, KA., Taylor, J., Donnai, D., & Reardon, W. (1997). Fluorescent in situ hybridization (FISH) for hemizygous deletion at the elastin locus in patients with isolated supravalvular aortic stenosis. *Journal of Medical Genetics*, **34**, 306–308.

Gagliardi, C., Bonaglia, M.C., Selicorni, A., Borgatti, R., & Giorda, R. (2003). Unusual cognitive and behavioural profile in a Williams syndrome patient with atypical 7q11.23 deletion. *Journal of Medical Genetics*, **40**, 526–30.

Giannotti, A.G., Tiberio, G., Castro, M., Virgilli, F., Collistro, F., Digilio, M.C., et al. (2001). Coeliac disease in Williams syndrome. *Journal of Medical Genetics*, **38**, 767–68.

Giddins, N.G., Finley, J.P., Nanton, M.A., & Roy, D.L. (1989). The natural course of supravalvular aortic stenosis and peripheral pulmonary artery stenosis in Williams syndrome. *British Heart Journal*, **62**, 315–19.

Gothelf, D., Farber, N., Raveh, N., Apter, A., & Attias, J. (2006). Hyperacusis in Williams syndrome: characteristics and associated neuroaudiologic abnormalities. *Neurology*, **66**, 390–95.

Greer, M.K., Brown, F.R. 3rd, Pai, G.S., Choudry, S.H., & Klein, A.J. (1997). Cognitive, adaptive and behavioural characteristics of Williams syndrome. *American Journal of Medical Genetics*, **74**, 521–25.

Hadenius, A.M., Hagberg, B., Hyttnes-Bensch, K., & Sjogen, I. (1962). The natural prognosis of infantile hydrocephalus. *Acta Paediatrica Scandinavica*, **51**, 117.

Hammond, P., Hutton,T.J., Allanson, J.E., Campbell, L.E., Hennekam, R.C.M., Holden, S., et al. (2004). 3D analysis of facial morphology. *American Journal of Medical Genetics Part A*, **126A**, 339–48.

Hallidie-Smith, K.A., & Karas, S. (1988). Cardiac anomalies in Williams-Beuren syndrome. *Archives of Disease in Childhood*, **63**, 809–813.

Heller, R., Rauch, A., Luttgen, S., Schroder, B., & Winterpacht, A. (2003). Partial deletion of the critical 1.5 Mb interval in Williams Beuren syndrome. *Journal of Medical Genetics*, **40**, e99.

Hirota, H., Matsuoka, R., Chen, X.-N., Salandanan, L.S., Lincoln, A., Rose, F.E., et al. (2003). Williams syndrome deficits in visual spatial processing linked to GTF2IRD1 and GTF2I on chromosome 7q11.23. *Genetics in Medicine*, **5**, 311–21.

Hobart, H.H., Morris, C.A., Mervis, C.B., Pani, A.M., Kistler, D.J., Rios, C.M., et al. (2010). Inversion of the Williams syndrome region is a common polymorphism found more frequently in parents of children with Williams syndrome. *American Journal of Medical Genetics Part C: Seminars in Medical Genetics*, **154C**, 220–28.

Hopyan, T., Dennis, M., Weksberg, R., & Cytrynbaum, C. (2001). Musical skills and the expressive interpretation of music in children with Williams-Beuren syndrome: pitch, rhythm, melodic imagery, phrasing and musical affect. *Child Neuropsychology*, **7**, 42–53.

Howald, C., Merla, G., & Digilio, M.C. (2006). Two high throughput technologies to detect segmental aneuploidies identify new Williams-Beuren syndrome patients with atypical deletions. *Journal of Medical Genetics*, **43**, 266–73.

Howlin, P., Davies, M., Udwin, O. (1998). Cognitive functioning in adults with Williams syndrome. *The Journal of Child Psychology and Psychiatry*, **39**, 183–89.

Imashuku, S., Hayashi, S., Kuriyama, K., Hibi, S., Tabata, Y., & Todo, S. (2000). Sudden death of a 21-year-old-female with Williams syndrome showing rare complications. *Pediatr International*, **42**, 322–24.

Johnson, L.B., Comesu, M., & Clarke, K.D. (2001). Hyperacusis in Williams syndrome. *The Journal of Otolaryngology*, **30**, 90–92.

Joseph, M.C., & Parrott, D. (1958). Severe infantile hypercalcaemia with special reference to the face. *Archives of Disease in Childhood*, **33**, 385–95.

Kaplan, P., Levinson, M., & Kaplan,B.S. (1995). Cerebral artery stenosis in Williams syndrome cause strokes in childhood. *Journal of Pediatrics*, **126**, 943–45.

Karmiloff-Smith, A., Grant, J., Berthoud, I., Davies, M., Howlin, P., & Udwin, O. (1997). Language and Williams syndrome: how intact is "intact"? *Child Development*, 68, 246–62.

Karmiloff-Smith, A., Grant, J., Ewing, S., Carette, M.J., Metcalfe, K., Donnai, D., et al. (2003). Using case study comparisons to explore genotype–phenotype correlations in Williams–Beuren syndrome. *Journal of Medical Genetics*, 40, 136–40.

Kennedy, J.C., Kaye, D.L., & Sadler, L.S. (2006). Psychiatric diagnoses in patients with Williams syndrome and their families. *Jefferson Journal of Psychiatry*, 20, 22–31.

Klein, A.J., Armstrong, B.L., Greer, M.K., & Brown, F.R.D. (1990). Hyperacusis and otitis media in individuals with Williams syndrome. *The Journal of Speech and Hearing Disorders*, 55, 339–44.

Klein-Tasman, B.P., & Mervis, C.B. (2003). Distinctive personality characteristics of 8-, 9-, and 10-year-olds with Williams syndrome. *Developmental Neuropsychology*, 23, 269–90.

Korenberg, J.R., Chen, X.N., Hirota, H., Lai, Z., Bellugi, U., Burian, D., et al. (2000). VI. Genome structure and cognitive map of Williams syndrome. *Journal of Cognitive Neuroscience*, 12 Suppl 1, 89–107.

Levitin, D.J., Cole, K., Chiles, M., Lai, Z., Lincoln, A., & Bellugi, U. (2004). Characterizing the musical phenotype in Williams syndrome. *Child Neuropsychology*, 10, 223–47.

Levitin, D.J., Cole, K., Lincoln, A., & Bellugi, U. (2005). Aversion, awareness, and attraction: investigating claims of hyperacusis in the Williams syndrome phenotype. *The Journal of Child Psychology and Psychiatry*, 46, 514–23.

Leyfer, O.T., Woodruff-Borden, J., Klein-Tasman, B.P., Fricke, J.S., & Mervis, C.B. (2006). Prevalence of psychiatric disorders in 4 to 16-year-olds with Williams syndrome. *American Journal of Medical Genetics Part B: Neuropsychiatric Genetics*, 141B, 615–22.

Lopez-Rangel, E., Maurice, M., McGillivray, B., & Friedman, J.M. (1992). Williams syndrome in adults. *American Journal of Medical Genetics*, 44, 720–29.

Marler, J.A., Elfenbein, J.L., Ryals, B.M., Urban, Z., & Netzeloff, M.L. (2005). Sensorineural hearing loss in children and adults with Williams syndrome. *American Journal of Medical Genetics Part A*, 138A, 318–27.

Marler, J.A., Wightman, F.L., Kistler, D.J., Roy, J.L., & Mervis, C.A. (2009). Auditory processing in Williams syndrome: does normal behavioural hearing indicate normal auditory function? *Frontiers in Human Neuroscience*. DOI:10.3389/conf.neuro.09.2009.07.022 [abstract presented at the 12th International Professional Conference on Williams syndrome] <http://www.frontiersin.org/Community/AbstractDetails.aspx?ABS_DOI=10.3389/conf.neuro.09.2009.07.022> accessed 28 June 2011.

Marriage, J. (1996). *Hyperacusis in Williams Syndrome*. PhD thesis, University of Manchester.

Marshall, C.R., Young, E.J., Pani, A.M., Freckmann, M., Lacassie, Y., Howald, C., et al. (2008). Infantile spasms is associated with deletion of the MAG12 gene on chromosome 7q11.23-q21.11. *American Journal of Human Genetics*, 83, 106–111.

Martens, M.A., Wilson, S.T., & Reutens, D.C. (2008). Williams syndrome: a critical review of the cognitive, behavioural and neuroatomic phenotype. *The Journal of Child Psychology and Psychiatry*, 49, 576–608.

Martin, N.D.T., Smith, W.R., Cole, T.J., & Preece, M.A. (2007). New height, weight and head circumference charts for British children with Williams syndrome. *Archives of Disease in Childhood*, 92, 598–601.

Martin, N.D., Snodgrass, G.J., & Cohen, R.D. (1984). Idiopathic infantile hypercalcaemia- a continuing enigma. *Archives of Disease in Childhood*, 59, 605–613.

Mason, T.B.A.I., & Arens, R. (2006). Sleep patterns in Williams-Beuren syndrome. In C.A. Morris, H.M. Lenhoff & P.P. Wang (Eds), *Williams–Beuren Syndrome: Research, Evaluation, and Treatment* (pp. 294–308). Baltimore, MD: Johns Hopkins University Press.

Mervis, C.B., & John, A.E. (2010). Cognitive and behavioural characteristics of children with Williams syndrome: implications for intervention approaches. *American Journal of Medical Genetics Part C: Seminars in Medical Genetics*, 154C, 229–48.

Mervis, C.B., Klein-Tasman, B.P., & Mastin, M.E. (2001). Adaptive behavior of 4- through 8-year-old children with Williams syndrome. *American Journal of Mental Retardation*, 106, 82–93.

Mervis, C.B., Robinson, B.F., Bertrand, J., Morris, C.A., Klein-Tasman, B.P., & Armstrong, S.C. (2000). The Williams syndrome cognitive profile. *Brain and Cognition*, **44**, 604–28.

Metcalfe, K.A. (2001). *Williams Syndrome and the Elastin Gene*. MD thesis, University of Wales.

Metcalfe, K., Simeonov, E., Beckett, W., Donnai, D., Tassabehji, M. (2005). Autosomal dominant inheritance of Williams-Beuren syndrome in a father and son with haploinsufficiency for FKBP6. *Clinical Dysmorphology*, **14**, (61), e65.

Morris, C.A., & Carey, J.C. (1990). Three diagnostic signs in Williams syndrome. *American Journal of Medical Genetics, Supplement*, **6**, 100–101.

Morris, C.A., Demsey, S.A., Leonard, C.O., Dilts, C., & Blackburn, B.L. (1988). Natural history of Williams syndrome: physical characteristics. *Journal of Pediatrics*, **113**, 318–26.

Morris, C.A., Leonard, C.O., Dilts, C., & Demsey, S.A. (1990). Adults with Williams syndrome. *American Journal of Medical Genetics, Supplement*, **6**, 102–107.

Morris, C.A., Mervis, C.B., Hobart, H.H., Gregg, R.G., Bertrand, J., Ensing, G.J., et al. (2003). GTF2I hemizygosity implicated in mental retardation in Williams syndrome: genotype–phenotype analysis of five families with deletions in the Williams syndrome region. *American Journal of Medical Genetics Part A*, **123A**, 45–59.

Morris, C.A., Thomas, I.T., & Greenberg, F. (1993). Williams syndrome : autosomal dominant inheritance. *American Journal of Medical Genetics*, **47**, 478–81.

Nakaji, A., Kawame, Y., Nagai, C., & Iwata, M. (2001). Clinical features of a senior patient with Williams syndrome. *Rinsho Shinkeigaku*, **41**, 592–98.

Niskar, A.S., Kieszak, S.M., Holmes, A., Esteban, E., Rubin, C., & Brody, D. (1998). Prevalence of hearing loss among children 6 to 19 years of age: the Third National Health and Nutrition Examination Survey. *Journal of the American Medical Association*, **279**, 1071–75.

O'Hearn, K., Landau, B. (2007). Mathematical skill in individuals with Williams syndrome: evidence from a standardised mathematics battery. *Brain and Cognition*, **64**, 238–46.

Osborne, L.R., Li, M., Pober, B., Chitayat, D., Bodurtha, J., Mandel, A., et al. (2001). A 1.5 million-base pair inversion polymorphism in families with Williams-Beuren syndrome. *Nature Genetics*, **29**, 321–25.

Pagon, R.A., Bennett, F.C., LaVeck, B., Stewart, K.B., & Johnson, J. (1987). Williams syndrome: features in late childhood and adolescence. *Paediatrics*, **80**, 85–91.

Pankau, R., Partsch, C.J., Gosch, A., Oppermann, H.C., & Wessel, A. (1992). Statural growth in Williams-Beuren syndrome. *European Journal of Pediatrics*, **151**, 751–55.

Pankau, R., Partsch, C.J., Winter, M., Gosch, A., & Wessel, A. (1996). Incidence and spectrum of renal abnormalities in Williams-Beuren syndrome. *American Journal of Medical Genetics*, **63**, 301–304.

Partsch, C.J., Dreyer, G., Gosch, A., Winter, M., Schneppenheim, R., Wessel, A., et al. (1999). Longitudinal evaluation of growth, puberty and bone maturation in children with Williams sydrome. *Journal of Pediatrics*, **134**, 82–89.

Partsch, C.J., Siebert, R., Caliebe, A., Gosch, A., Wessel, A., & Pankau, R. (2005). Sigmoid diverticulitis in patients with Williams-Beuren syndrome: relatively high prevalence and high complication rate in young adults with the syndrome. *American Journal of Medical Genetics*, **137**, 52–54.

Paterson, S.J., Girelli, L., Butterworth, B., & Karmiloff-Smith, A. (2006). Are numerical impairments syndrome specific? Evidence from Williams syndrome and Down's syndrome. *The Journal of Child Psychology and Psychiatry*, **47**, 190–204.

Perez-Jurado, L.A., Peoples, R., Kaplan, P., Hamel, B.C., & Francke, U. (1996). Molecular definition of the chromosome 7 deletion in Williams syndrome and parent-of-origin effects on growth. *American Journal of Human Genetics*, **59**, 781–92.

Plissart, L., Borghgraef, M., Volcke, P.,Van den Berghe, H., & Fryns, J.P. (1994). Adults with Williams-Beuren syndrome: evaluation of the medical, psychological and behavioural aspects. *Clinical Genetics*, **46**, 161–67.

Pober, B.R., Lacro, R.V., Rice, C., Mandell, V., & Teele, R.L. (1993). Renal findings in 40 individuals with Williams syndrome. *American Journal of Medical Genetics,* **46**, 271–74.

Pober, B.R., Wang, E., Caprio, S., Peteren, K.F., Brandt, C., Stanley, T., et al. (2010). High prevalence of diabetes and pre-diabetes in adults with Williams syndrome. *American Journal of Medical Genetics Part C: Seminars in Medical Genetics,* **154C**, 291–98.

Putman, C.M., Chaloupka, J.C., Eklund, J.E., & Fulbright, R.K. (1995). Multifocal intracranial occlusive vasculopathy resulting in stroke: an unusual manifestation of Williams syndrome. *American Journal of Neuroradiology,* **16**, 1536–38.

Sadler, L.S., Gingell, R., & Martin, D.J. (1998). Carotid ultrasound examination in Williams syndrome. *Journal of Pediatrics,* **132**, 354–56.

Sadler, L.S., Olitsky, S.E., & Reynolds, J.D. (1996). Reduced stereoacuity in Williams syndrome. *American Journal of Medical Genetics,* **66**, 287–88.

Sadler, L.S., Robinson, L.K., Verdaasdonk, K.R., & Gingell, R. (1993). The Williams syndrome: evidence for possible autosomal dominant inheritance. *American Journal of Medical Genetics,* **47**, 468–70.

Sammour, Z.M., Gomes, C.M., Duarte, R.J., Trigo-Rocha, F.E., & Srougi, M. (2006). Voiding dysfunction and the Williams-Beuren syndrome: a clinical and urodynamic investigation. *Journal of Urology,* **175**, 1472–76.

Scothorn, D.J., & Butler, M.G. (1997). How common is precocious puberty in patients with Williams syndrome. *Clinical Dysmorphology,* **6**, 91–93.

Selicorni, A., Fratoni, A., Pavesi, M.A., Bottigelli, M., Annaboldi, E., & Milan, D. (2006). Thyroid anomalies in Williams syndrome: investigation of 95 patients. *American Journal of Medical Genetics Part A,* **140A**, 1098–1101.

Sforzini, C., Milani, D., Fossali, E., Barbato, A., Grumieri, G., Bianchetti, M.G., et al. (2002). Renal tract ultrasonography and calcium homeostasis in Williams-Beuren syndrome. *Pediatric Nephrology,* **17**, 899–902.

Sheih, C.H.P., Liu, M.-B., Hung, C.-S., Yang, K.-H., Chen, W.Y., & Lin, C.-Y. (1989). Renal abnormalities in school children. *Pediatrics,* **84**, 1086–90.

Soper, R., Chaloupka, J.C., Fayad, P.B., Greally, J.M., Shaywitz, B.A., Awad, I.A., et al. (1995). Ischaemic stroke and intracranial multifocal cerebral arteriopathy in Williams syndrome. *Journal of Pediatrics,* **126**, 945–48.

Stagi, S., Bindi, G., Neri, A.S., Lapi, E., Losi, S., Jenuso, R., et al. (2005). Thyroid function and morphology in patients affected by Williams syndrome. *Clinical Endocrinology,* **63**, 456–60.

Stinton, C., Elison, S., & Howlin, P. (2010). Mental health problems in adults with Williams syndrome. *Am J Intellect Dev Disabil,* **115**, 3–18.

Stromme, P., Bjornstad, P.G., & Ramstad, K. (2002). Prevalence estimation of Williams syndrome. *Journal of Child Neurology,* **17**, 269–71.

Tassabehji, M., Metcalfe, K., Karmiloff-Smith, A., Carette, M.J., Grant, J., Dennis, N., et al. (1999). Williams syndrome: use of chromosomal microdeletions as a tool to dissect cognitive and physical phenotypes. *American Journal of Human Genetics,* **64**, 118–25.

Tew, B. (1979). The 'cocktail party syndrome' in children with hydrocephalus and spina bifida. *British Journal of Disorders of Communication,* **14**, 89–101.

Thomas, N.S., Durkie, M., Potts, G., Sandford, R., VanZyl, B., Youings, S., et al. (2006). Parental and chromosomal origins of microdeletion and duplication syndromes involving 7q11.23, 15q11-q13 and 22q11. *European Journal of Human Genetics,* **14**, 831–37.

Udwin, O., Davies, M., & Howlin, P. (1996). A longitudinal study of cognitive abilities and educational attainment in Williams syndrome. *Developmental Medicine and Child Neurology,* **38**, 1020–29.

Udwin, O., & Yule, W. (1991). A cognitive and behavioural phenotype in Williams syndrome. *Journal of Clinical and Experimental Neuropsychology,* **13**, 232–44.

Vaux, K.K., Wojtczak, H., Benirschke, K., & Jones, K.L. (2003). Vocal cord abnormalities in Williams syndrome: a further manifestation of elastin deficiency. *American Journal of Medical Genetics Part A,* **119A**, 302–304.

Wang, C.-C., Hwu, W.-C., Wu, E.-T., Lu, F., Wang, J.-K., & Wu, M.-H. (2007). Outcome of pulmonary and aortic stenosis in Williams-Beuren syndrome in an Asian cohort. *Acta Paediatrica,* **96**, 906–909.

Wessel, A., Gravenhorst, V., Buchhorn, R., Gosch, A., Partsch, C.-J., & Pankau, R. (2004). Risk of sudden death in the Williams-Beuren syndrome. *American Journal of Medical Genetics Part A,* **127A**, 234–37.

Wessel, A., Motz, R., Pankau, R., & Bursch, J.H. (1997). Arterial hypertension and blood pressure profile in patients with Williams-Beuren syndrome [article in German]. *Zeitschrift für Kardiologie,* **86**, 215–57.

Wessel, A., Pankau, R., Kececioglu, D., Ruschewski, W., & Bursch, J.H. (1994). Three decades of follow-up of aortic and pulmonary vascular lesions in the Williams-Beuren syndrome. *American Journal of Medical Genetics,* **52**, 297–301.

Williams, J.C.P., Barratt-Boyes, M.B., & Lowe, J.B. (1961). Supravalvular aortic stenosis. *Circulation,* **24**, 1311–18.

Winter, M., Pankau, R., Amm, M., Gosch, A., & Wessel, A. (1996). The spectrum of ocular features in the Williams-Beuren syndrome. *Clinical Genetics,* **49**, 28–31.

Wollack, J.B., Kaifer, M., LaMonte, M.P., & Rothman, M. (1996). Stroke in Williams syndrome. *Stroke,* **27**, 143–46.

Woodruff-Borden, J., Kistler, D.J., Henderson, D.R., Crawford, N.A., & Mervis, C.B. (2010). Longitudinal course of anxiety in children and adolescents with Williams syndrome. *American Journal of Medical Genetics Part C: Seminars in Medical Genetics,* **154C**, 277–90.

Chapter 5

Adult outcomes and integration into society

Chris Stinton and Patricia Howlin

Introduction

Since the identification of Williams syndrome (WS) by Williams, Lowe & Barratt-Boyes (1961), research into the disorder has increased dramatically. The key clinical features of WS are well recognised: transient hypercalcaemia, distinctive facial features, cardiovascular disease and developmental delay with an unusual profile of strengths and difficulties (see Chapter 4). However, much of what is known about the syndrome is derived from research focusing on children and adolescents or mixed child/adult samples. Relatively little is known about adults with WS or about the longer-term outcomes for these individuals. In other syndrome groups, abilities in childhood provide clues to outcomes in adult life. For example, children with autism spectrum disorders who have higher cognitive and linguistic abilities tend to have better social outcomes in adulthood than those with an IQ below 70 (Billstedt et al., 2005; Eaves & Ho, 2008; Howlin et al., 2004; Howlin, 1997). For individuals with WS, prognostic indicators have not been investigated and it remains unknown which, if any, factors might contribute to better outcomes for them in adulthood. Although there is some suggestion of accelerated ageing in WS, primarily because of certain circumscribed memory difficulties and physical characteristics such as premature ageing of the skin and greying of the hair (e.g. Cherniske et al., 2004), many individuals with WS will enter their fifth and sixth decades of life in relatively good health (Elison et al., 2010). Yet care often falls to ageing parents, who may struggle to maintain this role. It is clear that this position is untenable in the long term. Understanding the long-term outcomes for individuals with WS is crucial in determining and delivering appropriate provision and it is a critically under-researched area.

The aim of this chapter is to provide an overview of outcomes in adult life for individuals with WS, focusing on areas such as physical and mental health, social outcomes, and cognitive and linguistic functioning. Using data from cross-sectional and longitudinal cohorts, current research in the field highlights areas of promise and those of concern for the future of individuals with WS as they enter their early and middle adult years.

Trajectories of cognitive and linguistic abilities during adulthood
General intelligence (IQ)

Much of the research in WS has focused on cognitive profiles. The vast majority of individuals with WS have mild-to-moderate intellectual disability (Martens et al., 2008). Typical IQ scores fall between 40 and 90 (mean: low 60s), although a small number of people with WS have an IQ within the normal range (Howlin et al., 2010). Research using a variety of methodologies has shown that the cognitive functioning of individuals with WS remains stable throughout life. When individuals with WS are followed up over time, no significant differences are observed in IQ scores from childhood through to adulthood (Udwin et al., 1996; Howlin et al., 2010). Similarly, cross-sectional studies comparing younger and older adults with WS (<50 years versus >50 years: Devenny et al., 2004; 20s versus 30s versus 40+ years: Howlin et al., 2010) and correlational studies (Searcy et al., 2004) typically show no age-related differences in IQ. However, IQ scores alone do not provide an adequate measure of the cognitive profiles and in-depth research has highlighted subtle and complex patterns of strengths and weaknesses. For example, performance on tasks of phonological memory, face processing and receptive vocabulary is often relatively good (Brock et al., 2007; Paul et al., 2002; Setter et al., 2007; see also Chapters 8, 10, 11 and 14), whereas tests of number and spatial cognition as well as planning and problem solving present considerable difficulties (Ansari et al., 2007; Farran et al., 2003; Howlin et al., 1998; see also Chapters 9, 12, 13 and 16). In general, if and how these areas of functioning change over time is not yet fully understood.

Memory

While longitudinal studies of cognitive functioning in WS have typically focused on IQ, several aspects of memory have also been investigated (see also Chapter 8). On tasks in which individuals are required to recall strings of digits or items presented either as pictures or verbally (measures of explicit and auditory short-term memory), task performance typically increases with age during childhood and is followed by a period of stability and a decline in later life (Devenny et al., 2004; Krinsky-McHale et al., 2005; Mervis et al., 1999). This pattern is similar to that observed in the general population (Henry, 1994; Maylor et al., 1999). Similarly consistent with normal ageing are the results of tests of episodic memory (memory for events) in WS in which participants aged over 50 years are significantly poorer at recalling lists of learnt items than those aged under 50 years, although the age at which this decline appears to occur is somewhat younger than compared with the typically developing population (Devenny et al., 2004). Finally, performance on a test of implicit memory (unconscious recollection of information) does not seem to be influenced by increasing age (Krinsky-McHale et al., 2005). Serious decline in memory (as a result of dementia) has occasionally been reported for adults with WS, although it is unclear if there is an increased risk of dementia in this syndrome (Cherniske et al., 2004).

Receptive and expressive vocabulary

Research into the linguistic abilities of individuals with WS shows considerable age-related changes (see also Chapters 10 and 11). As children, expressive vocabulary tends to be in advance of receptive vocabulary (Arnold et al., 1985; Orellana et al., 2008); yet, by adulthood the reverse is often the case (Howlin et al., 2010). This may reflect developmental changes in language skills. Whereas the receptive-vocabulary skills of children with WS are equivalent to those of children with Down syndrome (DS), by adolescence and into adulthood individuals with WS show a significant advantage over individuals with DS (Klein & Mervis, 1999; Vicari et al., 2004). By later childhood, individuals with WS perform better on tests of receptive vocabulary than would be predicted by their mental age and they may even outperform typically developing children matched for nonverbal reasoning (e.g. Brock et al., 2007). In the main, continuing improvements in receptive-vocabulary skills are observed throughout adolescence and into adulthood (Howlin et al., 2010; Jarrold et al., 1998; Jarrold et al., 2001). However, as individuals with WS enter their 30s, development in this area seems to reach a plateau, at about the level of a typically developing child aged 10-11 years (Howlin et al., 2010). For expressive vocabulary, the early advantagethat is shown by individuals with WS between the ages of 2-4 years compared with those with DS does not last and by around 5 years there are no differences between the two groups (Vicari et al., 2004). By adulthood, expressive vocabulary seems to reach a peak at around the 7-8-year-old level and falls behind receptive-vocabulary skills (Howlin et al., 2010). Although there is some evidence from longitudinal research of a small decline in expressive-vocabulary skills between the ages of 20 years and 30 years, this is not supported by cross-sectional research (Howlin et al., 2010).

Despite various methodological issues that limit comparisons between different studies, most research involving adults with WS indicates that cognitive and linguistic abilities remain relatively stable over time from the late teens onwards, with little evidence either of decline or major change. This is in contrast to the developmental trajectories recorded for other groups of individuals with intellectual disability. For example, individuals with DS show a decline in adaptive functioning and in both verbal and nonverbal abilities with increasing age (e.g. Carr, 2005; Wishart, 1993). A significant decrease in both IQ and adaptive functioning is also characteristic of individuals with fragile X syndrome (e.g. Fisch et al., 1999; Fisch et al., 2002), although unlike DS, in which deterioration typically occurs in the third decade and onwards (Kittler et al., 2004), in fragile X syndrome the decline in abilities usually begins during childhood and adolescence (Fisch et al., 2002). Some other disorders show a less clear pattern of change. Thus, in autism spectrum disorders, although IQ scores have been reported to decline during childhood in some studies (e.g. Fisch et al., 2002), most follow-up studies indicate stability in nonverbal skills and slight increases in verbal ability with increasing age (e.g. Howlin et al., 2004).

Social functioning and independence in adult life

Throughout adult life, individuals with WS have high levels of behavioural and social problems that affect independence, self-help and daily living skills. As younger adults in their mid-20s, over two-thirds of individuals with WS remain highly dependent upon their families for support. Educational and employment attainments are low and external support networks are frequently inadequate (Davies et al., 1997; Howlin et al., 1998; Howlin & Udwin, 2006). By later adulthood (up to 50 years), some differences and improvements are observed (Elison et al., 2010). With regard to living arrangements, although older individuals are less likely to be still living with their parents, overall around

50% continue to do so, and over one-third of those aged 40 years or older remain living at home. Younger individuals are more likely to have attended mainstream schools than those now in their 40s to 60s, but employment levels remain very low, with only around 7-12% of adults with WS being in independent work.

Research also indicates that self-care skills are now somewhat better among younger individuals with WS (i.e. those in their 20s and 30s versus those in their 40s and 50s), with the majority of younger individuals being able to wash and dress themselves with minimal or no assistance and without regular reminders to carry out personal hygiene routines. Improvements in self-care skills tend to occur in the 20s and 30s, during which time there is a narrowing of the gap between cognitive functioning and daily living and socialisation skills (Elison et al., 2010; Howlin et al., 1998). Nevertheless, a small but significant proportion (3-24%) of adults with WS remains highly dependent upon others for assistance with basic self-care. This is particularly true for older individuals (those in their 40s and older). Between half and two-thirds of individuals with WS will continue to require some assistance in these areas throughout their adult lives and a small number will require almost constant supervision.

Overall, social functioning (the ability to make friends and the quality of friendships) shows similar patterns, with moderate improvements being reported over time. Nevertheless, very few individuals, of any age, are able to form close relationships and many are described as having significant problems making and maintaining friendships. Social disinhibition and lack of awareness of more subtle social rules are characteristic of individuals with WS (see Chapter 15) and remain a significant concern for the majority of parents and carers, many of whom are particularly worried about the risk of inappropriate, negative sexual experiences. In the adult study of Elison et al. (2010), approximately 16% of adults with WS had experienced some form of sexual assault, ranging in severity from being inappropriately touched by another person (9%) to rape (2%).

Behavioural problems also tend to show some improvements over time. The problems reported to cause most difficulties in daily life include distractibility, circumscribed interests, bossiness, attention seeking, stereotyped behaviours/rituals, inappropriate displays of annoyance (e.g. shouting, breaking things), overactivity and, occasionally, aggression towards others. Unusual and circumscribed interests and ritualistic behaviours often cause particular problems. Examples include taking apart electrical equipment such as televisions and radios, and obsessively collecting and hoarding objects such as holiday brochures and catalogues (Elison et al., 2010). Other common, although generally less disruptive, behaviours include excessive chatter, making inappropriate comments, and eating and sleeping difficulties. Areas that parents report as showing improvement over time include social and daily living skills and reductions in maladaptive behaviours such as temper tantrums and extreme anxiety (Elison et al., 2010).

Physical health during adult life

Much of the research on WS has focused on the associated physical complications, many of which arise from the elastin insufficiency caused by the genetic deletion on chromosome 7 (see Chapter 3). These include renal abnormalities, cardiovascular problems such as supravalvular aortic stenosis, hypertension (high blood pressure), gastrointestinal complications and urinary tract and joint problems (Pober & Morris, 2007; Chapter 4). In adulthood, parental/carer reports indicate that the predominant physical health problems are cardiovascular abnormalities, hypertension, kidney problems, bowel problems, scoliosis and joint problems such as pain and stiffness (Elison et al., 2010). Approximately half of adults with WS have dental problems such as malocclusion and cavities. Hypercalcaemia, although often a major symptom in childhood, is no longer a significant problem in adulthood and only 9% of individuals continue on a special diet for this as adults. Hyperacusis, which is reported very frequently (90%) during childhood in WS (Cunniff et al., 2001), is slightly less common for adults but remains a problem in the majority of individuals. Over 50% of adults in their 30s to 50s continue to experience health difficulties (cardiac, joint and bowel problems) that are characteristic of WS. Certain problems such as cardiovascular problems, hypertension and bowel problems are somewhat more frequent in older individuals (40-55 years) but there is no evidence of any significant age-related decline in health (Elison et al., 2010). Very detailed physical assessments (including magnetic resonance imaging investigations) have also confirmed high rates of weight disorders, sensorineural hearing loss, cardiovascular disease, hypertension, gastrointestinal symptoms, diabetes, subclinical hypothyroidism and deceased bone density (Cherniske et al., 2004; Chapter 4).

Mortality is high in adults with WS, with around 1-9 deaths per 100 people with WS aged 19-55 years (Elison et al., 2010). This compares with a death rate of 1.29 per 2000 among typically developing adults aged 25-34 years and of 2.46 per 2000 among those aged 35-44 years (Office of National Statistics, 2005). Reported causes of death for adults with WS include cardiovascular disease, non-Hodgkin lymphoma and septicaemia (Elison et al., 2010; Wessel et al., 2004). The risk of sudden death in adults with WS is estimated to be 25-100 times higher than that in the age-matched typically developing population (Wessel et al., 2004; Chapter 4).

Several of the physical characteristics noted in adults with WS (e.g. premature greying of hair, cataracts and hearing loss) might indicate accelerated ageing in WS (Cherniske et al., 2004). However, parental reports do not indicate any major deterioration in health, at least not between the ages of 19 and 55 years (Elison et al., 2010). Yet, despite regular contact with health professionals, only around half (55%) of families report satisfaction with the care their son/daughter receives. Even lower rates (25%) of family satisfaction are reported in reference to hospital consultations, often because of limited understanding of WS. Satisfaction with general practitioners, however, is higher (68%).

Concerns about inadequate medical care for individuals with WS in the USA resulted in the publishing of specific medical and clinical guidelines for monitoring and managing mental and physical health (Cunniff et al., 2001; Cherniske et al., 2004). In the UK, a clinical guideline for the management of physical and psychological issues of individuals with WS of all ages has been developed (Williams Syndrome Guideline Development Group, 2009), with the aim of providing up-to-date, UK-specific, evidence-based recommendations regarding their health needs.

Mental health during adult life

Although WS is typically associated with a range of positive behavioural characteristics such as friendliness and sociability, emotional and behavioural difficulties are common. These problems include inappropriate social behaviours (such as approaching strangers), preoccupations and obsessions, impulsivity and distractibility (Einfeld et al., 2001; Udwin et al., 1987). Particularly notable in WS are very high rates of anxiety, with up to 54% of individuals with WS reported as having anxiety of a severity that meets psychiatric diagnostic criteria (Cherniske et al., 2004; Dykens, 2003; Kennedy et al., 2006; Leyfer et al., 2006; Stinton et al., 2010). Although figures vary from study to study, the types of anxiety reported include specific phobias (35-54%), agoraphobia (24%), generalised anxiety disorder (12-24%), obsessive compulsive disorder (2-12%), separation anxiety (4-7%), post-traumatic stress disorder (0.8-5%), social phobia (1.7%) and panic disorder with/without agoraphobia (0.8-5%). The incidence of depression is reported as being around 10-14%, that of dysthymia lies at 10% and that of manic depression at 5%. Cases of attention deficit hyperactivity disorder (43-65%) and sexual impulse control disorders (5%) have also been reported (e.g. Cherniske et al., 2004).

Although mental health problems remain common during adulthood, the rates are typically lower than those reported in younger individuals. Research indicates that over a quarter (29%) of adults with WS meet the criteria for at least one psychiatric diagnosis (Stinton et al., 2010). As in children, the most common problems are anxiety-related; the incidence is 12% for specific phobia (e.g. storms, hospital, dentists, heights, wasps), 2% for social phobia and 1% for generalised anxiety disorder. A smaller number of anxiety-related disorders are more common in adults than in children with WS, particularly agoraphobia (4% in adults versus <1% in children) and panic disorder (3% for adults versus <1% for children). This seems to reflect the trajectory found in other people with intellectual disabilities, with rates of these types of problems twice as high in adults as in children (e.g. Cooper et al., 2007; Emerson, 2003). Other problems identified in adults with WS include depression (9%), hypomania (3%) and psychotic disorders such as schizophrenia (1-2%). Figure 5.1 shows the rates of mental health problems in adults with WS compared with those in other adults with intellectual disabilities (Cooper et al.,

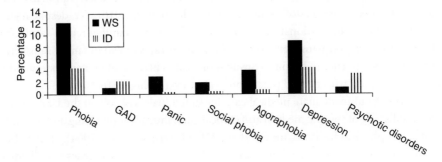

Fig. 5.1 (See also Plate 5) Mental health of adults with Williams syndrome versus adults with intellectual disabilities. Abbreviations: GAD = generalised anxiety disorder; ID = intellectual disabilities; WS = Williams syndrome.

2007; Moss et al., 2000; Stinton et al., 2010). A substantial proportion (10%) of adults with WS have more than one mental health problem—typically multiple anxiety disorders or anxiety disorders with depression.

Lower rates of some types of mental health problems among adults with WS compared with children may reflect age and family experience of anxiety over long periods of time. Thus, for some, stimuli that cause distress during childhood can become sources of interest during adulthood (e.g. fascinations with cleaning equipment such as vacuum cleaners and washing machines that had caused upset previously because of the noises that they made). In other cases, parents develop successful strategies of their own to reduce levels of anxiety, e.g. not giving too much advance warning about potentially worrying events or changes to regular routines. There is also evidence of the effectiveness of other treatment techniques for emotional and behavioural difficulties in WS. For example, functional analysis has shown that behavioural interventions (such as the use of ear plugs and modelling) can be effective in reducing pain and problem behaviours that occur in response to noise; behavioural strategies have also proved successful in treating food refusal (O'Reilly et al., 2000; O'Reilly & Lancioni, 2001). Further, cognitive behavioural intervention can improve awareness of behaviours and reduce ruminations and compulsions (Klein-Tasman & Albano, 2007).

The root causes of mental health problems in WS are unclear. Some promising results are reported in studies employing functional magnetic resonance imaging. In the typically developing population, individuals with specific phobias show increased amygdala activation in response to phobia-related stimuli. This increased activation is not seen in response to nonphobic stimuli or in controls who do not have specific phobias (Dilger et al., 2003). However, individuals with WS show increased amygdala reactivity, compared with typically developing controls, in response to threatening or fearful images (Muñoz et al., 2010). Almost without exception, other factors that have been demonstrated to be associated with mental health problems in other populations (e.g. age, degree of intellectual disability, family history of psychiatric disorders, negative life events and physical health) have, however, not been found to be significantly related to psychiatric morbidity in WS (Dodd & Porter, 2009; Kennedy et al., 2006; Stinton et al., 2010). This has led to suggestions that anxiety might be caused by or related to the specific WS genotype (Kennedy et al., 2006). However, not all individuals with WS experience high levels of anxiety and clearly such problems cannot be attributed to genetic factors alone. The cumulative effects of other social, environmental and individual factors (including personality type) that have been shown to be associated with mental health problems in other populations still require systematic study.

Provisions for adults with Williams syndrome

It is clear that the majority of individuals with WS will require support throughout their lives, particularly in relation to their physical and mental health, social functioning and independence. The need for health and social care services is evident (Elison et al., 2010; Stinton & Howlin, 2010). For example, in a typical 2-year period, adults with WS will visit their general practitioners seven times, although the range for individuals varies from 0 to 50 visits. Other commonly used services include dentistry, physiotherapy, hospital consultations and mental health services. A survey of parents/carers indicated that most (89%) were satisfied that the health and social care needs of the adults with WS were met. However, understanding of WS by professionals is variable, with around one-third of parents/carers reporting a generally good understanding among professionals, whereas others complain of poor or limited understanding of WS (Elison et al., 2010).

With regard to family support, Elison et al. (2010) found that although the majority (53%) of adults with WS continued to live with their parents, only one-third of families used respite care services. In general, this was because sufficient support was provided by family and friends or respite was not required because the adult with WS lived away from the parental home. However, a small proportion (10%) of families do not receive any respite care despite expressing a need for it. The majority of families who are in receipt of respite care are generally satisfied with this service, although dissatisfaction because of limited access (e.g. because of high demand and having to book in advance) or concerns about the standards of care in respite placements are issues for a minority of parents and carers (Elison et al., 2010).

In the UK, for the majority of adults with WS, daytime occupations consist of further education (25%) or voluntary employment (21%), with a small proportion (10%) having no occupation outside the home. Very few (6%) individuals are in paid full-time employment and typically jobs are low-skilled (e.g. gardening, stacking shelves in supermarkets) and poorly paid. For the majority of adults with WS, financial support is provided by families and via benefits, such as disability living allowance (78%), income support (56%) and housing benefit (13%). Satisfaction among families who received financial support was low, with fewer than half (48%) reporting that they were happy with the advice that they received from benefits agencies (Elison et al., 2010).

Parents/carers have proposed several ways in which they believe health and social care services could better meet the needs of adults with WS and support parents and carers (Stinton & Howlin, 2010). For example, the most common (46%) suggestion was for the professionals who come into contact with adults with WS to have more information about the syndrome, in particular in relation to common features such as anxiety and the discrepancy between verbal and other cognitive abilities. Other suggestions included: for parents to be provided with more feedback from clinical appointments; for financial assessors to understand that WS is a lifelong condition; for the person with WS to be listened to more; and for more information to be provided about healthy eating along with regular checks on weight.

In summary, although in some areas the longer-term outcomes are often positive and encouraging for individuals with WS and their families, there are considerable concerns with regard to the standards of health and social care available, particularly in terms of an understanding of WS among professionals. As a result of this, parents report a range of practical problems, such as difficulties claiming financial benefits, lack of specialist support in finding suitable employment and limited choice of residential placements. Other parental worries included accessing appropriate daytime activities. However, the most significant concern for parents/carers is in ensuring that adequate care provisions are in place for when they are no longer able to act as the primary carer because of their own age or health.

Improving outcomes for adults with Williams syndrome

Life expectancy for individuals with WS has increased dramatically over recent decades because of improvements in the recognition and early diagnosis of WS and the introduction of dietary and medical interventions that significantly reduce the effects of the physical abnormalities. However, knowledge about the particular educational and psychological profiles of these individuals and the provision of specialist programmes to meet their needs have lagged far behind medical interventions. Systematic studies of trajectories of development have an important role to play in improving the help and advice that is given to parents from the earliest years. For example, it is now evident that the sociability of individuals with WS, charming though this is in young children, can lead to difficulties from later childhood and adolescence when their indiscriminate approaches to other people can render them highly vulnerable. It is important for both parents and professionals to be aware of this and to ensure that basic 'keeping safe' rules are instilled as early as possible. Similarly, the special interests of some children can become increasingly pervasive and sometimes very disruptive as they grow older, and the early implementation of behavioural strategies to reduce the impact of such behaviours can help to avoid the later development of more serious problems.

Self-help and independence skills also tend to be out of keeping with cognitive levels, and consistent encouragement and support from parents, teachers and others to develop basic self-care and daily living skills, again from the earliest years, could help to reduce the disparity between skills in these areas.

The implications of recent psychological research for developing individually tailored teaching curricula for children with WS are becoming increasingly evident (Skwerer & Tager-Flusberg, 2011). However, it is doubtful whether many teachers of children with special needs are aware of this research or its importance for improving the learning and academic skills of individuals with WS. Thus, improving awareness of teachers about the specific profile of skills and deficits associated with WS is crucial for optimising educational progress.

Feedback from parents has also highlighted how lack of knowledge about the needs of individuals with WS continues throughout higher education, employment, and clinical, mental health and social services. Inadequate or inappropriate provision and intervention can have a profound effect on both people with WS and their families, often leading to an exacerbation of behavioural and emotional problems. Again, raising awareness of the very special needs of these individuals in professional and undergraduate training programmes is crucial.

Conclusion

Knowledge regarding adults with WS is at an early stage and an understanding of the longer-term needs of these individuals will become increasingly important to families, the individuals themselves and to health and social care services with whom they inevitable come into contact. Recent research has highlighted areas of promise in terms of cognitive and linguistic skills and some aspects of daily living skills. For example, unlike some other groups, such as individuals with DS or fragile X syndrome, most individuals with WS show stability and in some cases improvements in their abilities during adulthood. Moreover, some of the emotional and behavioural difficulties that are so common during childhood and adolescence tend to reduce somewhat during adulthood. While these areas show promise, problems such as physical and mental health difficulties do persist. Moreover, restricted opportunities in terms of occupation and accommodation coupled with generally poor skills in social functioning and independence remain a source of concern. Nevertheless, the fact that improvements are seen in some areas for adults with WS despite the absence of any specialist adult services indicates that further progress could be made if individuals were provided with better education, employment and social support than is available at present. In addition to improving the lives of individuals with WS, this additional assistance is likely to alleviate some of the concerns of parents about the future of their daughters and sons.

Editor commentary (Emily K. Farran & Annette Karmiloff-Smith)

This chapter discussed how physical and mental health, cognitive abilities and social skills, as well as environmental factors, impact the ability to integrate into society during adulthood in WS. The authors demonstrated that overall cognitive functioning does not change throughout adulthood in WS, a fact that stands in sharp contrast to many other syndromes, such as fragile X syndrome and DS, where premature cognitive decline is frequent. Nonetheless, even in WS decline varies across domains: short-term memory declines at a typical rate, whereas a premature decline is observed for episodic memory. The majority of individuals with WS live with their parents, with very few being in paid employment. Behavioural difficulties, such as socially inappropriate behaviour, preoccupations and obsessions, and mental health problems, such as anxiety, are common in WS. This highlights both cross-syndrome associations (e.g. obsessions are also a characteristic of autism) and dissociations. Mental health problems in WS are not related to family history of psychiatric disorders, negative life events and physical health, which implies a link to the WS genotype, although environmental factors such as parental strategies and behavioural intervention can have a positive effect.

The authors concluded by highlighting the fact that no syndrome is static, even in adulthood. This neuroconstructivist approach leads naturally to the idea that multidirectional interactions have the potential to improve outcomes, even in adulthood, in people with neurodevelopmental disorders through specialist programmes that take into account phenotypic differences as well as associations across syndrome groups. For example, although social difficulties are apparent in WS, DS and autism, intervention might concentrate on understanding facial communication cues in WS, subtle verbal communication cues in DS and social responsiveness in autism.

References

Ansari, D., Donlan, C., & Karmiloff-Smith, A. (2007). Typical and atypical development of visual estimation skills. *Cortex*, **43**, 758–68.

Arnold, R., Yule, W., & Martin, N. (1985). The psychological characteristics of infantile hypercalcemia - a preliminary investigation. *Developmental Medicine and Child Neurology*, **27**, 49–59.

Billstedt, E., Gillberg, C., & Gillberg, C. (2005). Autism after adolescence: population-based 13- to 22-year follow-up study of 120 individuals with autism diagnosed in childhood. *Journal of Autism and Developmental Disorders*, **35**, 351–60.

Brock, J., Jarrold, C., Farran, E.K., Laws, G., & Riby, D.M. (2007). Do children with Williams syndrome really have good vocabulary knowledge? Methods for comparing cognitive and linguistic abilities in developmental disorders. *Clinical Linguistics & Phonetics*, **21**, 673–88.

Carr, J. (2005). Stability and change in cognitive ability over the life span: a comparison of populations with and without Down syndrome. *Journal of Intellectual Disability Research*, **49**, 915–28.

Cherniske, E.M., Carpenter, T.O., Klaiman, C., Young, E., Bregman, J., Insogna, K., et al. (2004). Multisystem study of 20 older adults with Williams syndrome. *American Journal of Medical Genetics Part A*, **131A**, 255–64.

Cooper, S.A., Smiley, E., Morrison, J., Williamson, A., & Allan, L. (2007). Mental ill-health in adults with intellectual disabilities: prevalence and associated factors. *British Journal of Psychiatry*, **190**, 27–35.

Cunniff, C., Frias, J.L., Kaye, C.I., Moeschler, J., Panny, S.R., & Trotter, T.L. (2001). Health care supervision for children with Williams syndrome. *Pediatrics*, **107**, 1192–04.

Davies, M., Howlin, P., & Udwin, O. (1997). Independence and adaptive behavior in adults with Williams syndrome. *American Journal of Medical Genetics*, **70**, 188–95.

Devenny, D.A., Krinsky-McHale, S.J., Kittler, P.M., Flory, M., Jenkins, E., & Brown, W.T. (2004). Age associated memory changes in adults with Williams syndrome. *Neuropsychology*, **26**, 691–706.

Dilger, S., Straube, T., Mentzel, H.-J., Fitzek, C., Reichenbach, J., Hecht, H., et al. (2003). Brain activation to phobia-related pictures in spider phobic humans: an event-related functional magnetic resonance imaging study. *Neuroscience Letters*, **348**, 29–32.

Dodd, H.F., & Porter, M.A. (2009). Psychopathology in Williams syndrome: the effect of individual differences across the life span. *Journal of Mental Health Research in Intellectual Disabilities*, **2**, 89–109.

Dykens, E.M. (2003). Anxiety, fears, and phobias in persons with Williams syndrome. *Developmental Neuropsychology*, **23**, 291–316.

Eaves, L.C., & Ho, H.H. (2008). Young adult outcome of autism spectrum disorders. *Journal of Autism and Developmental Disorders*, **38**, 739–47.

Einfeld, S.L., Tonge, B.J., & Rees, V.W. (2001). Longitudinal course of behavioral and emotional problems in Williams syndrome. *American Journal on Mental Retardation*, **106**, 73–81.

Elison, E., Stinton, C., & Howlin, P. (2010). Health and social outcomes in adults with Williams syndrome: findings from cross-sectional and longitudinal cohorts. *Research in Developmental Disabilities*, **31**, 587–99.

Emerson, E. (2003). Prevalence of psychiatric disorders in children and adolescents with and without intellectual disability. *Journal of Intellectual Disability Research*, **47**, 51–58.

Farran, E.K., Jarrold, C., & Gathercole, S.E. (2003). Divided attention, selective attention and drawing: processing preferences in Williams syndrome are dependent on the task administered. *Neuropsychologia*, **41**, 696–87.

Fisch, G.S., Carpenter, N., Holden, J.J.A., Howard-Peebles, P.N., Maddalena, A., Borghgraef, M., et al. (1999). Longitudinal changes in cognitive and adaptive behavior in fragile X females: a prospective multicenter analysis. *American Journal of Medical Genetics*, **83**, 308–312.

Fisch, G.S., Simensen, R.J., & Schroer, R.J. (2002). Longitudinal changes in cognitive and adaptive Behavior scores in children and adolescents with the fragile X mutation or autism. *Journal of Autism and Developmental Disorders*, **32**, 107–114.

Henry, L.A. (1994). The relationship between speech rate and memory span in children. *International Journal of Behavioural Development*, **17**, 37–56.

Howlin, P. (1997). Prognosis in autism: do specialist treatments affect long term outcome. *European Child and Adolescent Psychiatry*, **6**, 55–72.

Howlin, P., Davies, M., & Udwin, O. (1998). Cognitive functioning in adults with Williams syndrome. *Journal of Child Psychology and Psychiatry*, **39**, 183–89.

Howlin, P., Elison, S., & Stinton, C. (2010). Cognitive, linguistic and adaptive functioning in Williams syndrome: trajectories from early to middle adulthood. *Journal of Applied Research in Intellectual disabilities*, **23**, 322–36.

Howlin, P., Goode, S., Hutton, J., & Rutter, M. (2004). Adult outcome for children with autism. *Journal of Child Psychology and Psychiatry*, **45**, 212–29.

Howlin, P., & Udwin, O. (2006). Outcome in adult life for people with Williams syndrome - results from a survey of 239 families. *Journal of Intellectual Disability Research*, **50**, 151–60.

Jarrold, C., Baddeley, A.D., & Hewes, A.K. (1998). Verbal and non-verbal abilities in the Williams syndrome phenotype: evidence for diverging developmental trajectories. *Journal of Child Psychology and Psychiatry*, **39**, 511–24.

Jarrold, C., Baddeley, A., Hewes, A., & Phillips, C. (2001). A longitudinal assessment of diverging verbal and non-verbal abilities in the Williams syndrome phenotype. *Cortex*, **37**, 423–31.

Kennedy, J.C., Kaye, D.L., & Sadler, L.S. (2006). Psychiatric diagnoses in patients with Williams syndrome and their families. *Jefferson Journal of Psychiatry*, **20**, 22–31.

Kittler, P., Krinsky-McHale, S.J., & Devenny, D.A. (2004). Sex differences in performance over 7 years on the Wechsler Intelligence Scale for Children - Revised among adults with intellectual disability. *Journal of Intellectual Disability Research*, **48**, 114–22.

Klein, B.P., & Mervis, C.B. (1999). Contrasting patterns of cognitive abilities of 9-and 10-year-olds with Williams syndrome or Down syndrome. *Developmental Neuropsychology*, **16**, 177–96.

Klein-Tasman, B.P., & Albano, A.M. (2007). Intensive, short-term cognitive behavioral treatment of OCD-like behavior with a young adult with Williams syndrome. *Clinical Case Studies*, **6**, 483–92.

Krinsky-McHale, S.J., Kittler, P., Brown, W.T., Jenkins, E.C., & Devenny, D.A. (2005). Repetition priming in adults with Williams syndrome: age-related dissociation between implicit and explicit memory. *American Journal on Mental Retardation*, **110**, 482–96.

Leyfer, O.T., Woodruff-Borden, J., Klein-Tasman, B.P., Fricke, J.S., & Mervis, C.B. (2006). Prevalence of psychiatric disorders in 4 to 16-year-olds with Williams syndrome. *American Journal of Medical Genetics Part B: Neuropsychiatric Genetics*, **141B**, 615–22.

Martens, M.A., Wilson, S.J., & Reutens, D.C. (2008). Williams syndrome: a critical review of the cognitive, behavioral, and neuroanatomical phenotype. *Journal of Child Psychology and Psychiatry and Allied Disciplines*, **49**, 576–608.

Maylor, E.A., Vousden, J.I., & Brown, G.D.A. (1999). Adult age differences in short-term memory for serial order: data and a model. *Psychology and Aging*, **14**, 572–94.

Mervis, C.B., Morris, C.A., Bertrand, J., & Robinson, B.F. (1999). Williams syndrome: findings from an integrated program of research. In H. Tager-Flusberg (Ed.), *Neurodevelopmental Disorders: Contributions to a New Framework from the Cognitive Neurosciences* (pp. 65–110). Cambridge, MA: MIT Press.

Moss, S., Emerson, E., Kiernan, C., Turner, S., Hatton, C., & Alborz, A. (2000). Psychiatric symptoms in adults with learning disability and challenging behaviour. *British Journal of Psychiatry*, **177**, 452–56.

Muñoz, K.E., Meyer-Lindenberg, A., Hariri, A.R., Mervis, C.B., Mattay, V.S., Morris, C.A., et al. (2010). Abnormalities in neural processing of emotional stimuli in Williams syndrome vary according to social vs. non-social content. *NeuroImage*, **50**, 340–46.

Office of National Statistics. (2005). *Deaths: Age and Sex, Numbers and Rates, 1976 Onwards (England and Wales): Population Trends* [dataset] <www.statistics.gov.uk/STATBASE/ssdataset. asp?vlnk=9552> accessed 11 July 2011.

O'Reilly, M.F., Lacey, C., & Lancioni, G.E. (2000). Assessment of the influence of background noise on escape-maintained problem behavior and pain behavior in a child with Williams syndrome. *Journal of Applied Behavior Analysis,* **33**, 511–14.

O'Reilly, M.F., & Lancioni, G.E. (2001). Treating food refusal in a child with Williams syndrome using the parent as therapist in the home setting. *Journal of Intellectual Disability Research*, **45**, 41–46.

Orellana, C., Bernabeu, J., Monfort, S., Rosello, M., Oltra, S., Ferrer, I.R., et al. (2008). Duplication of the Williams-Beuren critical region: case report and further delineation of the phenotypic spectrum. *Journal of Medical Genetics*, **45**, 187–89.

Paul, B.M., Stiles, J., Passaroti, A., Bavar, N., & Bellugi, U. (2002). Face and place processing in Williams syndrome: evidence for a dorsal-ventral dissociation. *Cognitive Neuroscience and Neuropsychology*, **13**, 1115–19.

Pober, B.R., & Morris, C.A. (2007). Diagnosis and management of medical problems in adults with Williams-Beuren syndrome. *American Journal of Medical Genetics Part C: Seminars in Medical Genetics*, **145C**, 280–90.

Searcy, Y.M., Lincoln, A.J., Rose, F.E., Klima, E.S., Bavar, N., & Korenberg, J.R. (2004). The relationship between age and IQ in adults with Williams syndrome. *American Journal on Mental Retardation*, **109**, 231–36.

Setter, J., Stojanovik, V., Van Ewijk, L., & Moreland, M. (2007). Affective prosody in children with Williams syndrome. *Clinical Linguistics and Phonetics*, **21**, 659–72.

Skwerer, D.P., & Tager-Flusberg, H. (2011). Williams syndrome. In P. Howlin, T. Charman & M. Ghaziuddin (Eds). *Handbook of Developmental Disorders* (pp. 97–98). London: Sage Publications.

Stinton, C., Elison, E., & Howlin, P. (2010). Mental health problems in adults with Williams syndrome. *American Journal on Intellectual and Developmental Disabilities*, **115**, 3–18.

Stinton, C., & Howlin, P. (2010). Adults with Williams syndrome: service use and parental satisfaction. *The Williams Syndrome Foundation Magazine*, **63**, 29.

Udwin, O., Davies, M., & Howlin, P. (1996). A longitudinal study of cognitive abilities and educational attainment in Williams syndrome. *Developmental Medicine and Child Neurology*, **38**, 1020–29.

Udwin, O., Yule, W., & Martin, N. (1987). Cognitive abilities and behavioral characteristics of children with idiopathic infantile hypercalcemia. *Journal of Child Psychology and Psychiatry and Allied Disciplines*, **28**, 297–309.

Vicari, S., Bates, E., Caselli, M.C., Pasqualetti, P., Gagliardi, C., Tonucci, F., et al. (2004). Neuropsychological profile of Italians with Williams syndrome: an example of a dissociation between language and cognition? *Journal of the International Neuropsychological Society*, **10**, 862–76.

Wessel, A., Gravenhorst, V., Buchhorn, R., Gosch, A., Partsch, C.J., Pankau, R. (2004). Risk of sudden death in the Williams-Beuren syndrome. *American Journal of Medical Genetics Part A*, **127A**, 234–37.

Williams, J.C., Lowe, J.B., & Barratt-Boyes, B.G. (1961). Supravalvular aortic stenosis. *Circulation*, **24**, 1311–18.

Williams Syndrome Guideline Development Group (2009). *Management of Williams Syndrome: a Clinical Guideline*. <http://www.dyscerne.org/dysc/digitalAssets/0/267_DRAFT_16_Dyscerne_website_FINAL. pdf> accessed 12 July 2011.

Wishart, J.G. (1993). The development of learning difficulties in children with downs syndrome. *Journal of Intellectual Disability Research*, **37**, 389–403.

Part 3

Domain-General Processes

Chapter 6

Attention

Kate Breckenridge, Janette Atkinson and
Oliver Braddick

Introduction

This chapter focuses on the analysis of developing processes of attention in early childhood, in the context of a model in which 'attention' comprises a number of distinct, but related, processes. In Chapter 13, a hypothesis on infants' increasing attentional abilities in the first year of life is put forward, linking early attentional systems with systems underpinning spatial cognition and actions. In this chapter, we consider the structure of attention beyond infancy, linking neurobiological subsystems to attentional ability for typically and atypically developing children. Firstly we briefly describe some of the theories of attention in typical development that have provided the basis for a model of development of attention throughout childhood and review existing data on how attention processes are affected in Williams syndrome (WS). We then describe a new test battery (the Early Childhood Attention Battery, or ECAB), based on this concept of multiple attention systems developed from neuropsychological and neuroimaging studies on adults. The ECAB was designed to extend research on the structure of the attention domain to younger (3-6 years) typically developing (TD) children than had hitherto been done, but also to provide a suitable tool for assessment of individuals with learning difficulties whose overall cognitive abilities and/or attentional capacities correspond to those seen in TD children aged 3-6 years. This enables analysis of attention in neurodevelopmental disorders within a neuroconstructivist framework involving cross-syndrome comparisons, consideration of the component functions of the attention domain and more extensive tracing of developmental trajectories, providing the means to give an individual profile for each child across different components of attention at different ages. Using the ECAB, we compare attentional disorders in WS and Down syndrome (DS). Finally, we attempt to summarise existing knowledge about attention within this framework.

Component subsystems of attention: typical development

To characterise the strengths and weaknesses of attention in WS and other neurodevelopmental disorders, the broad concept of attention needs to be analysed more specifically. It is widely accepted that attention and its underlying neural systems can be partitioned into subsystems. Atkinson and Braddick have proposed that infant subcortical attentional subsystems involving the superior colliculus underpin the attentional abilities of infants at birth; at a few months of post-term age, the cortex starts to function with cortical parieto-frontal networks underpinning switches of attention (Atkinson, 1984, 2000; Atkinson & Hood, 1997; Atkinson & Braddick, 2003; Chapter 13). In infants and children with brain abnormalities such as focal cortical lesions, inability to shift attention under competition (using the Fixation Shift paradigm) is a useful indicator of early attentional problems and can be used to predict future neural status in cognitive tasks (Atkinson et al., 1992; Hood & Atkinson, 1990; Braddick et al., 1992; Mercuri et al., 1996, 1997, 1999).

These early attentional cortical networks overlap strongly with networks controlling and planning visuocognitive spatial actions, which are considered to be part of the cortical dorsal stream. The theoretical concept of 'dorsal-stream vulnerability' is supported by data from studies of different neurodevelopmental disorders (genetically based or more environmentally based), showing correlations between attention deficits (in selective attention and executive function) and visual motion discrimination (dorsal stream) deficits in these children (see Braddick et al., 2003; Chapter 13).

Posner and Petersen (1990) proposed three specific subsystems of attention, based primarily on neuropsychological evidence from normal adults and patients with specific brain damage. They described an orienting subsystem, whose activity is reflected in spatial selective attention, a second subsystem for sustaining attention and a third system for top-down attentional control (or executive function). Fan et al. (2005) have provided neuroimaging evidence for distinct anatomical networks underlying these three systems. This work has provided a framework for subsequent models of attention based on these three subsystems.

A popular way to examine such models has been through patterns of performance across a range of attention tasks for the same individuals, using factor analysis to establish whether factor loadings support the proposed differentiation of attention functions. This approach has provided evidence for attentional subsystems in adults (e.g. Robertson et al., 1996; Mirsky et al., 1991). However, such a structure is the end point of a dynamic developmental process. Studies of attention in children are required to determine how valid this model might be across the lifespan and how the structure of subsystems emerges in development.

The measurement of individual elements of attention during childhood has been demonstrated in many studies, providing evidence for age-related improvements in selective attention (e.g. Trick & Enns, 1998; Scerif et al., 2004), in sustained attention (e.g. Levy, 1980; Aylward et al., 2002; Lin et al., 1999) and in the ability to switch attention flexibly between rules and inhibit prepotent responses (Gerstadt et al., 1994; Kirkham et al., 2003; Jones et al., 2003; Jacques & Zelazo, 2001). Indeed, some authors have gone on to demonstrate differences in developmental trajectories between different attention functions (e.g. McKay et al., 1994; Rueda et al., 2004; Kelly, 2000), supporting the notion of developmental differentiation between different domains of attention. Fewer studies, however, have directly approached the issue of separable attention functions via factor analysis, perhaps because of the inherent challenge of performing numerous tests with young children.

Attempts to investigate the hypothesis of separable, identifiable attention functions in school-age children include the work of Mirsky et al. (1991), Kelly (2000) and Manly et al. (2001). These studies have all used data sets from TD school-age children and provided support for an attention system in which distinct functions of selective/focused attention, sustained attention and executive aspects of attention could be identified. Although there are some inconsistencies, these studies provided support for attention as a multidimensional construct even in childhood. However, it is well known that considerable development of executive functions occurs during the early childhood/preschool years, and equivalent data for populations younger than 6 years were not available until the development of a new battery of attention tests, the ECAB.

The Early Childhood Attention Battery

The requirement to understand relatively complex tasks and the relatively long testing duration make test batteries such as the Test of Everyday Attention for Children (TEA-Ch; developed and used by Manly et al., 1999, 2001, in their factor analysis study) and other standardised tests of attention inappropriate for most children under 6 years, or indeed for children who are below this mental age by reason of neurodevelopmental delays.

The lack of standardised measures for investigating the different components of attention across the preschool age range and in neurodevelopmental disorders prompted the development of a new battery, the ECAB (Breckenridge, 2007; Breckenridge et al., submitted b), designed to be used for children with mental ages between 3 and 6 years. The ECAB is based on a variety of attention tests from the adult literature and from standardised tests for older children, such as the TEA-Ch, selected and simplified to be appropriate for the younger age group. From extensive piloting of a range of tests in a group of over 140 TD children aged between 2.5 and 6 years, eight measures were selected that corresponded as closely as possible to the tests of proven use with older children while maximising developmental sensitivity and age-appropriateness and minimizing nonattentional confounding variables. Table 6.1 lists these component subtests. Their value in providing an extension of existing measures to younger ages was supported by a strong correlation with TEA-Ch

Table 6.1 Component subtests of the Early Childhood Attention Battery and their proposed attentional underpinnings

Subtest	Attention component tested	Task requirements
Visual search	Selective attention	Identify target items from an array
Flanker task	Selective attention	Respond selectively to a central item, ignoring distractors
Visual sustained	Sustained attention	Maintain attention on visual stimuli to identify rare targets (5 minutes duration)
Auditory sustained	Sustained attention	Maintain attention on auditory stimuli to identify rare targets (5 minutes duration)
Dual sustained	Sustained attention	Monitor both visual and auditory stimuli to detect targets (2.5 minutes duration)
Verbal opposites	Attentional control	Respond to cat and dog pictures by giving the incorrect names
Counterpointing	Attentional control	Point to the opposite side of screen to where a target appears
Balloon sorting	Attentional control	Sort balloons according to changing rules (e.g. colour, shape)

scores in a subgroup of 19 children (aged 6 years 1 month to 7 years 1 month) who were tested with the TEA-Ch 7-15 months after their ECAB test.

Data from 154 TD children aged 3-6 years on the ECAB battery were examined using exploratory factor analysis to determine latent constructs underlying performance on the ECAB subtests. For the group as a whole, only two factors were apparent in the data, broadly reflecting sustained attention and selective response control. However, there was evidence for increasing differentiation of attention functions across this age range. Data from the younger children (aged 3-4.5 years) suggested two factors with substantial overlap between them, whereas data from the older children (4.5-6 years) suggested three factors very similar to those identified in adults and older children, corresponding to selective attention, sustained attention and executive control. There may be two alternative accounts of this developmental trajectory: either there is a genuine differentiation of some of the brain systems of attention with age or performance in the younger group is constrained by some overall limitation (e.g. memory, basic processing speed) that masks the contributions of distinct subsystems even if these are already present.

A major aim of this work on typical development was to provide a better framework for the understanding of atypical development of attention. This has been strongly influenced by the neuroconstructivist approach (see, for example, Karmiloff-Smith, 1998; Scerif & Karmiloff-Smith, 2005), which argues against identifying 'impaired' and 'intact' modules in neurodevelopmental disorders, pointing out that mature cognitive outcomes are the result of a dynamic developmental process. This approach implies a number of key considerations. First, even for scores in the normal range, children with neurodevelopmental disorders may achieve this performance through an atypical cognitive process. Second, performance in neurodevelopmental disorders is typically compared with controls matched on some measure of developmental age, meaning that even 'intact' functions are substantially impaired relative to chronological age. In either case, describing a function as 'intact' presents something of an inaccurate picture. Also, patterns of performance at one stage of development might not reflect the cognitive profile at an earlier or later stage. For example, levels of performance in a particular domain may be 'normal' in infancy but show a delay later in development. This highlights the need to trace the trajectories of functions in neurodevelopmental disorders, starting as early as possible. Such data will clarify whether patterns in neurodevelopmental disorders simply represent delay or whether they represent more complex deviations from the typical trajectory. Further, cognitive domains will need to be analysed in their component parts in order to map functional profiles of particular groups. Cross-syndrome comparisons of these profiles and trajectories are then needed to assess the specificity of an atypical profile.

Attention in Williams syndrome and other neurodevelopmental disorders

Some of the characteristics reported for children with WS, particularly in terms of the control of attention, resemble those described for adult patients with frontal-lobe lesions, including distractibility, impulsivity and difficulty in grasping the global aspects of a complex task or situation and in mastering new tasks. The frontal lobes in adults have been considered as a complex network of systems involved in the executive control of behaviour, including spatial planning, working memory, maintaining attention on the task in hand, cognitive flexibility in switching between tasks when necessary and inhibiting well-learnt responses that are inappropriate to the present situation (see, for example, Duncan et al., 1996; Goldman-Rakic, 1996; Robbins, 1996). These functions embrace the component of 'attentional control', one of the three components within the framework outlined earlier in this chapter. In this section, we give an overview of evidence on the three areas of attention in WS before turning in the subsequent section to recent data from an ECAB study that aimed to provide a direct comparison of the three.

Selective attention

A basic aspect of attentional processing, investigated in a number of WS studies, is selective spatial attention, which involves identifying, maintaining and switching the focus of processing between spatial locations. Control of selective attention can be determined either by an external sensory event ('exogenous attention') or by internally specified goals ('endogenous attention'). A simple aspect of this function is discussed in detail in Chapter 13, namely the control of the subcortical fixation reflex by cortical systems that allow disengagement from the current target and the transfer of attention to a competing target (Schiller, 1985). Young (under 6 years) children with WS show a deficit in this area, with fixation shifts under competition showing very long latencies compared with controls (Atkinson et al., 2003).

Studies by Brown et al. (2003) and Cornish et al. (2007) provide other examples suggesting early difficulties for children with WS in the selection of targets for visual attention. Visual search tasks provide a case where endogenous and exogenous controls of selective attention need to interact. Targets are typically specified by some sensory properties (e.g. size, colour), but the ability to find them efficiently depends on an endogenous strategy of moving the focus of attention systematically around the array. Difficulties of selective attention have been observed with toddlers with WS in a visual search task (Scerif et al., 2004), in which they made significantly more errors than matched controls. Specifically, errors tended to be erroneous responses to distractors, rather than repetitions on found targets, suggesting a problem with limiting selection and response to targets. There was an interesting contrast with children with fragile X syndrome, who made more perseveration errors on found targets, indicating that in this condition, performance is limited by a problem with inhibitory control.

Attentional control processes

If the ability to process incoming information is to be effectively deployed to meet relevant behavioural goals, it must be subject to top-down control. The inhibition of normally prepotent responses to allow a specific task to proceed is a general feature of the role of executive control processes based on the frontal lobe (see also Chapter 9). The simple example mentioned earlier (i.e. disengaging attention in order to shift fixation) uses the frontal eye fields rather than the prefrontal systems involved in more sophisticated behavioural control. A more advanced form of inhibitory control has been examined via the pointing/counterpointing task (Atkinson et al., 2003). This is an adaptation of the antisaccade task (e.g. Pierrot-Deseilligny et al., 1991), in which following the appearance of a central target, a target appears in a lateral position to the left or right. In the pointing task, the participants simply have to point to the appearing target as rapidly as they can; in the counterpointing task, they are required to point to the blank side of the screen opposite the newly appearing target. Children with WS aged over 4 years showed severe difficulties with this task, both in latencies and error rates (Atkinson et al., 2003), indicating poor inhibitory control in WS. The counterpointing task has been adapted as a component of the ECAB battery with similar results (see later in this chapter).

In the work reported in Atkinson et al. (2003), we tested the abilities of a large cohort of children with WS on a number of other tasks requiring the inhibitory control of prepotent responses. In the day/night task (Gerstadt et al., 1994), the response is verbal: the participant has to name a daylight scene, showing a sun, as 'night' and a night sky scene, showing a moon, as 'day'. Participants with WS performed relatively well on this task, in line with or often better than their overall verbal mental age. By contrast, in the detour box task (Hughes & Russell, 1993; Biro & Russell, 2001), the same group showed a marked deficit, whether considered in terms of chronological age or of verbal developmental age. This test requires the child to inhibit direct reaching for a ball and instead to retrieve it by an indirect operation. The WS group showed a progressive mastery of the task with increasing verbal developmental age (assessed through the British Picture Vocabulary Scale; Dunn et al., 1997), but this occurred with a sharp improvement at a developmental equivalent age of around 7 years rather than at 3.5 years as seen in typical development.

Overall, these results showed that children with WS have deficits in executive control processes, and the intercorrelations between the three tests (day-night, detour box and counterpointing) indicated a general 'frontal' factor in individuals' scores, even when the overall level of cognitive development indexed by the British Picture Vocabulary Scale was partialled out. However, the more striking result is the variation between tasks: a severe difficulty in inhibiting a prepotent response in spatial/motor domains (counterpointing and detour box) contrasting with the near-normal ability to inhibit a verbal response (day-night). Further evidence for such dissociation will also be reported later in this chapter from our results with the ECAB battery. A neuroimaging study (Mobbs et al., 2007) has shown that frontostriatal systems are underactivated by a response inhibition (go/no-go) task in WS compared with controls, but the test used did not differentiate between spatial and nonspatial inhibitory control. Interestingly, there has been some suggestion that children with DS also show a dissociation between different types of executive-function task, but that their deficits emerge primarily on tasks using verbal materials rather than visuospatial materials (Nadel, 2003). This would be consistent with deficits of control emerging out of interactions of executive control systems with task domains of relative difficulty.

Chapter 13 of this book discusses in more detail the processing of spatial and visuomotor information in WS and describes evidence for specific deficits in 'dorsal cortical stream' processing (i.e. processing for action control and the understanding of spatial relationships). The dorsal-stream problems in WS, it seems, are not only manifested in the spatial and visual processing mechanisms within the posterior brain (occipital and parietal lobes) but also in the processing of spatial information by frontal control systems. There is some evidence that segregated subsystems within the prefrontal cortex are involved in the control of spatial and nonspatial behaviours (Goldman-Rakic, 1996), although this is controversial (Owen et al., 1998). The pattern of deficit in WS may reflect either a deficit in the information transmitted to such systems, or differential processing capacities within them (perhaps as a developmental consequence of limited or disorganised input to them).

We should note that another important function intimately linked to executive control is working memory, which is needed to guide planned behavioural sequences and which is also a function of prefrontal cortex. This will not be further explored here, however, because a review of working memory processes in WS can be found in Chapter 8.

Sustained attention and cross-task/cross-syndrome comparisons

In their study on disengagement deficits in WS infants, Brown et al. (2003) observed that WS infants were no different from control infants in terms of sustained attention (measured by periods of interaction with toys). By contrast, infants with DS showed difficulties both with shifting fixation and with sustaining attention. Apart from this study, there is little other evidence on sustained attention in WS, although studies are beginning to draw together evidence from across the attention domain using cross-syndrome comparisons (see Chapter 18).

Cornish et al. (2007) have presented a collection of previously published and novel results, focusing on the development of aspects of attention in children with WS, DS and fragile X syndrome. In their first study, the authors compared orienting and inhibition processes in infants and toddlers with fragile X syndrome and WS, using a visual cuing paradigm. Whereas the fragile X syndrome children showed greatest difficulty in inhibiting saccades to a cue, the children with WS showed a pattern that seemed to reflect difficulty in disengaging attention, consistent with previous findings. The second study extended the results of Scerif et al.'s (2004) visual search experiment to include children with DS. In fact, the children with DS showed no difference in performance from MA-matched controls (the differences seen in WS and fragile X syndrome have already been described). The final study (Wilding et al., 2001) investigated attention performance in older children with DS and fragile X syndrome, using the map search and walk/don't walk tasks from the TEA-Ch and the sustained attention measure from the Wilding Attention Test for Children (Wilding et al., 2001). On the sustained attention measure, neither group was different from matched controls, but the DS group showed poorer performance on the selective attention measure, whereas the fragile X syndrome group performed worse on the executive control measure. Individuals with WS were not included in this study; however, before developing the ECAB, we examined performance of a small group of children with WS in this age range on tests from the TEA-Ch (Breckenridge, 2007). Results suggested impairments relative to mental age in selective attention, sustained attention and visuospatial inhibition tasks, but not verbal inhibition. However, this study raised issues regarding the impact of the nonattentional demands in some of these tests (particularly counting, a component of the sustained attention task), and so the full extent of impairments of attention performance in older children with WS remains to be determined.

Interestingly, Cornish et al. (2007) also compared children with different neurodevelopmental disorders in terms of correlations of task performance with age and found evidence for differing developmental trajectories that were syndrome-specific. This research highlights the interesting possibility that areas of particular impairment may alter over the course of development. For example, for children with DS, selective attention performance was comparable with that of MA-matched controls in toddlerhood but was significantly poorer than that of controls in mid–late childhood.

Careful consideration of the different component functions of the attention domain and of how these change over development has begun to provide a picture of how attention is affected in neurodevelopmental disorders. The next section in this chapter explores a significant new body of data from a study using the ECAB, which fills in some of the gaps in this picture, particularly in terms of the WS population.

Components of attention in children with Williams and Down syndrome assessed using the Early Childhood Attention Battery

The ECAB can provide comparative measures for WS and DS that are developmentally appropriate for children aged 5-15 years with these conditions while also enabling comparisons across component functions of the attention domain. Previous reports have suggested considerable attention problems in both of these groups. As well as the experimental studies briefly reviewed in the previous section (e.g. Atkinson et al., 2003; Brown et al., 2003; Cornish et al., 2007; Nadel, 2003; Scerif et al., 2004), children with WS or DS are frequently reported by parents and teachers to be more inattentive, distractible and hyperactive than TD peers (e.g. Greer et al., 1997; Pagon et al., 1987; Pueschel, 1990; Cuskelly & Dadds, 1992).

We have used the ECAB in a comparative study of 32 children with WS and 32 children with DS, matched overall in terms of mental age (MA) on selected subtests of the Wechsler Preschool and Primary Scale of Intelligence (WPPSI; Wechsler, 1989) and in terms of chronological age (see Table 6.2) (Breckenridge et al., submitted a). For each child, mental age was also used to derive age-scaled scores on each of the ECAB subtests, so that performance could be compared across groups and different aspects of attention. Figure 6.1 shows a plot of these age-scaled scores, in which a score of 10 indicates the expected mean score based on mental age.

The data in Figure 6.1 show that for both groups, overall scores were slightly below the norm of 10 (i.e. these attention functions show somewhat more impairment than expected from the overall cognitive level reflected in the WPPSI). Sustained attention was a relative strength for both groups, with performance at or above MA level on all subtests designed to measure this function. Auditory sustained attention was a particular strength for the DS group, with performance significantly better than in the WS group and better than

Table 6.2 Distribution of chronological and mental ages[a] of children included in the Early Childhood Attention Battery attention study (Breckenridge et al., submitted a)

Group	Chronological age		Mental age	
	Mean (years)	Range (years:months)	Mean (years)	Range (years:months)
Williams syndrome	8.45	5:0–15:11	4.89	3:10–5:11
Down syndrome	9.76	5:01–14: 07	4.51	3:01–5:11

[a] According to performance on selected subtests from the Wechsler Preschool and Primary Scale of Intelligence–Information, Block Design, Vocabulary and Picture Completion.

expected for their mental age. Although this will still generally represent a delay relative to chronological age, it was an area of particular proficiency relative to other skills. Relative strengths are arguably as important in understanding neurodevelopmental disorders as areas of relative impairment, and this result suggests that simple sustained attention is not particularly problematic in WS (at least relative to MA) and indeed may be a strength in DS. It is interesting that auditory sustained attention was somewhat better than visual sustained attention. One possible explanation is that maintaining visual attention requires the participant to fix attention on a particular spatial location; this control was apparently

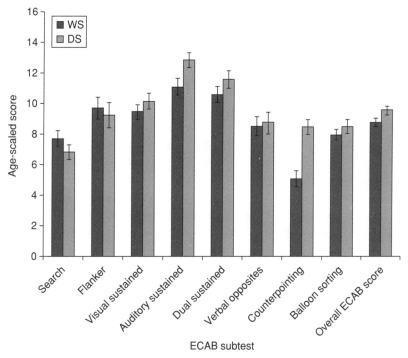

Fig. 6.1 Scores of Williams syndrome and Down syndrome groups (n=32 in each group) on individual subtests of the Early Childhood Attention Battery (ECAB). The overall score across subtests is shown in the far right column. The scores are scaled for mental age norms so that a score of 10 represents the expected mean score for a given mental age. The error bars show the standard error of the mean. Data from Breckenridge et al. (submitted a).

a potential problem for both groups and may be an aspect that relates to dorsal-stream deficits.

The visual search, counterpointing and balloon sorting tasks were significantly below MA level for both groups, as was the verbal opposites task for the WS group only. Visuospatial response control in the counterpointing task was a particular weakness for the WS group, consistent with the earlier findings of Atkinson et al. (2003), with performance being significantly worse than in the DS group. Both groups also showed significant deficits on the set-shifting task (Balloon Sorting), indicating problems of perseveration, consistent with impairments on the Wisconsin Card Sorting Task in adults with DS (Cornish et al., 2001).

Conclusions

One aim with the ECAB study was to provide information to further inform the growing picture of the developmental course of attention profiles in WS (and DS). In relating our findings to existing data, some developmental changes are apparent. The only infant data available on sustained attention in these two groups (Brown et al., 2003) showed deficits relative to MA-matched controls in DS but not in WS. It seems that by school age, both groups show sustained attention scores at or above MA level. It may well be the case that deficits may emerge on more complex tests of sustained attention, but basic vigilance skills at least seem to be relatively proficient at this stage of development. In the selective attention domain, when toddlers with WS and DS were compared directly on a visual search task (Cornish et al., 2007), the results again suggested deficits relative to MA in WS but not in DS. By contrast, by school age both groups in the ECAB study were showing performance below MA level on a visual search task. Interestingly, performance on the flanker task (another measure designed to assess selective focusing of attention) was at MA level for both groups, suggesting that selective attention impairments may be specific to situations where selection from a crowded array is required. Differences of this kind between tasks purporting to measure the same aspect of a domain suggest that even finer distinctions may be necessary to fully understand the profiles of functioning in neurodevelopmental disorders and to provide appropriate suggestions for intervention.

In Table 6.3, we have attempted to summarise existing data on attention in WS and DS across the lifespan. Of course, this summary may not be exhaustive and it contains studies that will not be directly comparable in terms of all relevant factors (e.g. selection criteria, sample sizes, mental age matching procedure). However it serves to broadly illustrate developmental trajectories in these domains. This summary also highlights areas where no data are yet available and where future research is required. For example, more formal studies comparing different attention functions in adolescents and adults with WS are needed to determine an end point for the developmental process in this group. However, some interesting patterns are apparent from areas where adequate data are available. Across infancy and childhood in WS, studies consistently show problems with selective attention and particular deficits in visuospatial control, even relative to mental age and on tasks that control for impairments in general processing abilities in the visuospatial

Table 6.3 Summary of the results from existing studies of attention in Williams syndrome and Down syndrome from infancy to adulthood

Phase of life	Attention function	Type of task	Performance[a]	
			WS	**DS**
Infancy/toddlerhood	Selective	Orienting/disengagement[1–3]	↓	=
	Sustained	Visual search[2,4]	↓	=
	Control	During play[3]	=	↓
			?	?
Early childhood	Selective	Visual search[5–6]	↓	↓
	Sustained	Flanker task[5]	=	=
	Control	Vigilance: visual[5]	=	=
		Auditory[5]	=	↑
		Dual-modality[5]	=	↑
		Inhibition: visuospatial[1,5]	↓	↓
		Verbal[1,5,7]	=	=
		Set-shifting[5,8]	↓	↓
Late childhood/ adolescence	Selective	Visual search[4,5,9]	↓	↓
	Sustained	Counting task[5]	↓	?
	Control	Vigilance task[4,9]	?	=
		Inhibition: visuospatial[4,5,9]	↓	=
		Verbal[5,9]	=	↓
Adulthood	Selective	Visual search[10]	?	↓
	Sustained	Counting task[10]	?	↓
	Control	Set-shifting (WCST)[10]	?	↓

Abbreviations: DS = Down syndrome; WCST = Wisconsin Card Sorting Task; WS = Williams syndrome.

[a] Upward-pointing arrows represent areas of improved performance relative to typically developing controls; equals signs represent performance equivalent to that of typically developing controls; downward-pointing arrows represent areas of poorer performance relative to typically developing controls; areas where no data are yet available are indicated with question marks.

Sources: [1] Atkinson et al., 2003; [2] Scerif et al., 2004; [3] Brown et al., 2003; [4] Cornish et al., 2007; [5] Breckenridge et al., submitted b; [6] Montfoort, et al. 2007; [7] Nadel, 2003; [8] Rowe, et al. 2006; [9] Munir et al., 2000; [10] Cornish, et al. 2001.

domain. By contrast, basic vigilance skills seem to be more in line with the overall level of developmental delay. In Chapter 13, we consider how events might interact in development in WS, particularly in terms of the possible consequences of disordered processing in the dorsal cortical stream. As we begin to build a picture of the profile of attention in WS and of how that profile might emerge and change over the course of development, we must consider how best this knowledge might be applied to the process of intervention and support for individuals with WS.

In summary, attention is a key area of cognitive competence that can be broadly defined as the ability to control our cognitive processing. However, neuropsychology, neuroimaging and psychometric analysis concur that it is not a unitary area; it has distinct subcomponents including the ability to select the current object of processing, the ability to maintain sustained processing for a specific goal and the executive ability to relate behaviour to current goals, ignore distractions, switch tasks when necessary and inhibit prepotent but irrelevant responses. These abilities, particularly the last, are closely connected to the broader concept of fluid intelligence (Duncan et al., 1996; Duncan, 2010). However, in individuals they can be assessed independently of general intelligence testing; our results and others show that in neurodevelopmental disorders, deficits may be revealed beyond those anticipated from the individual's overall mental age. These patterns of deficit are to some extent specific to particular syndromes and are linked to aspects of the cognitive profile outside the attentional domain (e.g. differential competence with linguistic versus spatial information). To understand the developmental trajectories of different syndromes and, ultimately, to relate these to the genetics and neurobiology of each disorder, it will be important to extend the data summarised in Table 6.3 and in our own work reported in this chapter, in particular to define further the age trajectories of the distinct aspects of attention. It is our hope that the ECAB tests we have described here will prove a valuable tool for this purpose, giving profiles for individual children. As well as promoting scientific understanding, the goal of such work should be to help individuals by characterising their patterns of strengths and deficits in greater detail. Such insights should aid devising programmes of rehabilitation and support that reflect these insights.

Editor commentary (Emily K. Farran & Annette Karmiloff-Smith)

Attention is one of the few cognitive systems that have been studied from infancy through stages of childhood and into adulthood in individuals with neurodevelopmental disorders. To this end, it provides an exemplary picture of the importance of the neuroconstructivist approach. In typical adults, three attentional subsystems (orienting attention, sustained attention, attentional control) have been identified at the behavioural level and subsequently linked to separable neural activation. The chapter showed that just two attentional subsystems are present in typical development at 3-4 years and that the three-component system of attention progressively emerges over the period from 4 years to 6 years. This exemplifies the neuroconstructivist stance that the adult end state is a product of gradual neurodevelopmental specialisation. Cross-syndrome comparisons illustrate how different neurodevelopmental disorders exhibit differing, atypical developmental trajectories of attention. For example, toddlers and young children with WS show deficits in selective attention and executive control but not in sustained attention. By contrast, we observe a deficit in DS in sustained attention and executive control but not selective attention. Yet, a different pattern emerges in the school-age years, and by adulthood, a fractionation emerges in WS between stronger performance on executive attention tasks that draw on verbal processing than on those tasks that draw on visuospatial processing, with the opposite profile obtained in DS. This chapter therefore provided a clear illustration of developmental specialisation of the brain in both typical and atypical development and represents an essential reference for a deeper understanding of any neurodevelopmental disorder, particularly those where atypical attentional mechanisms are reported such as attention deficit hyperactivity disorder, autism and fragile X syndrome. This chapter also serves as a preface to the discussions in Chapters 13 and 18 regarding the impact of attentional processing on the development of many domain-specific processes.

References

Atkinson, J. (1984). Human visual development over the first six months of life. A review and a hypothesis. *Human Neurobiology*, **3**, 61–74.

Atkinson, J. (2000). *The Developing Visual Brain*. Oxford: Oxford University Press.

Atkinson, J., & Braddick, O. (2003). Neurobiological models of normal and abnormal visual development. In M. De Haan & M.H. Johnson (Eds) *The Cognitive Neuroscience of Development* (pp. 43–71). Hove, Sussex: Psychology Press.

Atkinson, J., Braddick, O., Anker, S., Curran, W., & Andrew, R. (2003). Neurobiological models of visuospatial cognition in children with Williams syndrome: measures of dorsal-stream and frontal function. *Developmental Neuropsychology*, **23**, 141–74.

Atkinson, J., & Hood, B. (1997). Development of visual attention. In J.A. Burack & J.T. Enns (Eds), *Attention, Development, and Psychopathology* (pp. 31–54). New York, NY: Guildford Press.

Atkinson, J., Hood, B., Wattam-Bell, J. & Braddick, O.J. (1992). Changes in infants' ability to switch visual attention in the first three months of life. *Perception*, **21**, 643–53.

Aylward, G.P., Brager, P., & Harper, D.C. (2002). Relations between visual and auditory continuous performance tests in a clinical population: a descriptive study. *Developmental Neuropsychology*, **21**, 285–303.

Biro, S., & Russell, J. (2001). The execution of arbitrary procedures by children with autism. *Development and Psychopathology*, **13**, 97–110.

Braddick, O., Atkinson, J., Hood, B., Harkness, W., Jackson, G., & Vargha-Khadem, F. (1992). Possible blindsight in infants lacking one cerebral hemisphere. *Nature*, **360**, 461–63.

Braddick, O., Atkinson, J., & Wattam-Bell, J. (2003). Normal and anomalous development of visual motion processing: motion coherence and 'dorsal stream vulnerability'. *Neuropsychologia*, **41**, 1769–84.

Breckenridge, K. (2007). *The Structure and Function of Attention in Typical and Atypical Development*. PhD thesis, University of London.

Breckenridge, K., Braddick, O., Anker, S., Woodhouse, M., & Atkinson, J. (submitted a). Attention in Williams syndrome and Down's syndrome: performance on the new Early Childhood Attention Battery (ECAB).

Breckenridge, K., Braddick, O., Atkinson, J. (submitted b). The organisation of attention in typical development: a new preschool attention test battery.

Brown, J.H., Johnson, M.H., Paterson, S.J., Gilmore, R., Longhi, E., & Karmiloff-Smith, A. (2003). Spatial representation and attention in toddlers with Williams syndrome and Down syndrome. *Neuropsychologia*, **41**, 1037–46.

Cornish, K., Munir, F., & Wilding, J. (2001). A neuropsychological and behavioural profile of attention deficits in fragile X syndrome. *Revista de Neurologia*, **33**, S24–29.

Cornish, K., Scerif, G., & Karmiloff-Smith, A. (2007). Tracing syndrome-specific trajectories of attention across the lifespan. *Cortex*, **43**, 672–85.

Cuskelly, M. & Dadds, M. (1992). Behavioral problems in children with Down's syndrome and their siblings. *Journal of Child Psychology and Psychiatry*, **33**, 749–61.

Dunn, L.M., Dunn, L.M., Whetton, C., & Burley, J. (1997). *British Picture Vocabulary Scale Second Edition*. Windsor: NFER-Nelson.

Duncan, J. (2010). The multiple-demand (MD) system of the primate brain: mental programs for intelligent behaviour. *Trends in Cognitive Science*, **14**, 172–9.

Duncan, J., Emslie, H., Williams, P., Johnson, R., & Freer, C. (1996). Intelligence and the frontal lobe: the organization of goal-directed behavior. *Cognitive Psychology*, **30**, 257–303.

Fan, J., McCandliss, B.D., Fossella, J., Flombaum, J.I., & Posner, M.I. (2005). The activation of attentional networks. *NeuroImage*, **26**, 471–79.

Gerstadt, C.L., Hong, Y.J. & Diamond, A. (1994). The relationship between cognition and action: performance of children 3 1/2 - 7 years old on a Stroop-like day-night test. *Cognition*, **53**, 129–53.

Goldman-Rakic, P.S. (1996). The prefrontal landscape: implications of functional architecture for understanding human mentation and the central executive. *Philosophical Transactions of the Royal Society of London B*, **351**, 1445–53.

Greer, M.K., Brown, F.R., Pai, G.S., Choudry, S.H., & Klein, A.J. (1997). Cognitive, adaptive, and behavioral characteristics of Williams syndrome. *American Journal of Medical Genetics*, **74**, 521–25.

Hood, B., & Atkinson, J. (1990). Sensory visual loss and cognitive deficits in the selective attentional system of normal infants and neurologically impaired children. *Developmental Medicine and Child Neurology*, **32**, 1067–77.

Hughes, C., & Russell, J. (1993). Autistic children's difficulty with mental disengagement from an object: its implications for theories of autism. *Developmental Psychology*, **29**, 498–510.

Jacques, S., & Zelazo, P.D. (2001). The Flexible Item Selection Task (FIST): a measure of executive function in preschoolers. *Developmental Neuropsychology*, **20**, 573–91.

Jones, B.L., Rothbart, M.K., & Posner, M.I. (2003). Development of executive attention in preschool children. *Developmental Science*, **6**, 498–504.

Karmiloff-Smith, A. (1998). Development itself is the key to understanding developmental disorders. *Trends in Cognitive Sciences,* **2**, 389–98.

Kelly, T.P. (2000). The clinical neuropsychology of attention in school-aged children. *Child Neuropsychology*, **6**, 24–36.

Kirkham, N.Z., Cruess, L., & Diamond, A. (2003). Helping children apply their knowledge to their behavior on a dimension-switching task. *Developmental Science*, **6**, 449–76.

Levy, F. (1980). The development of sustained attention (vigilance) and inhibition in children: some normative data. *Journal of Child Psychology and Psychiatry*, **21**, 77–84.

Lin, C.C.H., Hsiao, C.K., & Chen, W.J. (1999). Development of sustained attention assessed using the Continuous Performance Test among children 6-15 years of age. *Journal of Abnormal Child Psychology*, **27**, 403–412.

Manly, T., Nimmo-Smith, I., Watson, P., Anderson, V., Turner, A., & Roberston, I.H. (2001). The differential assessment of children's attention: the Test of Everyday Attention for Children (TEA-Ch), normative sample and ADHD performance. *Journal of Child Psychology and Psychiatry*, **42**, 1065–81.

Manly, T., Roberston, I.H., Anderson, V., & Nimmo-Smith, I. (1999). *The Test of Everyday Attention for Children: TEA-Ch*. Bury St Edmunds: Thames Valley Test Company.

McKay, K.E., Halperin, J.M., Schwartz, S.T., & Sharma, V. (1994). Developmental analysis of three aspects of information processing: sustained attention, selective attention, and response organization. *Developmental Neuropsychology*, **10**, 121–32.

Mercuri, E., Atkinson, J., Braddick, O., Anker, S., Cowan, F., Rutherford, M., et al. (1997). Visual function in full-term infants with hypoxic-ischaemic encephalopathy. *Neuropediatrics*, **28**, 155–61.

Mercuri, E., Atkinson, J., Braddick, O., Anker, S., Nokes, L., Cowan, F., Rutherford, M., Pennock, J., & Dubowitz, L. (1996). Visual function and perinatal focal cerebral infarction. *Archives of Disease in Childhood*, **75**, F76–81.

Mercuri, E., Haataja, L., Guzzetta, A., Anker, S., Cowan, F., Rutherford, M., et al. (1999). Visual function in term infants with hypoxic-ischaemic insults: correlation with neurodevelopment at 2 years of age. *Archives of Disease in Childhood. Fetal and Neonatal Edition*, **80**, F99–F104.

Mirsky, A.F., Anthony, B.J., Duncan, C.C., Ahearn, M.B., & Kellam, S.G. (1991). Analysis of the elements of attention: a neuropsychological approach. *Neuropsychology Review*, **2**, 109–45.

Mobbs, D., Eckert, M.A., Mills, D., Korenberg, J., Bellugi, U., Galaburda, A.M., et al. (2007). Frontostriatal dysfunction during response inhibition in Williams syndrome. *Biological Psychiatry,* **62**, 256–61.

Montfoort, I., Frens, M.A., Hooge, I.T., Haselen, G.C., & van der Geest, J.N. (2007). Visual search deficits in Williams-Beuren syndrome. *Neuropsychologia*, **45**, 931–8.

Munir, F., Cornish, K.M., & Wilding, J. (2000). A neuropsychological profile of attention deficits in young males with fragile X syndrome. *Neuropsychologia*, **38**, 1261–70.

Nadel, L. (2003). Down's syndrome: a genetic disorder in biobehavioral perspective. *Genes Brain and Behavior*, **2**, 156–66.

Owen, A.M., Stern, C.E., Look, R.B., Tracey, I., Rosen, B.R., & Petrides, M. (1998). Functional organization of spatial and nonspatial working memory processing within the human lateral frontal cortex. *Proceedings of the National Academy of Sciences of the USA*, **95**, 7721–26.

Pagon, R.A., Bennett, F.C., Laveck, B., Stewart, K.B., & Johnson, J. (1987). Williams syndrome—features in late childhood and adolescence. *Pediatrics*, **80**, 85–91.

Pierrot-Deseilligny, C., Rivaud, S., Gaymard, B., & Agid, Y. (1991). Cortical control of reflexive visually-guided saccades. *Brain*, **114**, 1473–85.

Posner, M.I. & Petersen, S.E. (1990). The attention system of the human brain. *Annual Review of Neuroscience*, **13**, 25–42.

Pueschel, S.M. (1990). Clinical aspects of Down syndrome from infancy to adulthood. *American Journal of Medical Genetics*, **7**, 52–56.

Robbins, T.W. (1996). Dissociating executive functions of the prefrontal cortex. *Philosophical Transactions of the Royal Society of London B*, **351**, 1463–71.

Robertson, I.H., Ward, T., Ridgeway, V., & Nimmo-Smith, I. (1996). The structure of normal human attention: the Test of Everyday Attention. *Journal of the International Neuropsychological Society*, **2**, 525–34.

Rowe, J., Lavender, A., & Turk, V. (2006). Cognitive executive function in Down's syndrome. *British Journal of Clinical Psychology*, **45**, 5–17.

Rueda, M.R., Fan, J., McCandliss, B.D., Halparin, J.D., Gruber, D.B., Lercari, L.P., et al. (2004). Development of attentional networks in childhood. *Neuropsychologia*, **42**, 1029–40.

Scerif, G., Cornish, K., Wilding, J., Driver, J., & Karmiloff-Smith, A. (2004). Visual search in typically developing toddlers and toddlers with fragile X or Williams syndrome. *Developmental Science*, **7**, 116–30.

Scerif, G., & Karmiloff-Smith, A. (2005). The dawn of cognitive genetics? Crucial developmental caveats. *Trends in Cognitive Sciences*, **9**, 126–35.

Schiller, P.H. (1985). A model for the generation of visually guided saccadic eye movements. In D. Rose & V.G. Dobson (Eds) *Models of the Visual Cortex* (pp. 62–70). Chichester: John Wiley and Sons.

Trick, L.M., & Enns, J.T. (1998). Lifespan changes in attention: the visual search task. *Cognitive Development*, **13**, 369–86.

Wechsler, D. (1989). *Wechsler Pre-school and Primary Scale of Intelligence—Revised*. New York, NY: The Psychological Corporation.

Wilding, J., Munir, F., & Cornish, K. (2001). The nature of attentional differences between groups of children differentiated by teacher ratings of attention and hyperactivity. *British Journal of Psychology*, **92**, 357–71.

Chapter 7

Sleep-related learning

Dagmara Annaz and Anna Ashworth

Introduction

Quality and quantity of sleep are an essential part of health, cognition and well-being; yet, sleep disorders are disturbingly prevalent in neurodevelopmental disorders. The fragility of sleep and its variable sleep architecture between individuals still remains understudied. It is therefore unclear what mechanisms drive these differences. Sleep involves finely tuned multidimensional processes of biochemistry, genetics and psychological processes in response to external environmental cues. Thus, it is important to appreciate the complexity of the sleep state, which involves multiple levels of regulation and directly impacts on life. It is now time to move away from the static viewpoint of the sleep state, acknowledge the dynamic processes occurring during sleep and identify the impact of sleep on cognitive processing.

Sleep architecture

Our brains go through a variety of different activities during sleep. Sleep is subdivided into five stages (I to V), corresponding to different depths of sleep. As we drift off to sleep, we enter stage I of sleep, which usually lasts around 5-10 minutes. Stage I is marked by a slowing of electroencephalography (EEG) recordings as the fast alpha waves, characteristic of the drowsy wake state, are replaced by lower-frequency theta waves. This stage is considered a transition period between wakefulness and sleep and is also accompanied by slow, rolling eye movements. Stage II lasts for around 20 minutes and involves mixed-frequency brain waves with rapid bursts of rhythmic brain wave activity known as sleep spindles and intermittent high-amplitude K complexes (large positive and immediate negative deflections of the EEG signal). These electrophysiological markers have been associated with memory consolidation and learning. Stages III and IV of sleep are characterised by the slowest electrical waves in the delta frequency (4 Hz), which reflect synchronised depolarisation and hyperpolarisation in large populations of neurons (also termed slow-wave sleep [SWS] or deep sleep). SWS is characterised by a predominance of vagal activity with slowing and regularising of cardiorespiratory rates. Even though the person is deeply asleep, electromyography monitoring shows that tonic activity of the postural muscles is preserved, although in practice whole-body movement is almost entirely absent. It is, however, in this stage of sleep that parasomnias such as sleep walking may occur. Stage V, often known as rapid eye movement (REM) sleep, is when most dreaming occurs. This stage is characterised by increased brain activity, profound muscular hypotonia and increased sympathetic nervous system activation with irregularity of cardiac and respiratory rates. A distinctive feature of REM sleep is activation of cholinergic neurons to levels seen in the waking state.

Complex activity of hormones such as melatonin, cortisol and many others are secreted into the bloodstream during sleep. For example, growth hormone is related in part to repair processes that occur during sleep. A decrease in growth hormone release during sleep is linked to reduced muscle mass and strength, increased fat tissue and a weakened immune system, among other factors. Follicle-stimulating hormone and luteinising hormone, which are involved in maturational and reproductive processes, are among the hormones released during sleep. Melatonin plays a pivotal role as a major neuroendocrine modulator of circadian biorhythms. In addition to functioning as synchroniser of the biological clock, melatonin also exerts a powerful antioxidant activity and interacts with the immune system. Abnormally high levels of cortisol secretion during sleep have been associated with poorer performance on tasks of declarative memory, executive function and negative emotionality (Li et al., 2006; Scher et al., 2010).

Sleep and cognition

In recent years, a great body of literature has emerged debating the impact of sleep on daytime behaviours and cognition. It has become clear that sleep is essential for numerous functions, including health, mood and cognition, and that even a modest sleep disruption can have severe detrimental effects. In both adults and children, this can impact on daytime behaviour and the ability to maximise potential at school or work. In children, sleep disruption is often associated with symptoms observed in attention deficit hyperactivity disorder (ADHD). Parents often describe their tired children as 'bouncing off the walls'. This is clearly seen in children who snore. Snoring is the most common symptom of obstructive sleep apnoea syndrome (OSAS), which causes sleep disruption by decreasing oxygen levels in the blood (hypoxia) leading to arousal. On average, 27% of young children snore, but this improves with age to around 3-5% in children aged 9-14 years (see Gozal, 2008). Children who snore are reported to display deficits in daytime behaviours such as impaired attention, learning, memory and school performance, have a lower IQ and exhibit increased hyperactivity and problem behaviour. These deficits are often seen to improve after adenotonsillectomy (removal of the tonsils and adenoids), but with some residual long-lasting effects. This may reflect damage to the frontal lobes caused by prolonged apnoeic episodes and disruption to sleep architecture suffered during the critical growth stages of neural development, causing an information processing deficit (Andreou & Agapitou, 2007; Blunden et al., 2005; Gozal & Pope, 2001).

Clinicians disagree on whether daytime behaviour is most influenced by the sleep disruption caused by sleep-disordered breathing or by the hypoxia itself and by hypercarbia (increased circulation of carbon dioxide). Hypoxia refers to the abnormal drop in oxygen levels following apnoeic/hypopnoeic episodes. When this occurs during sleep, oxygen delivery to the brain is diminished. In rat models, this leads to cell death and reduced long-term potentiation, which can have significant long-term effects for neurocognition in the developing brain. This model is probably generalisable to humans.

In a review paper, Blunden and Beebe (2006) assessed the arguments for each case. A number of studies indicated that hypoxia is the aggravating factor for cognitive impairment in children, evidenced by the observation that children suffering mild levels of oxygen desaturation have associated deficits in neurocognitive and psychosocial domains, and also lower general intelligence, memory and attentional capacity, even without upper airway obstruction or respiratory arousals. Children have also been shown to make an improvement in vigilance and hyperactive behaviour following adenotonsillectomy. By contrast, impairments on sustained attention, vigilance, mental flexibility, memory, intelligence and school performance are most associated with disturbed sleep architecture and observable symptoms of sleep-disordered breathing, rather than hypoxia. Also, sleep problems that create sleep disruption or deficit, such as periodic limb movement disorder (PLMD), insufficient sleep syndrome, sleep fragmentation and experimental sleep disruption or restriction, create problematic cognitive and behavioural effects, even in the absence of sleep-disordered breathing. Blunden and Beebe (2006) concluded that sleep deprivation, sleep disruption and intermittent hypoxia may be independently sufficient to cause daytime deficits in vulnerable children. Further research could elucidate whether early intervention of OSAS could reverse the adverse cognitive effects because adenotonsillectomy is a relatively simple procedure that could have significant beneficial effects for learning and academic performance. This is an important consideration in neurodevelopmental disorders where OSAS is a particular problem, for example Down syndrome (DS). Snoring is relatively common in Williams syndrome (WS) compared with typical individuals (Annaz et al., 2011; Goldman et al., 2009).

In all children, bedtime struggles and early school start times often mean that children's sleep is restricted, and even a modest sleep restriction can significantly impact on daytime behaviour. Sadeh et al. (2003) investigated the neurobehavioural effects of extending or restricting the usual sleep pattern of children aged 9 or 11 years (39 boys, 38 girls) by 1 hour per night for three consecutive nights. Performance on working memory, motor speed, reaction time, vigilance, visual memory and attention tasks was tested. Children in the sleep extension group (n=21) adjusted their sleep by an average of 35 minutes, those in the sleep restriction group (n=28) by 41 minutes; 28 children failed to significantly adjust their sleep and so acted as a control group. As expected, sleep quality improved in the sleep-restricted group, whereas the opposite occurred in the extension group, because physiological compensatory mechanisms act to regulate sleep physiology. In spite of these mechanisms, children in the sleep-extended group improved their performances on a 'continuous performance reaction time' task and a 'digit span forward' task, whereas the sleep restriction group showed no change on these tasks. These improvements, seen even after only a modest extension of sleep, similar to normal life, were similar to, or greater than, the difference seen between the two age groups (9- and 11-year-olds) at baseline. In other words, the neurobehavioural improvements seen after a 35-minute extension in sleep are similar to those gained by 2 years of development, showing how sensitive children are to modest alterations of their natural sleep patterns. Working memory and attention difficulties have previously been linked with classroom behaviour and achievement (Gathercole & Alloway, 2006; Gathercole & Pickering, 2000), showing how such a modest alteration in sleep habits could have a significant effect in the classroom, especially in children with neurodevelopmental disorders.

In addition to impacting daytime behaviour, sleep is now also known to play a significant role in certain types of memory consolidation. Sleep-dependent learning is the phenomenon whereby information is preferentially consolidated during sleep, leading to improved performance following a retention interval of sleep. This is particularly evident in motor skill learning. For example, using a finger-tapping task where participants are requested to learn a short sequence with the nondominant hand (Karni et al., 1995), speed and accuracy were found to improve over time, especially when retesting occurred following a period of sleep (18.9% improvement) compared with wake (3.9% improvement) (Walker et al., 2002). This improvement was seen regardless of whether initial training takes place in the morning or evening. It is suggested that consolidation of motor memories requires plastic changes in the primary motor cortex. This may occur with cholinergic activity in the neocortex, seen during REM and wake, and is known to enhance attention, learning and memory consolidation and facilitate experience-dependent plasticity in the brain. Plasticity may also occur through reactivation of the brain. Positron emission tomography studies show that this reactivation is most pronounced during post-training REM sleep and occurs significantly more in participants who have trained on a task than in those who have not (Maquet et al., 2000). REM sleep may become increasingly necessary for procedural memory consolidation as task difficulty progresses, for example mirror tracing or word-stem priming as opposed to simple texture discrimination, where processing is thought to take place at pre-attentive levels (Gais et al., 2000). Declarative memory, on the other hand, relies on the hippocampus so may be more reliant on hippocampal consolidation mechanisms replaying most efficiently during SWS when there is little other interfering background electricity in the brain. This is evidenced with tasks such as word pair learning, where performance has been correlated positively with the percentage of non-REM (NREM) sleep and negatively with the percentage of REM sleep (Backhaus et al., 2008), and memory improves following SWS but not REM sleep (Plihal & Born, 1997).

Sleep disruption can therefore have a negative impact on learning because memories are preferentially consolidated during a full uninterrupted night's sleep. This makes it particularly important to assess sleep in children with WS and other neurodevelopmental disorders because their sleep problems could be having a detrimental impact on their daytime behaviour and learning, which are already subjected to lesser cognitive reserve owing to their conditions. It is therefore possible that some of the difficulties they find with cognitive skills could be alleviated if sleep problems could be treated, because the detrimental effects of sleep disruption can be reversed by good sleep hygiene.

Sleep in Williams syndrome

Although parents of children with WS informally report that their children have problems with sleep, research into the specific sleep problems in WS is scarce. However, with growing awareness, there are now several research groups investigating the issue. Early studies described settling problems and night waking (Udwin et al., 1987), as well as bed wetting and sleep anxiety (Sarimski, 1996).

More recently, polysomnography (PSG) in seven children with WS under 10 years of age has shown that these children spent a greater percentage of the sleep period in a wake state (10% compared with 4% in ten typical children; p<.05) and SWS (34% compared with 20%; p<.001) while spending a smaller percentage in stages I and II (41% compared with 59%; p<.001) (Arens et al., 1998).

In Arens et al.'s study (1998), children with WS were selected from an initial sample of 28 children and were diagnosed as having symptoms suggestive of a movement arousal disorder. As predicted, they showed a higher percentage of PLMD than typically developing (TD) controls (total number of leg movements: 158 versus 65; p<.001), with more arousals and awakenings because of leg movements. The authors note the significance of finding PLMD in all seven children; however, considering that these children had antecedently been screened and were only studied with PSG, if there was a possibility of a limb movement disorder, then it is not quite so surprising that all showed PLMD. What is perhaps surprising is that 16 of the original sample of 28 children were screened as having possible PLMD, which is considerably more than would be expected in TD children. However, these results should be taken with caution because children without PLMD risk factors were screened out of the tested subsample. Also, with such a small sample the results cannot be generalised, but they are certainly intriguing and require further investigation.

In a later PSG study of nine teenagers and young adults with WS (age range: 14-29 years, mean: 20.76), increased wake time and SWS were found compared with a healthy control group matched for chronological age and gender (Bódizs et al., 2009). The study also reported increased NREM and decreased REM durations and percentages, a shorter total sleep time and a lower sleep efficiency in participants with WS. Moreover, the authors observed increased uni- or bilateral leg movements, largely during NREM sleep, relative to controls and concluded that frequent periodic leg movements lead to sleep disruption in this group, hence supporting the findings of Arens et al. (1998).

The long sleep latencies and night wakings often described in WS are not only apparent in the PSG studies but also in actigraphy data, a form of activity monitoring using a wrist-worn accelerometer to assess sleep quality and quantity. We carried out a series of studies investigating sleep in children and adolescents with WS. In our studies, parental questionnaires and actigraphy (Annaz et al., submitted) were used to examine sleep patterns in children with WS aged 6 to 12 years. Questionnaire data (Children's Sleep Habits Questionnaire, Owens et al., 2000) from 64 children supported previous research findings that the main sleep problems in WS are long sleep latencies, sleep anxiety, bedtime resistance and night wakings. Some 97% of parents reported their children to have problems with sleep. None of the most frequently reported medical conditions associated with sleep disorders, such as recurrent ear infections, constipation, tonsillitis and epilepsy, were reported in this survey. However, asthma (12%) and allergies (20%) turned out to be strong predictors of sleep onset delay in the WS group.

The parental reports were supported by a follow-up actigraphy study of 22 children with WS (aged 6-12 years) and showed long sleep latencies—an average of 46 minutes—with six of these children taking more than 1 hour to get to sleep (Annaz et al., submitted). In the control group of 92 healthy children, it was found that any sleep problems decline with increased chronological age. This change was not evident in the WS group, indicating that sleep problems in WS decrease at a much slower rate and may be enduring into adulthood. We also found that 61% of children with WS complained of daytime tiredness, echoing the findings of Goldman et al. (2009), who found that in 23 young adults with WS, almost all reported feelings of tiredness and sleepiness during the day, with over one-third suffering excessive daytime sleepiness based on the Epworth Sleepiness Scale (Johns, 1991). Their actigraphy data suggested a disparity, showing that participants were achieving an adequate amount of sleep—an average of 7.6 hours—but their sleep efficiency was surprisingly low because of long sleep latencies and increased waking after sleep onset, with participants spending an average of 9 hours in bed in order to achieve only 7.6 hours of sleep. The disparity between feeling tired while having adequate sleep is possibly attributable to the sleep disruption caused by multiple factors common in WS, including nocturia, restless legs movement, sleep apnoea or other factors intrinsic to WS.

Sleep-related learning in WS

Little research has investigated the effects of sleep problems in WS. People with WS often have associated disorders such as ADHD, anxiety and other behavioural problems, which are known to be affected by sleep and improve when sleep problems are treated (e.g. O'Brien et al., 2003). Arens et al. (1998) treated five children with WS for PLMD with clonazepam, a drug known to relieve PLMD symptoms so allowing sleep patterns to return to normal in typical adults. Four of the treated children were reported to show an immediate and sustained improvement on sleep and daytime behaviour, with parents reporting less irritability during the day. Repeated PSG in three of these children 3-6 months after treatment showed a significant decrease in PLMD and PLMD-related arousals and awakenings, so that their sleep patterns were comparable with the control group. It is probable that fragmentation and altered sleep architecture in this group has an impact on daytime behaviour, as the authors found that clonazepam significantly reduced PLMD, arousals became fewer and shorter, and parents reported their children to be less irritable during the day.

Treating sleep problems in WS would probably also impact on sleep-dependent memory consolidation, attention and ability to learn during the day (for discussion of the attention and memory profiles characteristic of WS, see Chapters 6 and 8). We used the finger-tapping task to investigate the impact of sleep on motor memory (Annaz et al., submitted). In this task, participants use their left hand to repeatedly type a five-digit number sequence on a computer keyboard. Speed and accuracy are recorded and compared across time points (for further details on the task see Walker et al., 2002). Twelve children with WS aged 6-12 years (3 male, 9 female; mean age 8.6 years) were trained on the task in the evening and retested the following morning and afternoon. In line with previous studies, we found a dramatic overnight improvement in the control group but no evidence of sleep-related learning in WS, as illustrated in Figure 7.1. However, the lack of improvement in the WS

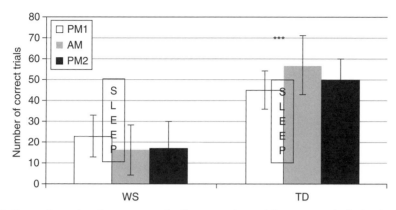

Fig. 7.1 Comparison of performance on the finger-tapping task between typically developing children and children with William syndrome. The error bars show the standard error of the mean. *** p<.001. Abbreviations: TD = typically developing; WS = Williams syndrome. Data from Annaz et al. (submitted).

group cannot be directly associated with sleep problems before we exclude possible problems with fine motor skills that are required to perform the finger-tapping task.

At the time of writing, we are not aware of any other publications on sleep-related learning in WS, but this is an area that requires thorough investigation because the sleep problems evident in WS could be at least in part responsible for many of the cognitive and behavioural deficits that these individuals experience. Sleep problems are often amenable to treatment, so alleviating the sleep problems in WS could have a hugely beneficial effect on their daytime functioning.

Sleep problems in other neurodevelopmental disorders

The neurological and physiological aspects of neurodevelopmental disorders have been well characterised in the wake state. Yet, although it is now well known that sleep problems are common in people with intellectual disabilities, there is relatively little information available characterising exact sleep patterns in these groups.

Autism

Sleep problems rank among one of the most concurrent clinical symptoms in children with autism, with estimates ranging from 40% to 80%. In a recent study using medical history and carer report, it was found that 83 of 160 (52%) children with autism spectrum disorder (ASD) had sleep problems, especially during early childhood, with the most common symptoms being frequent night waking and difficulty initiating sleep (Ming et al., 2008). Sleep problems were found to be associated with mood disorder and also with gastrointestinal problems, which in turn were associated with food intolerances because these could lead to bloating and bowel problems, leading to pain and increased night waking. The authors note anecdotal evidence of improving sleep problems by treating gastrointestinal dysfunction.

Parents of children with ASD tend to report settling problems and long sleep latencies, with some children taking over 1 hour to get to sleep, and night wakings, often lasting 2-3 hours, where children simply talk, laugh, scream or play with toys. Most children with ASD exhibit abnormal sleep–wake patterns, EEG activity and sleep architecture, although PSG studies disagree on the specifics, and differences could be attributable to patient population and methodology issues. Sleep problems are likely to be attributable to a complex interaction between physiological, psychological, environmental and sociological factors (see Cortesi et al., 2010). It is likely that circadian abnormalities play a role in sleep problems in ASD, as hormonal abnormalities have been found in a number of studies. For example, children with ASD have been found to have 42% decreased nocturnal melatonin compared with typical children (Tordjman et al., 2005). As with typical children, sleep problems in autism impact on daytime behaviours and, interestingly, are associated with more severe autistic traits (Schreck et al., 2003).

Down syndrome

It is well established that OSAS is common in the DS population, with prevalence rates estimated to be between 30% and 60%, whereas estimates of the prevalence of any sleep problems in DS are as high as 100% (Marcus et al., 1991). Craniofacial and upper airway abnormalities, obesity, tonsil and adenoid encroachment, and generalised underdevelopment (hypoplasia) of the upper airway have all been associated with OSAS, resulting in sleep fragmentation manifested in frequent awakenings, a higher percentage of wakefulness after sleep onset and therefore lower sleep efficiency.

In a longitudinal PSG study of 56 young children with DS, Shott et al. (2006) found abnormal PSG results in 32 (57%) children, defined by abnormal obstructive indexes (38%), abnormal carbon dioxide retention (hypercarbia; 30%) and/or hypoxia (20%). Some 61% of children had elevated arousal indexes. Parental sleep reports of their children's sleep were relatively inaccurate. In total, 35% of parents reported sleep problems, but only 36% of the children in this group had abnormal polysomnograms; by contrast, 69% of parents reported no sleep problems and yet 54% of their children had abnormal polysomnograms. The high incidence of OSAS and the inaccuracy of parent reports together necessitate that baseline PSG should be recommended for all children with DS. PSG also showed a lower percentage of REM sleep than would be expected in young children, a finding echoed by Miano et al. (2008), who also found increased stage 2 NREM and increased stage 1 NREM percentages compared with a healthy control group and a similar pattern of disrupted sleep architecture in children with fragile X syndrome.

Andreou et al. (2002) found that sleep apnoeas in young adults with DS significantly correlated with their scores on the Raven Progressive Matrices (Raven et al., 2003) test, which examines visuospatial skills. This in turn related to orientation on the Mini Mental State Examination (Folstein et al., 1975) of cognitive functioning, indicating that OSAS may be at least partly responsible for the difficulties that individuals with DS suffer with visuospatial skills and other behavioural or learning abilities.

Attention deficit hyperactivity disorder

Numerous studies show links between sleep disruption and ADHD symptoms. For example, O'Brien et al. (2003) found that in children with severe ADHD symptoms, OSAS was no worse than in a healthy control group (5% in each group). However, OSAS was present in 26% of children with mild ADHD symptoms, indicating that sleep-disordered breathing may impact on children's daytime behaviour, creating a hyperactive/inattentive behaviour phenotype similar to that seen in clinically diagnosed ADHD. Moreover, increased REM latency and decreased REM percentage were found in children with severe ADHD symptoms; yet, no differences in REM were found in children with mild ADHD symptoms compared with the control group. So although OSAS may be sufficient to cause ADHD-like symptoms, more severe ADHD is accompanied by specific differences in the sleep architecture. In addition, children attending sleep clinics for suspected sleep problems are likely to have ADHD (Chervin et al., 2006). Huang et al. (2007) found that treating sleep problems by adenotonsillectomy in children with ADHD not only relieved the symptoms of sleep-disordered breathing, but also led to an increase in REM sleep, SWS and total sleep time. It further led to better performance scores on a number of ADHD characteristics, such as social withdrawal, delinquency, internalising behaviour, physical symptoms, emotional distress and quality of life, as well as neuropsychological improvements on attention and reaction time tests. These positive outcomes were not seen to the same extent following treatment using methylphenidate, a commonly used treatment for ADHD. Hence, this is an important point, because improvements in attention and concentration indicate that children's performance at school improves following a relatively simple intervention.

Sleep management in neurodevelopmental disorders

The emergence of a 24-hour society and the increasing strain of modern living and its impact on family life have led to a gradual decline of good sleep hygiene habits for children and adults alike. Whether through a lack of bedtime routine or irregular bedtime and getting-up times, this could have a significant impact on children with developmental disabilities, whose fragile sleep patterns are easily disturbed. As outlined in this chapter, sleep problems can have a negative impact on daytime behaviour, learning, attention and other cognitive abilities, as well as problems with motor skills, such as coordination, and other health problems. It is therefore essential that good sleep hygiene is practised in children with neurodevelopmental disorders because their daytime functioning is already compromised because of their underlying condition. As a sleep loss of as little as 30 minutes can be enough to disrupt neuropsychological functioning in typical children (Sadeh et al., 2003), it is essential that parents are taught good sleep hygiene in order to give their children the greatest possible support and not exacerbate existing sleep problems. Good sleep habits include adding structure to the daytime and bedtime routines to act as *zeitgebers* (time cues) to reinforce circadian rhythms; removing tactile, visual, auditory and olfactory stimulation from the bedroom; scheduling regular bedtimes that do not fluctuate by more than 1 hour at weekends; and relaxing evening routines avoiding overstimulation (Jan et al., 2008). Children also need to learn aspects of when and how to fall asleep, and to unlearn bad habits. This could be particularly challenging for developmentally delayed children, who may not have the intellectual capacity to understand sleeping and so create problems such as bedtime resistance (Richdale & Wiggs, 2005).

In a recent survey of 63 children with WS, parents reported that almost one-third of children had used or currently use medication to get to sleep (Annaz et al., 2011). For almost one-third of these, the medication was melatonin, a hormone supplement often used to regulate circadian cycles. Although there is palpable evidence that melatonin supplementation is a well-tolerated pharmacotherapy to mitigate or eliminate the detrimental effects of poor sleep on children's mood, cognition and daytime function, its effectiveness in children with neurodevelopmental disorders remains inconclusive and has not been studied in WS as yet. In our study, parents reported temporary improvement or no improvement in sleep patterns after melatonin supplementation. Hence, controlled studies with measurement of melatonin secretion, careful developmental and behavioural history, and recordings of children's sleep patterns must be first obtained in order to treat children with disabilities for their sleep disorders.

We recommend that good sleep hygiene should be practised in children with WS, because a structured bedtime routine and suitable sleeping environment could alleviate problems with sleep anxiety and bedtime resistance so common in these children. Although behavioural techniques, tailored to the child's needs, can be effective with developmentally delayed children in order to aid appropriate bedtime routines, research in this area is in its infancy (for a review see Richdale & Wiggs, 2005). Also, good sleep hygiene alone may not be sufficient to treat sleep problems in neurodevelopmental disorders, but it provides a good basis for increasing the success of other interventions, such as behavioural management strategies, medication or treatment of OSAS by continuous positive airway pressure or adenotonsillectomy. This could greatly improve children's daytime functioning and improve quality of life for both the child and the parents.

Conclusion

Clearly, sleep is not only for the brain but also for the rest of the body. Integration of different approaches using parental reports, actigraphy, PSG and genetic and endocrine examination to determine the causality and disorder specificity of sleep disturbances should be considered in future studies. Cognitive studies of children with disorders such as WS should be considering sleep patterns of the child during their investigation because these may have a direct impact on performance scores. More studies on sleep and cognition are greatly needed. These should be carried out as early as from the fetal stage (e.g. Kozuma et al., 1993), through infancy and into adulthood by tracing sleep patterns and interactions between different functions. Notions such as interactivity, compensation, specialisation and localisation can be key in characterising in more depth how atypical sleep patterns affect at the cognitive and behavioural levels, with their implications for the consolidation of learning over developmental time (Annaz et al., 2008; Karmiloff-Smith, 1998).

Editor commentary (Emily K. Farran & Annette Karmiloff-Smith)

In this chapter, we learnt three striking facts that, when considered together, have enormous implications for our understanding of development in individuals with neurodevelopmental disorders. First, the authors reviewed evidence from WS, DS, ADHD and autism that indicated a high prevalence of sleep difficulties in these groups, which one can assume also extends across many other neurodevelopmental disorders. Second, lack of sleep can have a substantial negative impact on many domain-general processes, such as attention. Third, there are syndrome-specific types of sleep disturbance. If we take a neuronstructivist stance and consider the cascading impact that impaired attentional mechanisms can have on the development of domain-specific functions, discussed in Chapters 6 and 18, then an understanding of sleep and sleep-related learning is a key piece of the jigsaw of interacting systems that impact the developmental process.

Sleep is one component in a multilevel interaction, and thus sleep disruption in individuals with neurodevelopmental disorders can have a negative impact on the dynamics of brain development and cognitive processing, in tandem with the syndrome-specific constraints on development. In typical development, parts of the brain are more active during sleep than in wakefulness. Thus, sleep disruption also impacts learning because memories are preferentially consolidated during a full night's uninterrupted sleep. The chapter reported preliminary evidence that sleep-related learning is impaired in WS. This raises the intriguing possibility that aspects of the cognitive profile observed in WS, as well as in other groups that show sleep disturbance such as autism and ADHD, could in part relate to sleep disturbance. The chapter stressed that, given the relative ease at which sleep problems can be ameliorated, further research into the impact of sleep on learning on atypical groups is essential.

References

Andreou, G., & Agapitou, P. (2007). Reduced language abilities in adolescents who snore. *Archives of Clinical Neuropsychology, 22,* 225–29.

Andreou, G., Galanopoulou, C., Gourgoulianis, K., Karapetsas, A., & Molyvdas, P. (2002). Cognitive status in Down syndrome individuals with sleep disordered breathing deficits (SDB). *Brain and Cognition, 50,* 145–49.

Annaz, D., Hill, C.M., Ashworth, A., Holley, S., & Karmiloff-Smith, A. (2011). Characterization of sleep problems in school-aged children with Williams syndrome. *Research in Developmental Disabilities, 32,* 164–69.

Annaz, D., Hill, C.M., Ashworth, A., & Karmiloff-Smith, A. (submitted). Sleep and procedural memory consolidation in Williams syndrome.

Annaz, D., Karmiloff-Smith, A., & Thomas, M. (2008). The importance of tracing developmental trajectories for clinical child neuropsychology. In J. Reed & J. Warner Rogers (Eds), *Child Neuropsychology: Concepts, Theory and Practice* (pp. 7–18). Singapore: Wiley-Blackwell.

Arens, R., Wright, B., Elliott, J., Zhao, H., Wang, P.P., Brown, L.W., et al. (1998). Periodic limb movement in sleep in children with Williams syndrome. *The Journal of Pediatrics, 133,* 670–74.

Backhaus, J., Hoeckesfeld, R., Born, J., Hohagen, F., & Junghanns, K. (2008). Immediate as well as delayed post learning sleep but not wakefulness enhances declarative memory consolidation in children. *Neurobiology of Learning and Memory, 89,* 76–80.

Blunden, S., & Beebe, D. (2006). The contribution of intermittent hypoxia, sleep debt and sleep disruption to daytime performance deficits in children: consideration of respiratory and non-respiratory sleep disorders. *Sleep Medicine Reviews, 10,* 109–18.

Blunden, S., Lushington, K., Lorenzen, B., Martin, J., & Kennedy, D. (2005). Neuropsychological and psychosocial function in children with a history of snoring or behavioral sleep problems. *Journal of Pediatrics, 146,* 780–86.

Bódizs, R., Gombos, F., & Kovács, I. (2009). Sleep in Williams syndrome: from aperiodic leg movements to architectural, EEG spectral and spindling peculiarities. *Sleep Medicine*, **10 Supplement 2**, S48.

Chervin, R.D., Ruzicka, D.L., Giordani, B.J., Weatherly, R.A., Dillon, J.E., Hodges, E.K., et al. (2006). Sleep-disordered breathing, behavior, and cognition in children before and after adenotonsillectomy. *Pediatrics*, **117**, 769–78.

Cortesi, F., Giannotti, F., Ivanenko, A., & Johnson, K. (2010). Sleep in children with autistic spectrum disorder. *Sleep Medicine*, **11**, 659–64.

Folstein, M.F., Folstein, S.E., McHugh, P.R. (1975). "Mini-mental state". A practical method for grading the cognitive state of patients for the clinician. *Journal of Psychiatry Research*, **12**, 189–98.

Gais, S., Plihal, W., Wagner, U., & Born, J. (2000). Early sleep triggers memory for early visual discrimination skills. *Nature Neuroscience*, **3**, 1335–39.

Gathercole, S.E., & Alloway, T.P. (2006). Practitioner review: short-term and working memory impairments in neurodevelopmental disorders: diagnosis and remedial support. *Journal of Child Psychology and Psychiatry*, **47**, 4–15.

Gathercole, S.E., & Pickering, S.J. (2000). Working memory deficits in children with low achievements in the national curriculum at 7 years of age. *British Journal of Educational Psychology*, **70**, 177–94.

Goldman, S.E., Malow, B.A., Newman, K.D., Roof, E., & Dykens, E.M. (2009). Sleep patterns and daytime sleepiness in adolescents and young adults with Williams syndrome. *Journal of Intellectual Disability Research*, **53**, 182–88.

Gozal, D. (2008). Obstructive sleep apnea in children: implications for the developing central nervous system. *Seminars in Pediatric Neurology*, **15**, 100–106.

Gozal, D., & Pope Jr, D.W. (2001). Snoring during early childhood and academic performance at ages thirteen to fourteen years. *Pediatrics*, **107**, 1394–99.

Huang, Y.-S., Guilleminault, C., Li, H.-Y., Yang, C.M., Wu, Y.-Y., & Chen, N.H. (2007). Attention-deficit/hyperactivity disorder with obstructive sleep apnea: a treatment outcome study. *Sleep Medicine*, **1**, 18–30.

Jan, J.E., Owens, J.A., Weiss, M.D., Johnson, K.P., Freeman, R.D., & Ipsiroglu, O.S. (2008). Sleep hygiene for children with neurodevelopmental disabilities. *Pediatrics*, **122**, 1343–50.

Johns, M.W. (1991). A new method for measuring daytime sleepiness: the Epworth sleepiness scale. *Sleep* **14**, 540–5.

Karmiloff-Smith, A. (1998). Development itself is the key to understanding developmental disorders. *Trends in Cognitive Sciences*, **2**, 389–98.

Karni, A., Meyer, G., Jezzard, P., Adams, M.M., Turner, R., & Ungerleider, L.G. (1995). Functional MRI evidence for adult motor cortex plasticity during motor skill learning. *Nature*, **377**, 155–58.

Kozuma, S.N. Shinozuka, N., Kuwabara, Y., & Mizuno, M. (1993). A study on the development of sleepwakefulness cycle in the human fetus. *Early Human Development*, **29**, 391–93.

Li, G., Cherrier, M.M., Tsuang, D.W., Petrie, E.C., Colasurdo, E.A., Craft, S., et al. (2006). Salivary cortisol and memory function in human aging. *Neurobiology of Aging*, **27**, 1705–1714.

Maquet, P., Laureys, S., Peigneux, P., Fuchs, S., Petiau, C., Phillips, C., et al. (2000). Experience-dependent changes in cerebral activation during human REM sleep. *Nature Neuroscience*, **3**, 831–36.

Marcus, C.L., Keens, T.G., Bautista, D.B., von Pechmann, W.S., & Davidson Ward, S.L. (1991). Obstructive sleep apnea in children with Down syndrome. *Pediatrics*, **8**, 132–39.

Miano, S., Bruni, O., Elia, M., Scifo, L., Smerieri, A., Trovato, A., et al. (2008). Sleep phenotypes of intellectual disability: a polysomnographic evaluation in subjects with Down syndrome and Fragile-X syndrome. *Clinical Neurophysiology*, **119**, 1242–47.

Ming, X., Brimacombe, M., Chaaban, J., Zimmerman-Bier, B., & Wagner, G.C. (2008). Autism spectrum disorders: concurrent clinical disorders. *Journal of Child Neurology*, **23**, 6–13.

O'Brien, L., Holbrook, C.R., Mervis, C.B., Klaus, C.J., Bruner, J.L., Raffield, T.J., et al. (2003). Sleep and Neurobehavioral characteristics of 5- to 7-year old children with parentally reported symptoms of attention deficit/hyperactivity disorder. *Pediatrics,* 111, 554–63.

Owens, J.A., Spirito, A., & McGuinn, M. (2000). The Children's Sleep Habits Questionnaire (CSHQ): psychometric properties of a survey instrument for school-aged children. *Sleep,* 23, 1043–51.

Plihal, W., & Born, J. (1997). Effects of early and late nocturnal sleep on declarative and procedural memory. *Journal of Cognitive Neuroscience,* 9, 534–47.

Raven, J., Raven, J.C., & Court, J.H. (2003). *Raven's Progressive Matrices and Vocabulary Scales.* San Antonio, TX: Pearson Assessment.

Richdale, A., & Wiggs, L. (2005). Behavioral approaches to the treatment of sleep problems in children with developmental disorders: what is state of the art? *International Journal of Behavioral and Consultation Therapy,* 1, 165–90.

Sadeh, A., Gruber, R., & Raviv, A. (2003). The effects of sleep restriction and extension on school-age children: what a difference an hour makes. *Child Development,* 74, 444–55.

Sarimski, K. (1996). Specific eating and sleeping problems in Prader-Willi and Williams-Beuren syndrome. *Child Care, Health and Development,* 22, 143–50.

Scher, A., Hall, W.A., Zaidman-Zait, A., & Weinberg, J. (2010). Sleep quality, cortisol levels, and behavioral regulation in toddlers. *Developmental Psychobiology,* 52, 44–53.

Schreck, K.A., Mulick, J.A., & Smith, A.F. (2003). Sleep problems as possible predictors of intensified symptoms of autism. *Research in Developmental Disabilities,* 25, 57–66.

Shott, S.R., Amin, R., Chini, B., Heubi, C., Hotze, S., & Akers, R. (2006). Obstructive sleep apnea: should all children with Down syndrome be tested? *Archives of Otolaryngology–Head and Neck Surgery,* 132, 432–36.

Tordjman, S., Anderson, G.M., Pichard, N., Charbuy, H., & Touitou, Y. (2005). Nocturnal excretion of 6-sulphatoxymelatonin in children and adolescents with autistic disorder. *Biological Psychiatry,* 57, 134–38.

Udwin, O., Yule, W., & Martin, N. (1987). Cognitive abilities and behavioural characteristics of children with idiopathic infantile hypercalcaemia. *Journal of Child Psychology and Psychiatry,* 28, 297–309.

Walker, M.P., Brakefield, T., Morgan, A., Hobson, J.A., & Stickgold, R. (2002). Practice with sleep makes perfect: sleep-dependent motor skill learning. *Neuron,* 35, 205–211.

Chapter 8

Memory

Stefano Vicari and Deny Menghini

Introduction

Memory and learning have been extensively investigated in people with Williams syndrome (WS). Since the pioneering paper of Crisco et al. (1988), 115 papers on WS have been published that refer to memory in the title or include memory as a key word. These papers have demonstrated that memory in WS is atypical at numerous functional levels.

This chapter is dedicated to reviewing the recent literature and experimental studies regarding memory and learning development in people with WS. Following a developmental perspective, we will report strengths and impairments that characterise the end state of the memory profile in individuals with WS and mention (where data are available) how memory changes with development. Furthermore, consistent with a neuroconstructivist perspective, we will discuss the distinct memory profiles in WS in relation with the developmental interactions between genes, brain, environment and behaviour.

Before exploring the characteristics of memory in WS, we will briefly introduce relevant theories of memory. Memory is not considered a unique cognitive function but is organised into a series of functionally independent but interacting systems and subsystems. Following Atkinson and Shiffrin (1971), Squire (1987) distinguished between short-term memory (STM) and long-term memory (LTM). These two systems are characterised by differences in retention capacity (limited to only a few items for STM, practically unlimited for LTM), information coding (mainly phonological coding for STM, based on semantic processing of stimuli for LTM) and the mnesic-trace deterioration rate (lasting a few seconds without reiteration for STM, variable but relatively slow for LTM).

Baddeley and Hitch (1974) introduced a new concept for STM, namely that of working memory, which is defined as a limited-capacity system that temporarily stores information for subsequent further manipulation (Baddeley & Hitch, 1974; Baddeley, 1986). Working memory is not subserved by a unitary store but by the cooperation of two major systems. The first is a central executive system, a limited-capacity central processor able to temporarily store and process information from many modalities. The second major system of the working memory model consists of a number of peripheral limited-capacity systems called slave systems. They temporarily store and rehearse information belonging to a single modality when the flow of data surpasses the capacity of the central executive system.

The articulatory loop is a two-component slave system specialised for the temporary storage of verbal material. One component (the phonological store) is devoted to the passive maintenance of verbal information in a phonological code. The other component (articulatory rehearsal) prevents the decay of material stored in the phonological store by refreshing the memory trace. Moreover, it is involved in the re-coding of visually presented verbal material into a phonological format (Baddeley, 1986). The articulatory-loop model can account for two robust experimental findings in verbal span: the phonological-similarity effect and the word-length effect. The first effect refers to the phenomenon that strings formed by phonologically similar words (e.g. rat, bat, cat, mat) are more difficult to recall immediately after presentation than strings formed by phonologically dissimilar words (e.g. fish, girl, bus, hand). This finding is explained by the hypothesis that verbal material is held in an acoustic format in the phonological store and that, as a consequence, acoustically similar words form less distinctive memory traces. The word-length effect refers to the finding that memory span is longer for strings of short words (e.g. bus, pig, car, tree) than for lists of long words (e.g. banana, elephant, policeman, kangaroo) (Baddeley & Hitch, 1974). This finding is commonly interpreted as evidence of the contribution of articulatory rehearsal to the verbal span because long words take longer to be rehearsed than short words.

The visuospatial sketchpad (later named the visuospatial scratchpad) is the second peripheral slave system and it is specialised for the temporary storage of visual material. Although the functioning of this system has been far less investigated than that of the articulatory loop, there is reason to believe that an internal fractionation of structure and functioning occurs here as well. Indeed, clinical and experimental data support the hypothesis that temporary memories for visual object information (such as registering colours and shapes) and for the visuospatial location of objects are processed by different but functionally related subsystems (Della Sala & Logie, 2002; Logie, 1995; Vicari et al., 2003, 2006). In the model's current formulation, Baddeley (2001) has added another component, the episodic memory buffer, and has acknowledged the role of LTM in the functioning of the phonological loop and the visuospatial scratchpad.

Within the LTM domain, Squire's model distinguishes between explicit or declarative memory and implicit or procedural memory (Squire, 1987). Explicit memory is involved in intentional and/or conscious recall and recognition of experiences and information. Implicit memory is manifested as facilitation (i.e. performance improvement) in perceptual, cognitive and motor tasks without any conscious reference to previous experiences (for a review see Tulving & Schacter, 1990).

Verbal working memory

In contrast to the situation in other genetic syndromes with similar levels of intellectual functioning such as Down syndrome (DS), verbal STM is not severely impaired in adolescents and adults with WS. Indeed, the verbal STM of individuals with WS is usually appropriate for their mental age (Udwin & Yule, 1990; Vicari et al., 1996a) or higher (Klein & Mervis, 1999; Mervis et al., 1999). However, this verbal-STM profile may vary with development in the two syndromes. For example, Vicari et al. (2004) documented a selective WS advantage on a verbal-memory span (digit span) task only for participants older than 12 years but not for children younger than 8 years of age. By contrast, participants with DS exhibited a generalised impairment in verbal STM at all the ages investigated. This result is relevant because it points to different developmental trajectories in WS and DS, at least in terms of verbal-memory spans.

The relative advantage in verbal STM observed in adolescents with WS has been interpreted as consistent with the particular pattern exhibited by individuals with WS in the linguistic domain, in which phonological processing of words is relatively proficient but grammatical and semantic language is usually impaired, especially at adult ages (Chapters 10, 11 and 17; Mervis et al., 1999; Pezzini et al., 1999; Volterra et al., 1996; Vicari et al., 2004). Note that in children with WS, the acquisition of grammar is highly related to the efficiency of verbal STM, more than in typical development (Pléh et al., 2003; Robinson et al., 2003). This finding is particularly relevant because it indicates basic differences in how children with WS and typically developing (TD) controls acquire language.

Some studies on STM have investigated patterns of strengths and weaknesses in individuals with WS. In 1996, Barisinikov et al. reported the case of an individual with WS who showed phonological-similarity and word-length effects that were comparable with those displayed by a control group matched for chronological age (10-12 years). Vicari et al. (1996b) found similar results in a study that compared phonological-similarity, word-length and word-frequency effects in a verbal-span task among 10-year-old children with WS and TD controls (mean chronological age: 5 years) matched for nonverbal mental age. The performance of the participants with WS showed typical phonological-similarity and word-length effects, supporting the hypothesis of relatively strong phonological competencies in WS. However, the frequency effect in the WS group was reduced; although both groups repeated high-frequency words better than low-frequency words, the difference was significantly smaller in the WS group.

This possible dissociation between typical phonological encoding and the reduced contribution of lexical-semantic encoding mechanisms to word span in children with WS is particularly interesting in light of their pattern of linguistic abilities: various studies reported that children with WS have impaired lexical-semantic and grammar abilities and relatively proficient phonological processes (Grant et al., 1997; Karmiloff-Smith et al., 1997; Karmiloff-Smith et al., 1998; Mervis et al., 1999; Pezzini et al., 1999; Volterra et al., 1996). This linguistic pattern seems to be particularly pronounced in children younger than 8 years. Older children (above 12 years of age) have been shown to exhibit a relative strength in lexical abilities, but they still showed reduced grammatical abilities (Vicari et al., 2004).

Accordingly, the reduced frequency effect in children with WS may result from the rigid use of a phonological re-coding strategy for both high- and low-frequency words. However, contradictory findings attributable to methodological differences (e.g. related to the matching criteria and the choice of control groups) make it impossible to compare the results of these studies directly and to reach any definitive conclusions. Indeed, Majerus et al. (2003) confirmed the relative strength of phonological STM in four children with WS aged 10-12 years, but they failed to demonstrate more general preservation of phonological processing abilities in WS. Brock et al. (2005) demonstrated a similar frequency effect in children with WS as in TD children. Moreover, Laing et al. (2005)

studied 14 children and adults with WS whose chronological ages ranged from 10 years 11 months to 52 years. TD participants were matched to the WS group based on verbal STM and lexical abilities; a group of 13 TD children and 1 adult (average age: 9 years 2 months) was matched to the participants with WS on the basis of digit span scores, whereas a second group of 14 TD children (average age: 10 years 9 months) was matched on the basis of vocabulary scores. The results of this study documented that, similarly to the TD participants, children and adults with WS are able to access and make use of lexical semantics in a verbal-STM task.

In summary, the lexical influence on phonological STM in WS is still a controversial issue and it may become more evident at older ages. To contribute to clarifying this controversy, we recently administered two verbal-STM tasks to three different groups matched for mental age. Specifically, we recruited 15 adolescents with WS with a mean chronological age of 14 years 9 months, 13 adolescents with DS with a mean chronological age of 14 years 4 months and 14 TD children with a mean chronological age of 6 years 9 months. The adolescents with WS and the TD participants did not differ on the Peabody Picture Vocabulary Test (Dunn & Dunn, 1981), a traditional measure of lexical mental age. The two verbal-STM tasks administered were a nonword repetition task and a low-frequency words span task. Group differences were demonstrated in the nonword repetition task, with TD and WS individuals performing at a comparable level. However, the participants with DS obtained lower scores than the other two groups. A different pattern emerged in the low-frequency words span task, where the participants with WS obtained lower scores than the TD children and no differences were observed between the WS and DS groups. Thus, once again the WS group demonstrated their well-known verbal-STM abilities and the relative independence between their phonological abilities and their lexical-semantic competencies. Indeed, when this aspect was directly investigated by the word span task for low-frequency words, the individuals with WS performed worse than the TD children. Note also that the WS and TD participants were matched based on their lexical repertoire, which consequently cannot explain the results obtained.

In conclusion, the contribution of lexical-semantic competencies to solving verbal-STM tasks in adolescents with WS is reduced, compared with TD children matched for mental age. The execution of verbal-STM tasks may be supported by phonological abilities as documented by the phonological-similarity effect in the WS group.

Visuospatial working memory

The functioning of the visuospatial scratchpad (the slave system of the working memory model devoted to processing visual material) has been extensively investigated in people with WS. For example, Wang and Bellugi (1994) documented lower scores in individuals with WS than in those with DS on a visuospatial-STM task. Jarrold et al. (1999) confirmed this finding, which indirectly indicates that young adults with WS have a relative disadvantage for visuospatial relative to verbal span.

To examine the visuospatial domain, Vicari et al. (2006) compared individuals with DS and individuals with WS with TD mental-age-matched controls on two tests assessing the visual and spatial spans. The WS group had a mean chronological age of 19 years 8 months and a mean mental age of 6 years 11 months and was matched with a group of TD children with a mean chronological age of 6 years 10 months and a mean mental age of 6 years 11 months. The DS group had a mean chronological age of 15 years 10 months and a mean mental age of 5 years 2 months and was matched with a different TD group whose mean chronological age was 5 years 1 month and whose mean mental age was 5 years 2 months. The two tests involved studying the same complex, nonverbalisable figures and using the same response modality (pointing to targets on the screen). The crucial experimental variable was that in one case, the participants had to recall where the figure had appeared on the screen (task assessing the visuospatial span), whereas in the other case the participants had to recall the physical aspect of the figure (task assessing the memory span for visual objects). The results showed reduced performance on both tasks for people with DS. By contrast, those with WS exhibited specific difficulties in terms of their visuospatial STM but not in terms of their STM for visual objects. However, while the selective deficit in WS persisted even when perceptual abilities were taken into account (for discussion of visuospatial perception see Chapter 12), the individuals with DS no longer showed any deficits in either visuospatial STM or visual-object STM when their scores were adjusted for their level of perceptual ability. Indeed, after adjusting for the performance level on the visuoperceptual task, the performance of the DS and TD participants no longer differed on the two STM tasks.

Finally, Mandolesi and et al. (2009) investigated spatial working memory abilities in children with WS by using the radial-arm maze (RAM) task. The RAM task consists of a round central platform with eight arms radiating like the spokes of a wheel. Two different RAM paradigms were administered. In the free-choice paradigm, each child was allowed to explore the eight arms freely and retrieve the reward from the buckets located at the end of each arm. A trial was considered successful when all eight rewards were collected. Afterwards, the children were kept in the RAM for a short while to verify whether they continued their search for rewards. In other words, the experimenter observed whether the child revisited a previously explored arm and searched for a further reward in the bucket. After such an incorrect visit, the child was informed that the 'game' was over.

In the forced-choice paradigm, only four arms (e.g. arms 1, 3, 4, 7) were accessible; the remaining four arms were closed by a little chair at the proximal end of each arm. Different angles separated the opened arms to avoid the participants reaching the solution through the employment of a procedural strategy, for example performing only 45° angles. The child was placed by the experimenter on the central area of the maze and was allowed to explore the four open arms and collect the four accessible rewards. Afterwards, the child was guided out of the maze. He/she was kept in a separate place without seeing the maze. The child chatted with the experimenter for 120 seconds before the second phase of the task started. In the second phase, the child had free access to all arms, but only the four previously closed arms were rewarded because the other four rewards had already been collected. The success in visiting only the rewarded arms essentially depended on remembering the arms that had been visited previously, emphasising the working memory requirements and neglecting the search patterns. Thus, the free-choice paradigm was employed for analysing the aspects linked mainly to procedural and mnesic components, whereas the forced-choice paradigm served to disentangle components linked to spatial working memory from the procedural components.

The participants were 14 adolescents and young adults with WS (seven males and seven females) with a mean chronological age of 15 years 8 months and a mean mental age of 6 years 2 months. Fourteen TD children (seven males and seven females, mental age: 6 years 1 month) formed the control group.

The results evidenced a severe impairment of individuals with WS in solving both RAM paradigms, demonstrating—at least at the ages we investigated –deficits in the acquisition of procedural competencies and in spatial working memory processes. Overall, these results indicate that people with WS perform at their mental-age level on tasks assessing the working memory for verbal and visual information on objects but exhibit a reduced memory span for spatial information (see also Vicari et al., 2003).

Verbal explicit long-term memory

The few studies in the literature on the explicit LTM of individuals with WS report contra-dictory results. Vicari et al. (1996b) documented lower scores in a learning task involving delayed free recall of a word list among children with WS with a mean chronological age of 9 years 11 months and a mean mental age of 5 years 6 months, compared with a group of TD controls matched for mental age. Moreover, the authors found comparable recall of the last items on the list (recency effect) in the two groups, but reduced recall of the first items on the list (primacy effect) in the WS group. According to the classic dual-store interpretation of the serial-position curve for the immediate recall of word lists (e.g. Glanzer, 1972), the normal recency effect in the individuals with WS provides new support for the idea of their relatively proficient verbal STM (Vicari & Carlesimo, 2002, 2006). By contrast, the poor priming effect indicates difficulty in storing new verbal representations in the declarative LTM.

Results reported by Nichols et al. (2004) also support the hypothesis that language and auditory STM might be dissociated from verbal LTM in individuals with WS. However, Brock et al. (2006) reported contrasting findings. Their results showed that LTM per-formance in children with WS was comparable with that of TD children. Note, however, that the studies adopted different criteria to match the WS and TD groups (mental age in Nichols et al., 2004, and Vicari et al., 1996b, overall verbal-memory abilities in Brock et al., 2006), thus making it difficult to draw strong and definitive conclusions.

To investigate LTM in WS in more detail, we administered two different LTM tests that assessed word list learning and category word fluency (Vicari & Menghini, unpublished results). The word list learning task (Vicari, 2007) involved 15 words (nouns) denoting concrete but semantically unrelated objects. The test consisted of three consecutive trials of immediate free recall. During the trials, the examiner presented the 15 words orally and the participant had to immediately recall as many words as possible. We recruited 15 adolescents with WS with a mean chronological age of 14 years 9 months, 13 with DS with a mean chronological age of 14 years 4 months and 14 TD children with a mean chronological age of 6 years 9 months. The TD children improved their performance with each trial, confirming the presence of a learning effect in this group. By contrast, the performance in the WS group did not improve from the first to the second or from the second to the third trial, thus demonstrating a reduced learning effect in this group.

The second LTM task was the category word fluency task (Vicari, 2007), a traditional semantic-LTM task. In this test, the participants were requested to generate as many nouns within a specific category (animals, clothes, fruit or toys) as they could in 1 minute. TD children produced a higher number of words than the WS and DS groups, who in turn showed comparable performance on the task.

In summary, a relative impairment of verbal LTM emerged in individuals with WS and DS. However, different patterns of verbal-STM and -LTM abilities were found when the performances of different etiologic groups were compared. Whereas individuals with DS showed generalised impairment, those with WS exhibited a deficit only in LTM verbal abilities. As previously reported, verbal STM is mostly related to the phonological processing of words and verbal LTM mainly depends on semantic aspects of words to remember (for a review see Vicari & Carlesimo, 2002). Accordingly, the findings of a dissociation between STM and LTM in WS support the hypothesis of reduced semantic abilities but relatively proficient phonological abilities in this group.

Visuospatial explicit long-term memory

Explicit LTM for visuospatial information in the WS population has been much less investigated than LTM for verbal material. Vicari et al. (2005) compared the performance of WS and DS individuals on tests evaluating visual-object and visuospatial learning. Visual-object LTM (LTM for the physical characteristics of objects) and visuospatial LTM (LTM for position or motion in space) are mediated by different neural systems and therefore constitute two distinct aspects of the organisation of explicit LTM (Moscovitch et al., 1995). During the study phase of the visual-object task, 15 figures of common objects (e.g. a tree) were shown to the participants. During the test phase immediately following the study phase, four different versions of the same object (e.g. four trees) were depicted on each page. Only one of the four was the same as the target object in the study phase; the other three were physically different distracters. The study and test phases were presented three consecutive times. In the visuospatial learning task, the pages were divided into four quadrants and each figure was positioned in one of the quadrants. During the test phase, the target stimuli were presented and the participant was asked to indicate the position of the figure on an empty page divided into four quadrants. The entire task was administered three times.

Four groups comprised of 15 participants each were included: a WS group with a mean chronological age of 18 years 5 months and a mean mental age of 6 years 8 months and a control group comprised of TD children with a mean chronological age of 6 years 7 months; a DS group with a mean chronological age of 16 years 5 months and a mean mental age of 5 years 4 months and a control group of TD children with a mean chronological age of 5 years 6 months.

The results showed a decreased level of learning of visuospatial material but substantially typical learning of visual-object patterns among the participants with WS, compared with the TD children. The participants with DS showed the opposite profile, that is, typical learning of visuospatial sequences but impaired learning of visual-object patterns. The performance of the participants with WS indicates that the dissociation between the processing of visuospatial information (which is deficient) and the processing of visual information on objects (which is proficient)—described for perceptual (Atkinson et al., 1997; Atkinson et al., 2003) and working memory tasks (Vicari et al., 2003; 2006) in this population—extends to the LTM domain.

Note that what mainly distinguished the performance of the TD group from that of the WS group on the visuospatial task was the learning rate from the first to the third recognition trial. This finding is contrary to the reductionist hypothesis, which postulates deficient perceptual processing and/or working memory maintenance of visuospatial data as the origin of the LTM deficit in WS. Indeed, although the immediate recognition of items studied only once could also be heavily influenced by the proficiency in perceptual analysis and working memory processing, the reduced learning across successive trials seems to be a reliable index of a compromised ability to store new information in the LTM.

Researchers investigating performance on declarative-memory tasks have become increasingly interested in using a componential approach that distinguishes two different kinds of access to stored memories: recollection and familiarity. From a developmental perspective, it has been proposed that recollection emerges later than familiarity and shows more developmental changes. However, the relative contributions of recollection and familiarity to the recognition performance of individuals with intellectual disability have been scarcely investigated.

In a recent study, Costanzo et al. (2011) investigated the qualitative profile of declarative-LTM impairment in 13 participants with WS with a mean chronological age of 20 years 9 months and a mean mental age of 6 years 6 months matched to 13 TD children for mental age. Two different experimental paradigms to assess the contributions of familiarity and recollection were adopted. The first paradigm directly estimated the recollection and familiarity components of recognition by setting the two processes in opposition, in the inclusion and exclusion conditions of a process dissociation procedure task (according to Jacoby, 1991). The task involved 90 items selected from the Snodgrass and Vanderwart (1980) set of black-and-white line drawings. The 90 items were split into two test lists (one for the inclusion condition and one for the exclusion condition) that were comparable in terms of the item names' mean frequency of occurrence in the first vocabulary of Italian children.

During the study phase, the participants were shown a set of 15 coloured drawings (representing typical samples of the black-and-white line drawings in the test) and listened to a set of 15 words (the names of the black-and-white line drawings) spoken aloud by the examiner, and were asked to remember the items later. In the visual block, the participants were asked to name each item and then make a yes/no judgement about pleasantness. If they failed to name the item correctly, the participants were requested to repeat aloud the name produced by the examiner. In the auditory block, the participants were asked to repeat each word aloud and again make a yes/no judgement about pleasantness.

During the test phase (immediately after the study phase), the participants were shown the overall set of 45 black-and-white line drawings in random order. In the inclusion condition, which was given first, the participants were requested to respond 'old' to all items presented in the study phase, irrespective of the modality (visual or auditory) of presentation. Conversely, in the exclusion condition, which was given after the second study phase, the participants were asked to respond 'old' only to items that had been studied as coloured drawings and to respond 'new' to items studied in the auditory modality and to unstudied items.

The second paradigm contrasted the performance of participants on a declarative-memory task mainly relying on familiarity (single-item recognition) with the performance on a memory task requiring a larger contribution of recollection (between-item associative recognition) (Turriziani et al., 2004; Yonelinas, 2002).

The results from the two paradigms demonstrated a dissociation between recollection (reduced) and familiarity (proficient) in the WS group as compared with the mental-age-matched TD group. These are very new data and further studies are needed to clarify whether this finding is exclusively characteristic of people with WS or whether it is a profile shared with other syndromes characterised by intellectual disability.

Implicit long-term memory

In the last few years, research has been devoted to investigating the ability of individuals with intellectual disabilities to learn visuomotor and cognitive skills. Findings from Vicari et al. (2000, 2001) indicated differences in the skill learning abilities of individuals with WS and DS. Fourteen participants with DS with a mean chronological age of 21 years showed the same rate of implicit learning as a group of 20 TD children who were 5 years 9 months old and matched for mental age (Vicari et al., 2000). By contrast, 12 participants with WS with a chronological age of 11-19 years and a mean mental age of 6 years 5 months showed reduced procedural learning abilities compared with TD children matched for mental age (Vicari et al., 2001).

Don et al. (2003) reported contrasting findings. These authors investigated implicit learning in children and adults with WS and in a comparison group of TD controls matched for chronological age. The participants were tested in an artificial grammar learning paradigm and in a rotor pursuit task; the children and adults with WS showed evidence of implicit learning on both tasks.

In sum, the results from implicit memory studies of individuals with WS are inconsistent. To explore these contradictory findings, Vicari et al. (2007) conducted a direct comparison between WS and DS in a single study. One study group consisted of 32 adolescents with WS with a mean chronological age of 15.8 years and a mean mental age of 6.8 years. Another study group comprised 26 individuals with DS who had a mean chronological age of 17.1 years and a mean mental age of 6.4 years. The groups were comparable for chronological and mental age. Their performances on a traditional version of the serial reaction time test initially developed by Nissen and Bullemer (1987) were compared with those of a group of 49 TD children matched for mental age. The results documented that although the individuals with WS had faster reaction times than the DS and TD groups, two different reaction time curves were observed throughout the blocks: the TD and DS groups exhibited the U-shaped learning curve usually observed in this type of task, whereas the WS group failed to exhibit a learning curve. In other words, the individuals with DS were relatively proficient in implicit learning, whereas the adolescents with WS were severely impaired in this cognitive ability, at least at the ages investigated.

In summary, visual LTM is a relative strength in people with WS, whereas verbal and spatial LTM is impaired when compared with TD controls matched for mental age. Moreover, adolescents with WS show impaired implicit learning of new procedures.

Neurobiological perspectives

There is increasing evidence that the memory profile we have described in people with WS is the result of some specific characteristics of their anomalous brain development.

In general, as discussed in Chapter 2, brain imaging studies reported that adolescents and adults with WS have significant reductions in the volumes of total brain, white matter and grey matter (Chiang et al., 2007; Jernigan & Bellugi, 1990; Jernigan et al., 1993; Reiss et al., 2000, 2004).

The most consistent neuroimaging findings indicate the presence of occipital and parietal cortex abnormalities (Meyer-Lindenberg et al., 2004; Reiss et al., 2004; Eckert et al., 2005; Boddaert et al., 2006; Eisenberg et al., 2010). Another characteristic of the WS brain is a reduced volume in the posterior regions of the corpus callosum (Tomaiuolo et al., 2002; Luders et al., 2007). This hypoplasia of the corpus callosum may determine a defective callosal transfer of information, thus causing insufficient integration and coordination of the activity of the two cerebral hemispheres. On the basis of these observations, it seems plausible that the reduced posterior regions of the brain and corpus callosum may have a role in the occurrence of the visuospatial STM and LTM deficits among adolescents with WS. Moreover, the more pronounced difficulty in retaining visuospatial material reported in individuals with WS could be related to a particularly delayed maturation of the dorsal visual system (Eckert et al., 2005; Meyer-Lindenberg et al., 2004; Reiss et al., 2004). In accord with this hypothesis, diffusion tensor imaging studies found an increased fractional anisotropy in the superior longitudinal fasciculus in WS individuals relative to TD participants (Hoeft et al., 2007), indicating that the underling white-matter tracts subserving the dorsal stream of visual processing may also be aberrant.

On the other hand, an atypical cytoarchitecture of the primary auditory cortex (Holinger et al., 2005), a reduced leftward asymmetry of the planum temporale (Eckert et al., 2006a) and an increased volume of the superior temporal gyrus have been observed in participants with WS (Reiss et al., 2004; Campbell et al., 2009). Some of these findings have been related to their relatively proficient performance in verbal-STM tasks (Reiss et al., 2004).

In addition, differences between people with WS and TD individuals were found in the volume/morphology of the cerebellum, hippocampus, putamen/globus pallidus and thalamus (Meyer-Lindenberg et al., 2005; Reiss et al., 2000, 2004; Schmitt et al., 2001;

Campbell et al., 2009). The difficulties reported in visuomotor skill learning in WS could be related to a deficient maturation of striatal circuits, the thalamus and the cerebellum, which are known to be critical for implicit memory.

However, although there is increasing knowledge of the neuroanatomical differences between people with WS and TD individuals, neuroimaging studies often reported inconsistent results on the anatomical correlates accounting for the cognitive profile observed in WS (for example, see Meyer-Lindenberg et al., 2004; Reiss et al., 2004; Haas et al., 2009; Menghini et al., 2011). The different findings across neuroimaging studies may be interpreted as an expression of heterogeneity in the brain morphology within WS, which could account for the fact that there is some variability in the cognitive profiles of people with WS. In addition, there are some methodological aspects that may determine inconsistencies across neuroanatomical studies, especially when automated methods such as voxel-based morphometry (Ashburner & Friston, 2005) are employed.

Furthermore, we are only now beginning to see studies on genetic syndromes that provide the rare opportunity to observe the effects of a small number of genes on brain development (see also Chapter 3). Recent studies have been conducted to investigate the interactions between genes, the brain and behaviour by probing the molecular and genetic influences on the typical neurodevelopmental trajectory (Thompson et al., 2001; Fan et al., 2003). However, research on neurodevelopmental disorders provides a unique opportunity to link genetic alteration with specific cognitive profiles and brain development. In particular, developmental studies are informative because they allow us to understand how a change in the trajectory of development may lead to a cascade of cognitive and behavioural deficits.

This is a very fascinating topic with great potential for understanding the effects of genes on brain morphology, brain function and behaviour, and for interpreting the atypical development observed among people with intellectual disability.

Conclusion

Memory is usually impaired in people with WS and the impairment occurs at different levels of memory articulation. For example, within the STM domain, people with WS show relatively proficient articulatory-loop functioning and an impairment of the visuospatial scratchpad, at least in terms of the spatial component. In terms of LTM, performance in WS is characterised by a relative strength in manipulating visual material and by impairments in verbal and spatial memory. Moreover, adolescents with WS are impaired in the implicit learning of new procedures.

The memory profile in WS, as in other syndromes, may be interpreted as the expression of a complex interplay between genes, biology and the environment. The parallel evaluation of scores on neuropsychological tests and of morphovolumetric and neurofunctional data in WS seems a promising avenue for localising and investigating the neural circuits underlying atypical memory development in different syndrome groups, and allows researchers to explicitly link genes and gene expression to the development of neural circuits.

Editor commentary (Emily K. Farran & Annette Karmiloff-Smith)

This chapter explored the memory profile of individuals with WS. Cross-syndrome comparisons with individuals with DS yielded distinct profiles for each group. The working memory profiles of each group related to the overall cognitive profiles of each group (in WS the cognitive profile is characterised by stronger verbal than visuospatial abilities, with the opposite being the case in DS). Taking a neuroconstructivist approach, the chapter demonstrated that the discrepancy between better verbal than visuospatial working memory in WS is an emergent product of development. This is in agreement with the developmental pattern of verbal and visuospatial abilities described by Jarrold et al. (2001) and suggests that the rate of development of verbal working memory is faster than that of visuospatial working memory. Analytical investigation demonstrated further differentiation between poorer visuospatial memory than visual-object memory in WS, which is reminiscent of the profile observed within the visuospatial domain (see Chapter 12). Within the verbal-memory domain, an atypical reliance on phonological processing over semantic processing is observed in WS. This parallels the profile observed within the development of language (see Chapter 11).

Bidirectional impacts between memory and verbal ability were highlighted. First, a reliance on phonological processing in WS supports verbal-STM performance in WS, albeit in an atypical manner, but not verbal LTM, which is relatively impaired. In the other direction, the chapter suggested an impact of memory processing on the developmental trajectories of language, in which lexical processing in WS shows a higher reliance on phonological processing than on semantic processing, compared with typical development. Domain-general memory processes, therefore, both influence and are influenced by domain-specific processes in WS, although relatively little is known about the developmental trajectories of these interactions.

Given the widespread impact of the domain-general process of attention on development (Chapter 6), it is likely that the impact of memory processing is also far-reaching. This has implications for our understanding of the impaired memory processes observed across many neurodevelopmental disorders such as specific language impairment, development dyscalculia and fragile X syndrome, to name but a few.

References

Ashburner, J., & Friston, K.J. (2005). Unified segmentation. *NeuroImage*, **26**, 839–51.

Atkinson, J., Braddick, O., Anker, S., Curran, W., Andrew, R., Wattam-Bell, J., et al. (2003). Neurobiological models of visuospatial cognition in children with Williams syndrome: measures of dorsal-stream and frontal function. *Developmental Neuropsychology*, **23**, 139–72.

Atkinson, J., King, J., Braddick, O., Nokes, L., Anker, S., & Braddick, F. (1997). A specific deficit of dorsal stream function in Williams syndrome. *NeuroReport*, **8**, 1919–22.

Atkinson, R.C., & Shiffrin, R.M. (1971). The control of short-term memory. *Scientific American*, **225**, 82–90.

Baddeley, A.D. (1986). *Working Memory*. London: Oxford University Press.

Baddeley, A.D. (2001). Is working memory still working? *American Psychologist*, **56**, 849–64.

Baddeley, A.D., & Hitch, G. (1974). Working memory. In G.H. Bower (Ed.), *The Psychology of Learning and Motivation*, vol. **8** (pp. 47–90). New York, NY: Academic Press.

Barisinikov, K., Van Der Linden, M., & Poncelet, M. (1996). Acquisition of new words and phonological working memory in Williams syndrome: a case study. *Neurocase, 2,* 395–404.

Boddaert, N., Mochel, F., Meresse, I., Seidenwurm, D., Cachia, A., Brunelle, F., et al. (2006). Parieto-occipital grey matter abnormalities in children with Williams syndrome. *NeuroImage, 30,* 721–25.

Brock, J., Brown, G.D.A., & Boucher, J. (2006). Free recall in Williams syndrome: is there a dissociation between short and long term memory? *Cortex, 42,* 366–75.

Brock, J., McCormack, T., & Boucher, J. (2005). Probed serial recall in Williams syndrome: lexical influences on phonological short-term memory. *Journal of Speech, Language, and Hearing Research, 48,* 360–371.

Campbell, L.E., Daly, E., Toal, F., Stevens, A., Azuma, R., Karmiloff-Smith, A., et al. (2009). Brain structural differences associated with the behavioural phenotype in children with Williams syndrome. *Brain Research, 1258,* 96–107.

Chiang, M.C., Reiss, A., Lee, A., Bellugi, U., Galaburda, A., Korenberg, J., et al. (2007). 3D pattern of brain abnormalities in Williams syndrome visualized using tensor-based morphometry. *NeuroImage, 36,* 1096–1109.

Costanzo, F., Vicari, S., & Carlesimo, G.A. (2011). Familiarity and recollection in Williams syndrome. *Cortex.* [EPub ahead of print 22 June 2011].

Crisco, J.J., Dobbs, J.M., & Mulhern, R.K. (1988). Cognitive processing of children with Williams syndrome. *Developmental Medicine and Child Neurology, 30,* 650–66.

Della Sala, S., & Logie, R.H. (2002). Neuropsychological impairments of visual and spatial working memory. In A.D. Baddeley, B. Wilson & M. Kopelman (Eds), *Handbook of Memory Disorders* (pp. 271–92). Chichester: John Wiley and Sons.

Don, A.J., Schellenberg, E.G., Reber, A.S., DiGirolamo, K.M., & Wang, P.P. (2003). Implicit learning in children and adults with Williams syndrome. *Developmental Neuropsychology, 23,* 201–25.

Dunn, L.M., & Dunn, L.M. (1981). *Peabody Picture Vocabulary Test—Revised.* Circle Pines, MN: American Guidance Service.

Eckert, M., Hu, D., Eliez, S., Bellugi, U., Galaburda, A., Korenberg, J., et al. (2005). Evidence for superior parietal impairment in Williams syndrome. *Neurology, 64,* 152–53.

Eckert, M.A., Galaburda, A.M., Karchemskiy, A., Liang, A., Thompson, P., Dutton, R.A., et al. (2006a). Anomalous sylvian fissure morphology in Williams syndrome. *NeuroImage, 33,* 39–45.

Eisenberg, D.P., Jabbi, M., & Berman, K.F. (2010). Bridging the gene-behavior divide through neuroimaging deletion syndromes: velocardiofacial (22q11.2 deletion) and Williams (7q11.23 deletion) syndromes. *NeuroImage, 53,* 857–69.

Fan, J., Fossella, J., Sommer, T., Wu, Y., & Posner, M.I. (2003). Mapping the genetic variation of executive attention onto brain activity. *Proceedings of the National Academy of Sciences of the USA, 100,* 7406–7411.

Glanzer, M. (1972). Storage mechanisms in recall. In G.H. Bower (Ed.), *The Psychology of Learning and Motivation: Advances in Research and Theory,* vol. **5** (pp. 129–93). New York, NY: Academic Press.

Grant, J., Karmiloff-Smith, A., Gathercole, S.A., Paterson, S., Howlin, P., Davies, M., et al. (1997). Phonological short-term memory and its relationship to language in Williams syndrome. *Cognitive Neuropsychiatry, 2,* 81–99.

Haas, B.W., Mills, D., Yam, A., Hoeft, F., Bellugi, U., & Reiss, A. (2009). Genetic influences on sociability: heightened amygdala reactivity and event-related responses to positive social stimuli in Williams syndrome. *Journal of Neuroscience, 29,* 1132–39.

Hoeft, F., Barnea-Goraly, N., Haas, B.W., Golarai, G., Ng, D., Mills, D., et al. (2007). More is not always better: increased fractional anisotropy of superior longitudinal fasciculus associated with poor visuospatial abilities in Williams syndrome. *Journal of Neuroscience, 27,* 11960–65.

Holinger, D.P., Bellugi, U., Mills, D.L., Korenberg, J.R., Reiss, A.L., Sherman, G.F., et al. (2005). Relative sparing of primary auditory cortex in Williams syndrome. *Brain Research, 1037,* 35–42.

Jarrold, C., Baddeley, A.D., & Hewes, A.K. (1999). Genetically dissociated components of working memory: evidence from Down's and Williams syndrome. *Neuropsychologia, 37,* 637–51.

Jernigan, T.L., & Bellugi, U. (1990). Anomalous brain morphology on magnetic resonance images in Williams syndrome and Down syndrome. *Archives of Neurology, 47,* 529–33.

Jernigan, T.L., Bellugi, U., Sowell, E., Doherty, S., & Hesselink, R. (1993). Cerebral morphologic distinctions between WS and DS. *Archives of Neurology, 50,* 186–91.

Jacoby, L.L. (1991). A process dissociation framework: separating automatic from intentional uses of memory. *Journal of Memory and Language, 30,* 513–41.

Jarrold, C., Baddeley, A.D., Hewes, A.K., & Phillips, C. (2001). A longitudinal assessment of diverging verbal and non-verbal abilities in the Williams syndrome phenotype. *Cortex, 37,* 423–31.

Karmiloff-Smith, A., Grant, J., Berthoud, I., Davies, M., Howlin, P., & Udwin, O. (1997). Language and Williams syndrome: how intact is "intact"? *Child Development, 68,* 274–90.

Karmiloff-Smith, A., Tyler, L.K., Voice, K., Sims, K., Udwin, O., Howlin, P., et al. (1998). Linguistic dissociation in Williams syndrome: evaluating receptive syntax in on-line and off-line tasks. *Neuropsychologia, 36,* 343–51.

Klein, B.P., & Mervis, C.B. (1999). Contrasting patterns of cognitive abilities of 9-and 10- year olds with Williams syndrome or Down syndrome. *Developmental Neuropsychology, 16,* 177–96.

Laing, E., Grant, J., Thomas, M., Parmigiani, C., Ewing, S., & Karmiloff-Smith, A. (2005). Love is . . . an abstract word: the influence of lexical semantics on verbal short-term memory in Williams syndrome. *Cortex, 41,* 169–79.

Logie, R.H. (1995). *Visuo-spatial Working Memory.* Hove: Lawrence Erlbaum.

Luders, E., Di Paola, M., Tomaiuolo, F., Thompson, P.M., Toga, A.W., Vicari, S., et al. (2007). Callosal morphology in Williams syndrome: a new evaluation of shape and thickness. *Neuroreport, 18,* 203–207.

Majerus, S., Barisnikov, K., Vuillemin, I., Poncelet, M., & Van der Linden, M. (2003). An investigation of verbal short-term memory and phonological processing in four children with Williams syndrome. *Neurocase, 9,* 390–401.

Mandolesi, L., Addona, F., Foti, F., Menghini, D., Petrosini, L., & Vicari, S. (2009). Spatial competences in Williams syndrome: a radial arm maze study. *International Journal of the Developmental Neuroscience, 27,* 205–213.

Mervis, C.B., Morris, C.A., Bertrand, J., & Robinson, B.F. (1999). Williams syndrome: findings from an integrated program of research. In H. Tager-Flusberg (Ed.), *Neurodevelopmental Disorders* (pp. 65–110). Cambridge, MA: MIT Press.

Meyer-Lindenberg, A., Kohn, P., Mervis, C., Kippenhan, J., Olsen, R., Morris, C., et al. (2004). Neural basis of genetically determined visuospatial construction deficit in Williams syndrome. *Neuron, 43,* 623–31.

Meyer-Lindenberg, A., Mervis, C., Sarpal, D., Koch, P., Steele, S., Kohn, P., et al. (2005). Functional, structural, and metabolic abnormalities of the hippocampal formation inWilliams syndrome. *Journal of Clinical Investigation, 115,* 1888–95.

Moscovitch, C., Kapur, S., Kohler, S., & Houle, S. (1995). Distinct neural correlates of visual long-term memory for spatial location and object identity: a positron emission tomography study in humans. *Proceedings of the National Academy of Sciences of the USA, 92,* 3721–25.

Nichols, S., Jones, W., Roman, M.J., Wulfeck, B., Delis, D.C., Reilly, J., et al. (2004). Mechanisms of verbal memory impairment in four developmental disorders. *Brain and Language, 88,* 180–89.

Nissen, M.J., & Bullemer, P. (1987). Attentional requirements of learning: evidence from performance measures. *Cognitive Psychology, 19,* 1–32.

Pezzini, G., Vicari, S., Volterra, V., Milani, L., & Ossella, M.T. (1999). Children with Williams syndrome: is there a unique neuropsychological profile? *Developmental Neuropsychology, 15,* 141–55.

Pléh, C., Lukács, A., & Racsmány, M. (2003). Morphological patterns in Hungarian children with Williams syndrome and the rule debates. *Brain and Language, 86,* 377–83.

Reiss, A., Eckert, M., Rose, F., Karchemskiy, A., Kesler, S., Chang, M., et al. (2004). An experiment of nature: brain anatomy parallels cognition and behavior in Williams syndrome. *Journal of Neuroscience, 24,* 5009–5015.

Reiss, A., Eliez, S., Schmitt, J., Straus, E., Lai, Z., Jones, W., et al. (2000). IV. Neuroanatomy of Williams syndrome: a high-resolution MRI study. *Journal of Cognitive Neuroscience, 12,* 65–73.

Robinson, B.F., Mervis, C.B., & Robinson, M. (2003). The role of verbal short-term memory and working memory in acquisition of grammar by children with Williams syndrome. *Developmental Neuropsychology, 23,* 13–31.

Schmitt, J.E., Eliez, S., Bellugi, U., & Reiss, A.L. (2001). Analysis of cerebral shape in Williams syndrome. *Archives of Neurology, 58,* 283–87.

Snodgrass, J.G., & Vanderwart, M. (1980). A standardized set of 260 pictures: norms for name agreement, image agreement, familiarity, and visual complexity. *Journal of Experimental Psychology, Human and Learning, 6,* 174–215.

Squire, L.R. (1987). *Memory and Brain,* Oxford: Oxford University Press.

Tomaiuolo, F., Di Paola, M., Caravale, B., Vicari, S., Petrides, M., & Caltagirone, C. (2002). Morphology and morphometry of the corpus callosum in Williams syndrome: a magnetic resonance imaging analysis. *NeuroReport, 13,* 1–5.

Thompson, P., Cannon, T.D., Narr, K.L., van Erp, T., Poutanen, V.-P., Huttunen, M., et al. (2001). Genetic influences on brain structure. *Nature, 4,* 1–6.

Tulving, E., & Schacter, D.L. (1990). Priming and human memory systems. *Science, 247,* 301–306.

Turriziani, P., Fadda, L., Caltagirone, C., & Carlesimo, G.A. (2004). Recognition memory for single items and for associations in amnesic patients. *Neuropsychologia, 42,* 426–33.

Udwin, O., & Yule, W. (1990). Expressive language of children with Williams syndrome. *American Journal of Medical Genetics, Supplement, 6,* 108–114.

Vicari, S. (2007). *PROMEA: Prove di Memoria e Apprendimento per l'età evolutiva.* Florence: Giunti OS.

Vicari, S., Bates, E., Caselli, M.C., Pasqualetti, P., Gagliardi, C., Tonucci, F., et al. (2004). Neuropsychological profile of Italians with Williams syndrome: an example of a dissociation between language and cognition? *Journal of International Neuropsychological Society, 10,* 862–76.

Vicari, S., Bellucci, S., & Carlesimo, G.A. (2000). Implicit and explicit memory: a functional dissociation in persons with Down syndrome. *Neuropsychologia, 38,* 240–51.

Vicari, S., Bellucci, S., & Carlesimo, G.A. (2001). Procedural learning deficit in children with Williams syndrome. *Neuropsychologia, 39,* 665–77.

Vicari, S., Bellucci, S., & Carlesimo, G.A. (2003). Visual and spatial working memory dissociation: evidence from a genetic syndrome. *Developmental Medicine and Child Neurology, 45,* 269–73.

Vicari, S., Bellucci, S., & Carlesimo, G.A. (2005). Visual and spatial long-term memory: differential pattern of impairments in Williams and Down syndromes. *Developmental Medicine and Child Neurology, 47,* 305–311.

Vicari, S., Bellucci, S., & Carlesimo, G.A. (2006). Evidence from two genetic syndromes for the independence of spatial and visual working memory. *Developmental Medicine and Child Neurology, 48,* 126–31.

Vicari, S., Brizzolara, D., Carlesimo, G.A., Pezzini, G., & Volterra, V. (1996a). Memory abilities in children with Williams syndrome. *Cortex, 32,* 503–514.

Vicari, S., & Carlesimo, G.A. (2002). Children with intellectual disabilities. In A. Baddeley, B. Wilson, & M. Kopelman (Eds), *Handbook of Memory Disorders* (pp. 501–518). Chichester: John Wiley and Sons.

Vicari, S., & Carlesimo, G.A. (2006). Short-term memory deficits are not uniform in Down and Williams syndromes. *Neuropsychological Review, 16,* 87–94.

Vicari, S., Carlesimo, G.A., Brizzolara, D., & Pezzini, G. (1996b). Short-term memory in children with Williams syndrome: a reduced contribution of lexical-semantic knowledge to word span. *Neuropsychologia*, **34**, 919–25.

Vicari, S., Verucci, L., & Carlesimo, G.A. (2007). Implicit memory is independent from IQ and age but not from etiology: evidence from Down and Williams syndromes. *Journal of Intellectual Disability Research*, **51**, 932–41.

Volterra, V., Capirci, O., Pezzini, G., Sabbadini, L., & Vicari, S. (1996). Linguistic abilities in Italian children with Williams syndrome. *Cortex*, **32**, 663–77.

Wang, P.P., & Bellugi, U. (1994). Evidence from two genetic syndromes for dissociation between verbal and visual-spatial short-term memory. *Journal of Clinical Experimental Neuropsychology*, **16**, 317–22.

Yonelinas, A.P. (2002). The nature of recollection and familiarity: a review of 30 years of research. *Journal of Memory and Language*, **46**, 441–517.

Chapter 9

Executive function and motor planning

Kerry D. Hudson and Emily K. Farran

Introduction

Executive function encompasses a number of cognitive processes that allow for goal-directed processing of novel or complex situations. Executive functions can be subdivided into two categories: metacognitive executive functions and emotional/motivation executive functions (Ardila, 2008). The first category, metacognitive executive functions, represent behaviour typically measured in neuropsychological tasks such as mental set-shifting (switching attention between tasks), inhibition of a prepotent response (deliberate suppression of a dominant response) and monitoring/updating of representations in working memory (active manipulation of information held in working memory) (Miyake et al., 2000). These abilities are largely grounded in the dorsolateral prefrontal cortex (Fuster, 2002). The second category, emotional/motivation executive functions, involve control of affective impulses, such as tailoring behaviour in order to be socially appropriate. These abilities are driven by ventromedial areas of the prefrontal cortex that link to limbic areas and the orbitofrontal prefrontal cortex (Fuster, 2002), and can be assessed by affect-laden tasks such as those involving gambling or rewards.

In typically developing (TD) children, executive-function abilities develop rapidly during the first year of life, with a second spurt in development of executive function between 3 and 7 years of age (Riggs et al., 2006) and further refinement in adolescence owing to pruning of frontal neural systems (Luna et al., 2010). Pruning increases functional prefrontal connections by removing weaker synaptic connections and retaining and strengthening the remaining synapses that are frequently activated. Relatively little attention has been given to executive function in Williams syndrome (WS), although evidence suggests that executive function is impaired. In this disorder, components of executive function are largely studied in isolation and in either adults or children. Such an approach risks gleaning task-dependent results that mask overall executive-function ability and do not reveal developmental changes. Assessment of attention and inhibition is also complicated by comorbidity; it has been reported that 65% of individuals with WS aged 4-16 years meet the criteria for diagnosis with attention deficit hyperactivity disorder (ADHD) (Leyfer et al., 2006).

Tasks that involve the generation of a motor plan for action are also impaired in WS, although this can be commensurate with general levels of motor development (Elliott et al., 2006). Motor development therefore is a limiting factor in the execution of motor plans, and it is difficult to determine the extent to which difficulty executing a motor plan relates to motor ability or an individual's ability to generate a motor plan. Generation of a motor plan represents a complex interaction of cognitive, visual and proprioceptive information. One must select the effector to conduct the action and determine the target for that action (e.g. using a hand to reach and grasp an object), which typically involves activation of the dorsal premotor area (Hoshi & Tanji, 2007; Sober & Sabes, 2003; see also Chapter 13 for discussion of dorsal-stream activation and motor control). TD adults can actualise sophisticated motor plans and TD children improve motor planning ability with development (Haywood & Getchell, 2009).

This chapter will assess inhibition (such as inhibition of a prepotent response) and its influence on social functioning and evaluate how the cascading developmental effects of poor planning ability impact wider functioning on other aspects of cognition such as performance on visuospatial tasks. Studies that have investigated the interplay between multiple executive functions will also be examined to resolve the mixed evidence relating to executive dysfunction in WS. Motoric planning will be discussed in terms of walking, stair-descent and reaching studies that reveal evidence for poor motor planning in WS. The chapter will highlight how the use of neuroimaging techniques and analysis of movement in real-world situations has advanced our understanding of executive function and motor planning in typical development as well as in groups with neurodevelopmental disorders including WS.

Inhibition of irrelevant impulses and stimuli

Go/no-go task

Suppression and inhibition of irrelevant impulses and stimuli greatly aids daily functioning (Garavan et al., 1999). Experimentally, inhibition can be assessed by the go/no-go task, in which participants are presented with a series of letters and are required to press a button as each letter appears, but are instructed not to press the button on presentation of an 'X', for example. Participants must sustain attention throughout the task and inhibit the prepotent button-push response on recognition of the target 'X'.

Sinzig et al. (2008) used the go/no-go task to show that children with ADHD made more errors than TD controls matched for chronological age (mean chronological age: 13 years, standard deviation: 3 years) and children with autistic spectrum disorder (ASD) with or without comorbid ADHD. Within the ASD groups, those with comorbid ADHD made more errors than those without ADHD, and they also made more errors than TD controls. The go/no-go task is therefore sensitive to subtle phenotypic differences across different groups with neurodevelopmental disorders, specifically in relation to attentional control.

Mobbs et al. (2007) used functional magnetic resonance imaging to investigate the neural activation involved in inhibition as measured by the go/no-go task in adults with WS and age-matched TD controls. Seven of 18 participants with WS performed at chance on this task. The remaining participants with WS showed a slower response time during the task, but the accuracy of the responses was comparable with that among controls. Both groups exhibited a speed-accuracy trade-off; inhibiting the button-press was associated with longer response times and therefore participants' response times were greater in order to ensure accuracy. Note, however, that Menghini et al. (2010) showed that despite making more errors, individuals with WS did not have greater response times than mental-age-matched controls (mean age: 6 years 11 months). This discrepancy in whether group differences are observed for accuracy or response time probably relates to differences in the participant exclusion criteria.

Mobbs et al.'s (2007) WS group exhibited reduced activation in the dorsolateral prefrontal cortex and the dorsal anterior cingulate cortex (regions associated with attentional control) and in the striatum (involved in motor planning), compared with the control group. Individuals with WS therefore had difficulty recruiting frontostriatal circuits for behavioural inhibition. The WS group showed increased activation in the medial precuneus and posterior cingulate cortex relative to controls. Reduced activation in these areas has been implicated in poor response inhibition in ADHD (Rubia et al., 2005). Mobbs et al. (2007) suggest that increased activation in these areas in WS may reflect a compensatory mechanism for reduced frontostriatal functioning. This interestingly alludes to the plastic nature of the brain in order to maintain behavioural functioning despite atypical brain function. It seems that during development in WS, alternative pathways have developed to overcome frontostriatal dysfunction, although this progression has not been formally assessed in WS. Deficits in attention are seen in ADHD and WS, but they result from different levels of activation in the same brain areas. This provides a useful avenue for cross-syndrome research to elucidate brain–behaviour interactions.

Counterpointing, detour-reaching and day/night tasks

Atkinson et al. (2003) used three inhibition tasks (counterpointing, detour-reaching and day/night tasks) to assess inhibition in children with WS relative to age-matched TD children. As these behavioural inhibition tasks are typically associated with frontoparietal activation, it was predicted that WS performance would be impaired. In the counterpointing tasks, the participants were asked to point to the opposite side of a screen to which a target was presented, whereas in a pointing condition the participants pointed directly at the target. The control children performed at ceiling when pointing and counterpointing. The WS group (aged 5-15 years) pointed to the correct side of the screen in all pointing trials and in 88% of the counterpointing trials; this rate was significantly lower than that achieved by controls. The WS group was also slower than the TD group on counterpointing trials and relied on the verbalisation of actions or made late movement corrections. The WS group therefore used compensatory measures; verbal strategies might have enabled inhibitory mechanisms to be applied at a later stage in the execution of the point, thus scaffolding counterpointing performance. The use of verbal strategies is not atypical (Matuga, 2003), and thus it would be interesting to determine how the pattern observed in WS compares with a younger control group of TD children for whom counterpointing performance is not at ceiling.

In the detour-reaching task, the participants can see a coloured ball through a window in a box, and the ball can be reached through a circular aperture. If children reach through this aperture, the ball falls out of sight in the box. The ball can be reached more indirectly by pulling a lever that pushes the ball into a tray that can be reached. The lever can be disabled (by the experimenter) and in this case a light illuminates on the box and children must press a switch in order to reach through the circular aperture to collect the ball without it falling. The latter condition is more cognitively demanding because there is no explicit link between pressing the switch and accessing the ball. TD children master this level of the task at 3 years 6 months. This is 1 year later than the condition using the lever. Children with WS (aged 3-13 years) performed well on the lever condition but showed many errors in the switch condition, such that 31% of participants failed to complete the task. Overall, 42% of children with WS failed to reach levels of TD children aged 3 year 6 months in the switch condition. Children with ASD also struggled to inhibit the prepotent reaching response to obtain the ball in the switch condition, making more errors than children with moderate learning difficulties matched for verbal ability (Hughes & Russell, 1993). This supports Sinzig et al.'s (2008) suggestion that difficulties with inhibition in ASD are perhaps attributable to unreported ADHD symptoms. These studies suggest that difficulty with inhibition tasks is qualitatively different in neurodevelopmental disorders such as ASD, WS and ADHD. Poor inhibition results from differing neural activation in neurodevelopmental disorders and thus from subtly distinct manifestations of disinhibtion (e.g. the dissociation of activation in the medial precuneus and posterior cingulate cortex in WS and ADHD).

The day/night task is a variation of the Stroop task (Stroop, 1935) and is suitable for use with children. Cards are shown with a line-drawing of a moon in a starry sky or a sun in a cloudy sky. Participants must inhibit the association between the sun and daytime and between the moon and night time and say the opposite name upon presentation of a card (e.g. saying 'day' when presented with a picture of the moon). Atkinson et al. (2003) showed that participants with WS performed at an age-appropriate level or above, with little evidence of poor inhibitory control. The WS group was accurate on 86% of control (no inhibition) trials and 83% of experimental trials, indicating that the prepotent association of the images on the cards with 'day' and 'night' could be inhibited.

The relatively strong performance on this task may be related to task demands and reflects the uneven cognitive profile in WS; while this task has a verbal component, the counter-pointing and detour-reaching box tasks are heavily reliant on spatial processing. In the day/night task, the rule can be vocalised in order to improve performance, an effect that has been documented in TD groups (Russell et al., 1999). As discussed earlier, participants with WS also made use of verbal strategies to circumvent spatial difficulties in the counterpointing task. Individuals with WS therefore used relative strengths (language) in order to scaffold weaker areas of cognition. Indeed, deficits in verbal self-regulation (speech used to direct behaviour) in ASD have been linked to poor performance in day/night tasks (Joseph et al., 2005).

Menghini et al. (2010) used a day/night-like task. In contrast to Atkinson et al. (2003), they showed evidence of poor performance in individuals with WS relative to mental-age-matched controls, but performance on a Stroop task was not significantly different from that of controls. This indicates that inhibition of responses is not necessarily typical in WS, even when verbal responses are required in the absence of spatial task demands. These studies suggest that use of verbalisation strategies may represent an adaptive approach to overcoming difficulties with tasks that tap frontoparietal function and aid performance in spatial tasks. Taken together, disinhibition is observed in a range of neurodevelopmental disorders, but is attributable to qualitatively different underlying impairments as evidenced by task-dependent patterns of deficits.

Inhibition and emotional/motivation executive functions

Early in development, executive-function ability in TD children is closely related to socio-emotional functioning. Children who are difficult to manage in a classroom can benefit from interventions that target executive function in order to improve social functioning, indicating an interplay between cognitive and emotional development (Riggs et al., 2006). This relationship between socio-emotional functioning and executive function is also observed in WS.

A defining feature of the WS cognitive profile, evident from a young age, is hypersociability and a propensity to approach strangers (Doyle et al., 2004; Udwin et al., 1998). Individuals with WS rate unfamiliar faces as highly approachable and show increased gaze frequency in infancy (Frigerio et al., 2006; Mervis et al., 2003; see also Chapter 15). Hypersociability is not unique to WS and has been reported in individuals with Down syndrome (DS) (Porter et al., 2007), although this can be masked by poor verbal ability and an inability to maintain an interaction. Hypersociability is also seen in individuals with amygdala damage (Holland & Gallagher, 2004) in which connections to the frontal lobe for emotion regulation and decision-making are disrupted, which reduces social inhibition. Porter et al. (2007) proposed that hypersociability in WS and DS may result from amygdala dysfunction, environmental influence owing to increased salience of social stimuli (such as the greater attention paid to faces by individuals with WS and DS) or frontal-lobe dysfunction. By assessing social approach and emotion recognition, Porter et al. (2007) concluded that hypersociability in both syndromes was best explained by frontal-lobe dysfunction. This is because patients with frontal-lobe dysfunction show abnormal social approach and emotion recognition behaviour, but are aware that this behaviour is inappropriate. This also describes behaviour that was observed in the WS and DS groups. This suggests that hypersociability may have its roots in poor response inhibition and, thus, that deficits in executive function range beyond impacting cognitive skills but also affect socio-emotional functioning in daily living.

Rhodes et al. (2010) related executive-function ability to behavioural measures of social functioning in participants with WS (age range: 11-29 years). Planning and set-shifting correlated highly with difficulties with attention, conduct and emotional regulation. This highlights the wider impact of executive dysfunction throughout development in neurodevelopmental disorders and implies that interventions that address poor inhibition could have cascading positive effects on many aspects of development.

Planning

Planning is an important executive function, and describes the ability to establish and sequence subgoals towards achieving an outcome. Difficulties in planning may affect a range of abilities in WS such as performance in visuospatial-construction tasks and planning of drawings. Drawing ability in WS is typified by production of the local elements of a model but a lack of global cohesion. The lack of cohesion might represent not only a visuospatial deficit but also a failure to adequately plan the integration of parts. Booth et al. (2003) examined graphic planning in ASD, ADHD and TD children and suggested that poor planning of part placements can result from excessive focus on local-level detail in atypical groups and disorganised hierarchical placement of parts in TD children. However, recent work (Hudson & Farran, 2009; Hudson & Farran, 2011) has shown that the pattern and level of graphic planning ability for simple shapes in WS is similar to that of a TD 6-year-old, but that individuals with WS have a low threshold for complexity such that planning breaks down for relatively complex figures (Hudson & Farran, 2011). Further research is therefore needed to understand the role of planning in drawings by those with neurodevelopmental disorders and whether this changes across the lifespan.

Interaction between task complexity and performance in block construction tasks

Hoffman et al. (2003) proposed that the difficulties observed in WS when solving block construction tasks could be explained by a deficit in planning and sequencing movements in order to copy the model. The ability to successfully complete this task is reliant upon segmentation of the model into its component blocks and the integration of these parts to form a whole that corresponds to the model. Individuals with WS are reported to select the correct component blocks to replicate a model but fail at the integration stage and do not form a cohesive representation of the configuration of the parts (e.g. Bellugi et al., 2000). This compares to superior performance in autism, which is accounted for by strong segmentation skills in this group (Shah & Frith, 1993). Patterns of performance in WS are also reported as an inverse of those of TD and DS groups, in which global-level detail takes precedence over local features (Bellugi et al., 2000; Brosnan et al., 2004). In addition, errors may be exacerbated by the slow and sequential approach to solving the task seen in WS groups (Hoffman et al., 2003).

Hoffman et al. (2003) presented simple (only single coloured blocks) and complex (one- and two-coloured blocks in which the colours were divided at oblique and vertical/horizontal orientation) computerised block constructions comprising two, three, four, six or nine blocks. Participants with WS altered the strategies employed between simple and complex puzzle-solving tasks, which suggests that the increased demands placed on the ability to comprehend spatial relations in complex tasks impacts upon the use of executive skills. The WS group solved the simple puzzles strategically, checking the model and the replication frequently to plan part placements. When puzzles became complex, participants with WS verbalised their anticipated failure to replicate the model prior to completion and looked less frequently between the model and the copy. The model was inspected once and the parts were quickly placed, with a final look to the model. There was little evidence of checking between the model and the copy in order to determine the accuracy of the replication, as seen in the simple puzzles (for further evidence of this pattern, see Hudson & Farran, submitted). Performance was weak relative to simple puzzle completion, particularly on puzzles with many blocks. This indicates that individuals with WS show poor planning when tasks are complex but can plan efficiently when presented with simple constructions.

A similar effect of complexity has been observed when individuals with WS draw intersecting and embedded figures. Drawing and construction becomes less strategy-driven than in nonverbal ability-matched TD controls when figures contain many, compared with fewer, spatial relations (Hudson & Farran, 2011).

This interaction between task complexity and performance provides an interesting insight into the inter-relationship between visuospatial cognition and executive-function abilities in WS. It is perhaps too simplistic to explain visuospatial ability in WS in terms of a propensity towards local-level features of visual scenes (see Chapter 12 for further discussion of visuospatial cognition) without also considering the engagement of executive-function ability.

Assessment of multiple aspects of executive function in William syndrome

Research into executive function in WS has recently begun to assess the relationship between executive-function abilities rather than examination of executive functions in isolation. Menghini et al. (2010) assessed attention, planning, shifting and inhibition and Rhodes et al. (2010) investigated set-shifting and planning. Menghini et al. (2010) used a wide range of tasks such as planning, working memory, and attention and inhibition tasks with a WS group (age range: 11-35 years) and controls matched for mental age (mental age range: 5-8 years). There was mixed evidence of poor attention in WS; visual selective and auditory sustained attention were poor, whereas auditory selective and visual sustained attention were not significantly different from those in controls matched for mental age. Visual selective attention is likely to have been impaired in WS because of the spatial task demands. Participants had to group pairs of items that were in close proximity and interpretation of spatial relations may have been problematic for the WS group (Farran, 2005). Therefore, there is disparity between differing types of attention ability in WS, with performance at or below the level expected for the mental age.

Planning was assessed by Menghini et al. (2010) using the Tower of London task, in which participants must replicate a sequence of movements of balls on pegs according to specified rules. The WS group solved fewer puzzles than the control group, but in a comparable time. Poor planning may have resulted from inadequate inhibition of responses because individuals with WS made impulsive moves rather than determining future moves towards the end-state positions. Poor mental imagery in WS (Farran et al., 2001; Vicari et al., 2001) may also have led to lower performance than expected for mental age, because of the inability to visualise the outcome of different moves to complete the puzzles. In a computer-based version of this task (Rhodes et al., 2010), the WS group made more moves to complete puzzles than controls matched for verbal ability and chronological age. However, thinking times in the WS group were comparable with those of TD children matched for verbal ability. Planning ability as evidenced by problem-solving tasks is therefore poor in WS. This may be exacerbated by the impact of wider cognitive and executive dysfunction.

Participants with WS took longer than controls in a trail-making task that assessed set-shifting behaviour (Menghini et al., 2010). Trail-making is achieved by drawing a line between alternating letters and numbers on a page, for example 'A', '1', 'B', '2'. The finding by Menghini et al. suggests that set-shifting (between letters and numbers) in WS is poor when spatial relations need to be interpreted and produced. However, there was no difference between groups when set-shifting was assessed using a verbal task. In the verbal set-shifting task, the participants were required to produce pairs of words belonging to specified categories, but to interleave the pairs; for example, if the categories were items of furniture and animals, the participants could respond 'chair, rabbit, table, elephant'.

Rhodes et al. (2010) used a computerised analogue of the Wisconsin Card Sorting Test in order to assess set-shifting. Individuals with WS (age range: 11-29 years) demonstrated poorer performance than TD participants matched for chronological age and gender or TD participants matched for verbal ability. This task is associated with a heavy load on attention and visual discrimination abilities, which is likely to have made the task particularly difficult for the WS group. In agreement with the results reported by Menghini et al. (2010), poor performance in set-shifting was seen where there was little verbal load. The poorer performance relative to the verbal-matched group is perhaps not surprising owing to verbal ability being a relative strength in WS when contrasted with relatively poor visuospatial and executive-function skills (Jarrold et al., 1998). It is therefore likely that the visuospatial cognition in the WS group was lower than that of the controls. This underlines the importance of matching for abilities that are likely to subserve performance in experimental tasks where matching is used; for example Raven's Coloured Progressive Matrices (Raven, 1993) are frequently used for matching participants in visuospatial tasks (see Van Herwegen et al., 2011). Indeed, a more developmental approach would be to explore the relationship between visuospatial and/or verbal maturation and task performance in the WS group and to compare this with typical development within the same developmental range (see Chapter 1).

Summary of executive function in WS

As a whole, these studies illustrate the diffuse nature of executive-function performance in WS. It seems apparent that where verbal ability can be employed to solve tasks, individuals with WS perform at the level expected for their mental age, but that in tasks that rely on an understanding of spatial relations, performance is poor. This difficulty is borne out in drawing tasks, where replication of multiple spatial relations between parts of an image can render drawings unrecognisable (Hudson & Farran, 2011).

Assessing the relationship between executive-function abilities in WS highlights the disparity between tasks that measure different executive functions and tap into distinct domains in WS, but also in other neurodevelopmental disorders. Andersen and Cui (2009) have suggested that the interplay between executive functions such as attention and planning are implicated in sequencing and generating movements. The lateral intraparietal region allocates attention and guides the occulomotor system when planning saccades (Corbetta et al., 1998). Therefore, if executive function is atypical, this may constrain motor functioning (such as saccadic eye movements or reaching behaviour) and, in turn, interaction with the environment, leading to further atypical neural development and cortical specialisation.

Motor planning

Wolpert et al. (1995) proposed two internal models that determine motor plans of action. These models identify when a mismatch between vision and action occurs. At a cortical level, the intraparietal sulcus and mediolateral cerebellum work in a functional loop in order to estimate motor states during movement execution (Blakemore & Sirigu, 2003). Generation and execution of a motor plan therefore represents a complex process of prediction, action and correction of movements (see also Chapter 13). Individuals with WS commonly show a delay in achieving developmental motor milestones (Carrasco et al., 2005). Supported walking is typically achieved by 11 months in TD infants but does not occur until 18 months in children with WS. Into adulthood, 68% of people with WS report difficulties with walking, particularly over uneven surfaces and while descending stairs and slopes (Withers, 1996). In addition, 92% of individuals with WS show a deficit in motor planning (Semel & Rosner, 2003). Along with perceptual difficulties, poor motor planning is probably the root of atypical walking behaviour in WS. Research into gross motor function in WS is hampered by orthopaedic and biomechanical symptoms such as instability of joints that alter gait patterns (Elliott et al., 2006; Hocking et al., 2008).

Cerebellar dysfunction and motor planning

A recent theory posits that cerebellar dysfunction in WS may be the basis of motor and some perceptual difficulties seen in the syndrome (Hocking et al., 2008). Enlargement of the cerebellar vermis is commonly reported in neuroimaging studies of individuals with WS across the lifespan (Jones et al., 2002). This suggests that this neuroatypicality is stable across development and allows for mapping of brain–behaviour links. Cerebellar involvement is also suggested in a range of neurodevelopmental disorders that manifest motor control abnormalities, such as general developmental delay (Webb et al., 2009), ASD (Gowen & Miall, 2005), fragile X syndrome (Huber, 2006) and fetal alcohol syndrome (Riikonen et al., 1999), in which the cerebellum is either atrophied or enlarged. In typical development, the dentate nuclei and lateral portions of the cerebellar hemispheres mediate motor planning, particularly in multijoint movements and fine motor control (Fredericks, 1996). The cerebellum is therefore a potential candidate to explain difficulties in walking, stair descent and fine motor control in neurodevelopmental disorders.

Walking and stair-descent cross-syndrome comparisons

Walking is highly demanding of executive functions such as planning and task monitoring because steady gait relies on correct sequencing and execution of a motor plan and constant monitoring of body position and foot location. To avoid falling, one must also monitor the surface that is walked on and potential obstacles, further increasing both motor and executive demands to update one's position in space and the intended location. Reliance on visual cues for walking has been suggested as the root of gait abnormalities in children with developmental coordination disorder (Deconinck et al., 2006).

Hocking et al. (2009) provided the first systematic investigation of gait characteristics in adults with WS. Walking was typified by variable, slow, broad-based steps that resembled gait hypokinesia owing to irregular stride length but not step frequency. Performance IQ (from the Wechsler Adult Intelligence Scale Third Edition [WAIS-III]; Wechsler, 1997) correlated with stride length when walking at the preferred, slowed or fast speed, and processing speed (from WAIS-III) was related to stride length when walking slowly.

Holtzer et al. (2006) have related executive function (attention and problem-solving) to gait velocity in TD older adults and have argued against a view that walking is largely an automatic process. In WS, a dorsal-stream deficit further impacts upon walking because of difficulty in planning and controlling walking through the use of online visuomotor integration (Atkinson et al., 1997).

Spatiotemporal patterns of gait in Parkinson disease can be successfully improved by internal and external cueing (Morris et al., 1996). In Parkinson disease, basal ganglia disruption leads to a shortening of steps attributable to inadequate motor plan generation (by providing phasic cues to the supplementary motor area) and execution that is disrupted by atypical spatial processing (Almeida & Lebold, 2010).

Hocking et al. (2010) manipulated executive and visual cues used while WS, DS and TD (age- and gender-matched) adult participants walked. The participants were instructed to walk at their preferred speed and use internal and external cuing to increase their normal stride length by 20% because stride length in WS and DS was typically short. The participants were internally cued by specifically attending to increasing the stride length. External cueing was achieved during walking by stepping on markers placed on the floor set at distances greater than the preferred stride length. The ability to adapt preferred gait patterns is a core ability in order to navigate uneven surfaces and descend stairs, both of which are commonly difficult for people with WS. Processing of internal cues is a complex task that relies on continual updating of motor plans and visual cues. External cueing reduced motor and executive demands because it facilitated movement planning by providing visual cues for walking. Individuals with WS found increasing their stride length problematic with both internal and external cues because their preferred stride lengths were short. When using internal cues, the gait speed decreased and the gait variability increased in WS; when using external cues, the gait speed and the cadence (steps per minute) were reduced. When using internal cues, one must allocate attention to internal and external environmental states. It is possible that this exceeds attentional resource limits during walking in WS. Furthermore, frontoparietal and executive dysfunction in WS may affect internally cued gait through a failure to inhibit walking with preferred spatiotemporal patterns. WS performance contrasted with that in the DS and TD groups, who showed no significant difference between baseline and cued walking ability, indicating that individuals with DS are relatively less impaired at cued walking than people with WS. This highlights the importance of cross-syndrome comparisons to reveal subtle differences in motor execution and provides an avenue for remediation strategies in neurodevelopmental disorders associated with difficulties in motor execution, such as WS and DS.

Difficulty and hesitancy with stair descent are seen in a range of neurodevelopmental disorders such as WS (Van der Geest et al., 2005; Cowie et al., in press), ASD and sensory-processing disorder (a disorder characterised by a difficulty in the integration of visual and motor information throughout development) (May-Benson et al., 2009). Stair descent in WS may be atypical because of difficulties interpreting depth cues in order to guide movement (Van der Geest et al., 2005). If depth processing is aberrant, motor plans based upon this information will not be sufficient to allow for a smooth descent of stairs. Depth cues from steps are not always apparent and instead these cues must be deduced by perceptual features such as boundaries between textures and interposition of steps. Stepping down on stairs is therefore a complex motor and cognitive task. TD children as young as 3 years old can successfully use visual information in order to plan a smooth descent of steps (Cowie et al., 2010). The generation of a motor plan to control descent therefore relies on the integration and processing of a number of cues in order to accommodate appropriate sequencing and execution of movements. Individuals with WS report that walking aids such as sticks can be used to guide stepping down. This may provide useful haptic (as opposed to visual) depth cues in order to permit motor programmes to be planned. The laboured step-by-step approach to stair descent in WS is probably a manifestation of reliance upon short-term motor plans with short end-state points (going down step by step rather than looking at the staircase as a whole).

Reaching

We reach for objects every day with little thought of the complex integration of biomechanical and perceptual cues that are required to complete the action. Atypical reaching is seen in autism (Mari et al., 2003) and developmental coordination disorder (Johnston et al., 2002), in which planning and execution of reaches results in awkward, slow movements. Correct sequencing of movements required to make a reach relies on online visuomotor control using the dorsal visual stream.

A deficit in dorsal-stream functioning may underlie some atypical reaching behaviour in WS (see Chapter 13). Atkinson et al. (1997) assessed dorsal- and ventral-stream processing in children with WS and TD children and adults. The participants posted a card though a slot (dorsal task) or orientated a mannequin's hand to post a card (ventral task). In the ventral task, 55% of the participants with WS orientated the mannequin's hand similarly to TD controls and the remaining participants with WS produced greater orientation errors than controls. TD adults and older children showed fewer orientation errors in the dorsal task compared with TD 4-year-olds and 82% of the WS group (the remaining 18% orientated similarly to adults who had developed typically). Unlike the TD participants, the individuals with WS adopted an awkward arm position when posting the card. The card was rotated in an incorrect direction and orientation, such as flat against the postbox. This results from poor visuomotor integration to plan the correct trajectory and orientation for the hand.

The goal is the same in both dorsal and ventral tasks: a hand must be orientated in order to align the card and slot. The additional demands of integrating visual flow with the dorsal stream led to poor and often erroneous performance in the WS group. Errors in orientating the hand may also reflect the inability to generate a motor plan for the correct orientation of the hand. TD adults and children can readily accommodate both reaching and locomotive moments to account for end-state comfort (Cowie et al., 2010). Initial movements may be awkward in order to achieve a final comfortable position. The findings of Atkinson et al. (1997) may reflect the inability of the WS group to plan for end-state comfort.

Elliott et al. (2006) sought to establish whether the deficits in visuomotor tasks in WS were linked to the visual regulation of movement or a dysfunction in movement planning. The study examined adults with WS, neurodevelopmental disorders (DS or unspecified aetiology) and TD controls. The participants completed a computerised aiming task in which a computer mouse was placed on tracks to permit movement on only a single axis away from the body midline. The participants moved the mouse from a home location to one of three targets. The mouse cursor either remained in view during movement (vision condition) or disappeared when it had left the home location (no-vision condition).

The participants in the neurodevelopmental disorder groups exhibited greater response times than the TD controls. This increase resulted from greater time spent planning and executing the reaching movement in both conditions. The neurodevelopmental disorder groups differed kinematically from TD adults in the fluency and velocity of their movements, which were slowed with discontinuous trajectories. The discontinuity of the movements could reflect both inefficient updating of proprioceptive information about the location of the hand and poor online planning for adjustments to the movement on the basis of errors and mismatches to the original plan. The participants were able to reach the target with practice, indicating that in neurodevelopmental disorders, slow and regularly updated practising of movements aids learning in motor programmes.

The WS group had difficulty with initial movement execution when aiming to far targets, with a lower peak velocity that was slowed and poorly scaled relative to the neurodevelopmental disorder group. This indicates ineffective movement planning prior to onset of the reach motion because account has not been taken of the intended end state and the means to reach this point. Individuals with WS therefore seem to continually generate motor plans for smaller end-state points before meeting a target. This may be a compensatory strategy to overcome dorsal-stream difficulties. Reaching behaviour in WS therefore provides useful insight into motor planning, indicating that planning is atypical and may be adaptive, based on cognitive and biomechanical constraints.

Conclusions

More research is needed to better understand executive function and motor planning in WS across the lifespan. Much research focuses on single abilities in isolation and at single time points, without an appreciation of the progression of abilities with development. Diamond (2000) has argued that deficits in executive function might originate from motor planning impairments owing to the role of the cerebellum and prefrontal cortex. This suggests that atypicality in these areas early in development might impact upon the development of executive function and motor ability. With the wider use of developmental trajectory approaches in future research, facets of executive function and motor planning ability could be related to typical and atypical groups as well as between domains. This approach should be used in combination with a methodology that assesses relative ability across combinations of executive-function tasks, because research to date has revealed disparate performance in executive-function tasks even when they are purported to assess the same abilities. Mervis and John (2010) argued that executive-function ability may be consistent with the overall WS cognitive profile; tasks that can be verbally mediated lead to better performance than those with motor or spatial components. The performance in WS groups can be aided by verbalising strategies as a compensatory measure for poor executive-function ability. The use of compensatory strategies may be a result of neural restructuring to bypass atypical pathways. Neuroimaging and genetic techniques allow for WS to provide an insight into the interaction of genes, behaviour and the brain using a neuroconstructivist approach.

Editor commentary (Emily K. Farran & Annette Karmiloff-Smith)

The term 'executive function' encompasses a range of domain-general processes such as attention switching, working memory and inhibition of a prepotent response, as well as emotional processes such as affective impulses. Typical developmental trajectories of executive function do not reach an adult end state until mid-adolescence, meaning that the opportunity for atypical multilevel interactions is far-reaching. In this chapter, we learnt that executive functions, as well as motor planning, are impaired in WS. Multilevel analyses of WS and ADHD demonstrate that poor response inhibition is associated with increased or decreased activation of the same areas of the brain, respectively, emphasising the neuroconstructivist stance that similar behaviour does not necessarily stem from the same associations at the neural level. We also observed that, similar to the memory profile (Chapter 8), the profile of executive functions in people with WS is not simply delayed, but is influenced by their cognitive profile of stronger verbal than nonverbal abilities, such that performance is poorer on tasks that are predominantly spatial in nature, compared with those that can be solved using verbal strategies. Motor planning is also impaired in WS. This has been linked to the atypical structure of the cerebellum (see Chapter 2), which has been implicated in both executive functions and motor planning. Cross-syndrome comparisons across other neurodevelopmental disorders that show cerebellar abnormalities, such as fragile X syndrome and fetal alcohol syndrome, will help to determine the nature of neural and behavioural integration between executive processes and motor planning.

References

Almeida, Q.J., & Lebold, C.A. (2010). Freezing of gait in Parkinson's disease: a perceptual cause for a motor impairment? *Journal of Neurology, Neurosurgery and Psychiatry*, **81**, 513–18.

Andersen, R.A., & Cui, H. (2009). Intention, action planning, and decision making in parietal-frontal circuits. *Neuron*, **63**, 568–83.

Ardila, A. (2008). On the evolutionary origins of executive functions. *Brain and Cognition*, **68**, 92–99.

Atkinson, J., Braddick, O., Anker, S., Curran, Q., Adrew, R., Wattam-Bell, J., & et al. (2003). Neurobiological models of visuospatial cognition in children with Williams syndrome: measures of dorsal-stream and frontal function. *Developmental Neuropsychology, 23*, 139–72.

Atkinson, J., King, J., Braddick, O., Nokes, L., Anker, S., & Braddick, F. (1997). A specific deficit of dorsal stream function in Williams syndrome. *NeuroReport*, **8**, 1919–22.

Bellugi, U., Lichtenberger, L., Jones, W., Lai, Z., & St. George, M. (2000). The neurocognitive profile of Williams syndrome: a complex pattern of strengths and weaknesses. *Journal of Cognitive Neuroscience*, **12 Supplement 1, 7–29.

Blakemore, S.-J., & Sirigu, A. (2003). Action prediction in the cerebellum and in the parietal lobe. *Experimental Brain Research*, **153**, 239–45.

Booth, R., Charlton, R., Hughes, C., & Happé, F. (2003). Disentangling weak coherence and executive dysfunction: planning drawing in autism and attention-deficit/hyperactivity disorder. *Philosophical Transactions of the Royal Society B: Biological Sciences*, **358**, 387–92.

Brosnan, M.J., Scott, F.J., Fox, S., & Pye, J. (2004). Gestalt processing in autism: failure to process relationships and implications for contextual understanding. *Journal of Child Psychology and Psychiatry*, **45**, 459–69.

Carrasco, X., Castillo, S., Aravena, T., Rothhammer, P., & Aboitiz, F. (2005). Williams syndrome: pediatric, neurologic and cognitive development. *Pediatric Neurology*, **32**, 166–72.

Corbetta, M., Akbudak, E., Conturo, T.E., Snyder, A.Z., Ollinger, J.M., Drury, H.A., et al. (1998). A common network of functional areas for attention and eye movements. *Neuron*, **21**, 761–73.

Cowie, D., Atkinson, J., & Braddick, O. (2010). Development of visual control in stepping down. *Experimental Brain Research, 202*, 181–88.

Cowie, D., Braddick, O., & Atkinson, J. (in press). Visually guided locomotion in children with Williams syndrome. *Developmental Science*.

Deconinck, F.J.A., Clercq, D.D., Savelsbergh, G.J.P., Coster, R.V., Oostra, A., Dewitte, G., et al. (2006). Visual contribution to walking in children with Developmental Coordination Disorder. *Child: Care, Health and Development*, **32**, 711–22.

Diamond, A. (2000). Close interrelation of motor development and cognitive development and of the cerebellum and prefrontal cortex. *Child Development*, **71**, 44–56.

Doyle, T.F., Bellugi, U., Korenberg, J.R., & Graham, J. (2004). 'Everybody in the world is my friend': hypersociability in young children with Williams syndrome. *American Journal of Medical Genetics*, **124**, 263–73.

Elliott, D., Welsh, T.N., Lyons, J., Hansen, S., & Wu, M. (2006). The visual regulation of goal-directed reaching movements in adults with Williams syndrome, Down syndrome, and other developmental delays. *Motor Control*, **10**, 34–54.

Farran, E.K. (2005). Perceptual grouping ability in Williams syndrome: evidence for deviant patterns of performance. *Neuropsychologia*, **43**, 815–22.

Farran, E.K., Jarrold, C. & Gathercole, S.E. (2001). Block design performance in the Williams syndrome phenotype: a problem with mental imagery? *Journal of Child Psychology and Psychiatry*, **42**, 719–28.

Fredericks, C.M. (1996). Disorders of the cerebellum and its connections. In C.M. Fredericks & L.K. Saladin (Eds), *Pathophysiology of the Motor Systems: Principles and Clinical Presentations* (pp. 445–66). Philadelphia, PA: F.A. Davis Company.

Frigerio, E., Burt, D.M., Gagliardi, C., Cioffi, G., Martelli, S., Perrett, D.I., et al. (2006). Is everybody always my friend? Perception of approachability in Williams syndrome. *Neuropsychologia*, **44**, 254–59.

Fuster, J.M. (2002). Frontal lobe and cognitive development. *Journal of Neurocytology*, **31**, 373–85.

Garavan, H., Ross, T.J., & Stein, E.A. (1999). Right hemispheric dominance of inhibitory control: an event-related functional MRI study. *Proceedings of the National Academy of Sciences of the USA*, **96**, 8301–8306.

Gowen, E., & Miall, R. (2005). Behavioural aspects of cerebellar function in adults with Asperger syndrome. *The Cerebellum*, **4**, 279–89.

Haywood, K.M., & Getchell, N. (2009). *Life Span Motor Development*, 5th edn. Champaign, IL: Human Kinetics Publishers.

Hocking, D.R., Bradshaw, J.L., & Rinehart, N.J. (2008). Fronto-parietal and cerebellar contributions to motor dysfunction in Williams syndrome: a review and future directions. *Neuroscience and Biobehavioral Reviews*, **32**, 497–507.

Hocking, D.R., McGinley, J.L., Moss, S.A., Bradshaw, J.L., & Rinehart, N.J. (2010). Effects of external and internal cues on gait function in Williams syndrome. *Journal of the Neurological Sciences*, **291**, 57–63.

Hocking, D., Rinehart, N., McGinley, J., & Bradshaw, J. (2009). Gait function in adults with Williams syndrome. *Experimental Brain Research,* **192**, 695–702.

Hoffman, J.E., Landau, B., & Pagani, B. (2003). Spatial breakdown in spatial construction: evidence from eye fixations in children with Williams syndrome. *Cognitive Psychology*, **46**, 260–301.

Holland, P.C., & Gallagher, M. (2004). Amygdala-frontal interactions and reward expectancy. *Current Opinion in Neurobiology*, **14**, 148–55.

Holtzer, R., Verghese, J., Xue, X., & Lipton, R.B. (2006). Cognitive processes related to gait velocity: results from the Einstein aging study. *Neuropsychology*, **20**, 215–23.

Hoshi, E., & Tanji, J. (2007). Distinctions between dorsal and ventral premotor areas: anatomical connectivity and functional properties. *Current Opinion in Neurobiology*, **17**, 234–42.

Huber, K.M. (2006). The fragile X–cerebellum connection. *Trends in Neurosciences*, **29**, 183–85.

Hudson, K.D., & Farran, E.K. (September 2009) *Graphic Planning Ability in Williams syndrome.* Presented at the British Psychological Society Developmental Section Conference 2009, Nottingham.

Hudson, K.D., & Farran, E.K. (2011). Drawing the line: drawing and construction strategies for simple and complex figures in Williams syndrome and typical development. *British Journal of Developmental Psychology.* **29**, 687–705.

Hudson, K., & Farran, E.K. (submitted). Looking around houses: Attention to a model when drawing complex shapes in Williams syndrome and typical development. *British Journal of Developmental Psychology.*

Hughes, C., & Russell, J. (1993). Autistic children's difficulty with mental disengagement from an object: its implications for theories of autism. *Developmental Psychology*, **29**, 498–510.

Jarrold, C., Baddeley, A.D., & Hewes, A.K. (1998). Verbal and nonverbal abilities in the Williams syndrome phenotype: evidence for diverging developmental trajectories. *Journal of Child Psychology and Psychiatry*, **39**, 511–23.

Johnston, L.M., Burns, Y.R., Brauer, S.G., & Richardson, C.A. (2002). Differences in postural control and movement performance during goal directed reaching in children with developmental coordination disorder. *Human Movement Science,* **21**, 583–601.

Jones, W., Hesselink, J., Courchesne, E., Duncan, T., Matsuda, K., & Bellugi, U. (2002). Cerebellar abnormalities in infants and toddlers with Williams syndrome. *Developmental Medicine & Child Neurology*, **44**, 688–94.

Joseph, R.M., McGrath, L.M., & Tager-Flusberg, H. (2005). Executive dysfunction and its relation to language ability in verbal school-age children with Autism. *Developmental Psychology*, **27**, 361–78.

Leyfer, O.T., Woodruff-Borden, J., Klein-Tasman, B.P., Fricke, J.S., & Mervis, C.B. (2006). Prevalence of psychiatric disorders in 4 to 16-year-olds with Williams syndrome. *American Journal of Medical Genetics Part B: Neuropsychiatric Genetics*, **141B**, 615–22.

Luna, B., Padmanabhan, A., & O'Hearn, K. (2010). What has fMRI told us about the development of cognitive control through adolescence? *Brain and Cognition*, **72**, 101–113.

Mari, M., Castiello, U., Marks, D., Marraffa, C., & Prior, M. (2003). The reach-to-grasp movement in children with autism spectrum disorder. *Philosophical Transactions of the Royal Society of London. Series B: Biological Sciences,* **358**, 393–403.

Matuga, J.M. (2003). Children's private speech during algorithmic and heuristic drawing tasks. *Contemporary Educational Psychology,* **28**, 552–72.

May-Benson, T.A., Koomar, J.A., & Teasdale, A. (2009). Incidence of pre-, peri-, and post-natal birth and developmental problems of children with sensory processing disorder and children with autism spectrum disorder. *Frontiers in Integrative Neuroscience,* **3**, 1–12.

Mervis, C.B., & John, A.E. (2010). Cognitive and behavioral characteristics of children with Williams syndrome: implications for intervention approaches. *American Journal of Medical Genetics Part C: Seminars in Medical Genetics,* **154C**, 229–48.

Mervis, C.B., Morris, C.A., Klein-Tasman, B.P., Bertrand, J., Kwitn, S. Appelbaum, L.G., et al. (2003). Attentional characteristics of infants and toddlers with Williams syndrome during triadic interactions. *Developmental Neuropsychology,* **23**, 243–68.

Menghini, D., Addona, F., Costanzo, F., & Vicari, S. (2010). Executive functions in individuals with Williams syndrome. *Journal of Intellectual Disability Research,* **54**, 418–32.

Miyake, A., Friedman, N., Emerson, M.J., Witzki, A.H., Howerter, A., & Wager, T.D. (2000). The unity and diversity of executive functions and their contributions to complex '"frontal lobe" tasks: a latent variable analysis. *Cognitive Psychology,* **41**, 49–100.

Mobbs, D., Eckert, M.A., Mills, D., Korenberg, J., Bellugi, U., Galaburda, A.M., et al. (2007). Frontostriatal dysfunction during response inhibition in Williams syndrome. *Biological Psychiatry,* **62**, 256–61.

Morris, M.E., Iansek, R., Matyas, T.A., & Summers, J.J. (1996). Stride length regulation in Parkinson's disease: normalization strategies and underlying mechanisms. *Brain,* **119**, 551–68.

Porter, M.A., Coltheart, M., & Langdon, R. (2007). The neuropsychological basis of hypersociability in Williams and Down syndrome. *Neuropsychologia,* **45**, 2839–49.

Raven, J.C. (1993). *Coloured progressive matrices.* Oxford: Information Press.

Rhodes, S.M., Riby, D.M., Park, J., Fraser, E., & Campbell, L.E. (2010). Executive neuropsychological functioning in individuals with Williams syndrome. *Neuropsychologia,* **48**, 1216–26.

Riggs, N.R., Jahromi, L.B., Razza, R.P., Dillworth-Bart, J.E., & Mueller, U. (2006). Executive function and the promotion of social-emotional competence. *Journal of Applied Developmental Psychology,* **27**, 300–309.

Riikonen, R., Salonen, I., Partanen, K., & Verho, S. (1999). Brain perfusion SPECT and MRI in foetal alcohol syndrome. *Developmental Medicine & Child Neurology,* **41**, 652–59.

Rubia, K., Smith, A.B., Brammer, M.J., Toone, B., & Taylor, E. (2005). Abnormal brain activation during inhibition and error detection in medication-naïve adolescents with ADHD. *American Journal of Psychiatry,* **162**, 1067–75.

Russell, J., Jarrold, C., & Hood, B. (1999). Two intact executive capacities in children with autism: implications for the core executive dysfunctions in the disorder. *Journal of Autism and Developmental Disorders,* **29**, 103–112.

Semel, E.M., & Rosner, S.R. (2003). Perceptual and motor performance. In E.M. Semel & S.R. Rosner, *Understanding Williams Syndrome: Behavioural Patterns and Interventions* (pp. 108–186). Mahwah, NJ: Lawrence Erlbaum.

Shah, A., & Frith, U. (1993). Why do autistic individuals show superior performance on the Block Design task? *Journal of Child Psychology and Psychiatry,* **34**, 1351–64.

Sinzig, J., Morsch, D., Bruning, N., Schmidt, M., & Lehmkuhl, G. (2008). Inhibition, flexibility, working memory and planning in autism spectrum disorders with and without comorbid ADHD-symptoms. *Child and Adolescent Psychiatry and Mental Health,* **2**, 4–16.

Sober, S.J., & Sabes, P.N. (2003). Multisensory integration during motor planning. *Journal of Neuroscience,* **23**, 6982–92.

Stroop, J.R. (1935). Studies of interference in serial verbal reactions. *Journal of Experimental Psychology*, **18**, 643–62.

Udwin, O., Howlin, P., Davies, M., & Mannion, E. (1998). Community care for adults with Williams syndrome: how families cope and the availability of support networks. *Journal of Intellectual Disability Research*, **42**, 238–45.

Van der Geest, J.N., Lagers-van Haselen, G.C., van Hagen, J.M., Brenner, E., Govaerts, L.C.P., de Coo, I.F.M. et al. (2005). Visual depth processing in Williams–Beuren syndrome. *Experimental Brain Research*, **166**, 200–209.

Van Herwegen, J., Farran, E.K., Annaz, D. (2011). Item and error analysis on Raven's Coloured Progressive Matrices in Williams Syndrome. *Research in Developmental Disabilities*, **32**, 93–99.

Vicari, S., Bellucci, S., & Carlesimo, G.A. (2001). Procedural learning deficit in children with Williams syndrome. *Neuropsychologia*, **39**, 665–77.

Webb, S.J., Sparks, B.-F., Friedman, S.D., Shaw, D.W.W., Giedd, J., Dawson, G., et al. (2009). Cerebellar vermal volumes and behavioral correlates in children with autism spectrum disorder. *Psychiatry Research: Neuroimaging,* **172**, 61–67.

Wechsler. (1997). *Wechsler Adult Intelligence Scale Third Edition.* San Antonio, TX: The Psychological Corporation.

Withers, S. (1996). A new clinical sign in Williams syndrome. *Archives of Disease in Childhood*, **75**, 89.

Wolpert, D.M., Ghahramani, Z., & Jordan, M.I. (1995). An internal model for sensorimotor integration. *Science*, **269**, 1880–82.

Part 4

Domain-Specific Processes

Part 4a

Verbal Domain

Chapter 10

Precursors to language and early language

Carolyn B. Mervis and Angela E. John

Introduction

The focus of this chapter is on precursors to language acquisition and the acquisition of language by toddlers, preschool children and early primary-school children who have Williams syndrome (WS). In the first report of the psychological characteristics of individuals with WS, von Arnim and Engel (1964) described children with this syndrome as having 'an unusual command of language' (p.367) despite severe intellectual disability. This depiction of individuals with WS as having normal or near-normal language abilities in the face of very significant intellectual disability has continued to make headlines both in the popular press (e.g. Cowley, 2003; Dobbs, 2007; Finn, 1991) and among academic pundits (e.g. Jackendoff, 1994; Piattelli-Palmarini, 2001; Pinker, 1999).

WS came to the attention of behavioural researchers through the pioneering work of Bellugi and her colleagues (Bellugi et al., 1988), who argued—consistent with von Arnim and Engel's (1964) statement—that WS provided a paradigmatic case of the independence of language from cognition and thus clear evidence for the modularity of language. Bellugi et al. (1988) reported on three adolescents with WS who comprehended and produced complex linguistic constructions (e.g. reversible passives, embedded relative clauses, conditionals, tag questions). At the same time, they were unable to conserve either number or quantity, cognitive abilities that had been argued to be necessary for the comprehension of complex syntactic constructions (Beilin, 1975). These adolescents also were reported to use 'unusual vocabulary' (Bellugi et al., 1988, p.182) and to have vocabulary abilities that were higher than expected for their mental age (MA).

Over the last two decades, researchers have more comprehensively studied the language and cognitive abilities of individuals with WS. The results of studies of adolescents and adults have indicated that rather than being associated with severe intellectual disability, WS is characterised by overall intellectual abilities in the borderline-to-moderate intellectual disability range (Howlin et al., 1998; Howlin et al., 2010; Searcy et al., 2004) with a characteristic pattern of relative strengths in language (particularly vocabulary) and verbal short-term memory and considerable weakness in visuospatial construction (e.g. Mervis et al., 2000). At the same time, rather than language skills being independent of cognition, they are strongly correlated with nonverbal cognitive abilities. For example, Mervis (1999) found significant and strong correlations between receptive vocabulary, receptive grammar, nonverbal reasoning, visuospatial construction, verbal short-term memory and verbal working memory. Partial correlational analyses indicated that the relations between language and visuospatial-construction abilities were mediated primarily by nonverbal reasoning and verbal working memory.

Studies of adolescents and adults with WS have also yielded a characteristic pattern of language strengths and weaknesses. The area of greatest strength is concrete vocabulary. When researchers include multiple standardised assessments in their batteries, the highest mean standard score is consistently for the Peabody Picture Vocabulary Test (PPVT; e.g. Dunn & Dunn, 1981, 1997, 2007; adapted as the British Picture Vocabulary Scale in the UK, e.g. Dunn et al., 1997), which measures concrete receptive vocabulary (e.g. Brock et al., 2007; Mervis & John, 2010b). Bellugi and her colleagues (e.g. Bellugi et al., 1988; Bellugi et al., 2000) reported the same pattern, but for age equivalents. Interestingly, the finding that PPVT age equivalents are higher than nonverbal age equivalents also has been reported for adults with Down syndrome (DS) (e.g. Glenn & Cunningham, 2005; however, see Bellugi et al., 2000, for contradictory findings). Problems in interpreting findings based on age equivalents are discussed in Mervis and Robinson (2005). The grammatical abilities of adolescents and adults with WS are at the level expected for overall level of intellectual ability (Mervis, 2006; see Chapter 11 for reviews) and pragmatics is an area of considerable weakness. Laws and Bishop (2004) reported that 79% of adolescent and adult participants with WS (but only 50% of participants with DS) met the criterion for pragmatic language impairment on the Children's Communication Checklist (Bishop, 1998).

In the remainder of this chapter, we briefly summarise the findings from research on the intellectual abilities of toddlers and young children with WS as measured by performance on standardised assessments. We then describe the findings from research on the early language phenotype of WS, focusing on results related to prelinguistic and early language development in the areas of vocabulary (lexicon), grammar and pragmatics. Two central themes will emerge. First, despite the initial claims regarding the independence of language from cognition, WS provides strong evidence for their interdependence throughout development. Second, there is considerable continuity in the pattern of strengths and weaknesses across development, with the adult pattern apparent in early childhood.

General intellectual ability

The cognitive profile associated with WS is most apparent when intellectual abilities are assessed by the Differential Ability Scales (DAS: Elliott, 1990; DAS-II: Elliott, 2007) (Mervis & John, 2010a, 2010b). The mean DAS-II GCA (General Conceptual Ability; similar to IQ) score for 120 children and adolescents with WS aged 4-17 years who had classic deletions was 64.56 (standard deviation: 12.33, range 31-96) (Mervis & John, 2010a). The performance on the Verbal cluster (mean standard score: 74.06) and/or the Nonverbal Reasoning cluster (mean standard score: 78.89) was significantly better than performance on the Spatial cluster (mean standard score: 54.82) for 86% of the children. Verbal short-term memory performance (DAS-II Recall of Digits Forward subtest; mean standard score: 72.06) was consistent with performance on the Verbal and Nonverbal

Reasoning clusters. The same pattern of strengths and weaknesses was found across the full age range studied.

This pattern of performance is also evidenced in toddlers and young preschool children with WS on the Mullen Scales of Early Learning (MSEL; Mullen, 1995). The MSEL includes four scales—Visual Reception (measuring primarily nonverbal reasoning), Fine Motor (measuring fine motor skills and visuospatial construction), Receptive Language and Expressive Language (also measuring verbal short-term memory)—that may be combined to give the Early Learning Composite (ELC). The mean ELC for 144 children aged 2.01-4.96 years was 61.45 (standard deviation: 11.31, range: 49 [lowest possible ELC] to 96) (Mervis & John, 2010a). Performance on the Fine Motor scale (mean T score: 21.18, in contrast to the general-population mean of 50 ± 10) was considerably lower than that on the Visual Reception (mean T score: 29.51), Receptive Language (mean T score: 29.45) and Expressive Language (mean T score: 32.60) scales. This pattern also holds for 1-year-olds (Mervis & John, unpublished data).

In summary, across both the DAS-II and the MSEL, the mean level of overall performance of young children with WS is in the mild-intellectual-disability range. However, this over-all standard score does not accurately represent the children's abilities. Instead, perform-ance on average is in the borderline range for language, nonverbal reasoning and verbal short-term memory and in the moderate disability range for visuospatial construction, the same pattern as we reported earlier for adolescents and adults.

Precursors to lexical development

The onset of language development is delayed for almost all children with WS (Mervis & Becerra, 2007). Mervis et al. (2003) followed the early vocabulary development of 13 children with WS longitudinally using the MacArthur–Bates Communicative Development Inventory (CDI; Fenson et al., 1993, 2007) Words and Sentences form. At the time children entered the study, their expressive vocabularies (spoken and/or signed) included fewer than six words (mean: one word). Age of acquisition of a 10-word expressive vocabulary was below the 5th percentile for all participants; for all but one child, age of acquisition of 50- and 100-word expressive vocabularies was also below the 5th percentile. The median age of acquisition of a 100-word expressive vocabulary was 37 months (range: 26-68 months) compared with a mean of 18 months (5th percentile: 28 months) for typically developing (TD) children (Fenson et al., 2007).

At least three types of language-relevant abilities that are acquired during the prelin-guistic period by TD children have been shown to be delayed in children with WS: onset of canonical babble (or, more generally, early phonological development), segmentation of words from continuous speech, and comprehension and production of pointing gestures (and, more generally, engagement in triadic joint attention). Research on each of these topics is briefly described in this section. Delays in these areas, in addition to global developmental delay, have been argued to contribute to the children's language delay. The long-term impact of delay for each type of ability probably differs, as will be described.

The first type of ability for which delays have been identified is the onset of canonical babble (or, more generally, phonological development). Masataka (2001), in a longitudinal study of eight very young children with WS, demonstrated that all early motor and language milestones were considerably delayed. Nevertheless, the pattern of relations between the language-relevant abilities studied was similar to that previously found by Eilers et al. (1993) for both full-term and preterm TD children. In particular, all of the children with WS demonstrated the onset of rhythmic hand banging (mean: 74.5 weeks) before or at the same time as the onset of canonical babble (mean: 76.5 weeks), and the onset of canonical babble consistently occurred well before the onset of first words (defined as the child's age at the session in which his or her cumulative spontaneous or imitated expressive vocabulary reached 25 words; mean: 98.5 weeks). Masataka argued that rhythmic hand banging provides the motor substrate for canonical babble and that without canonical babble, the production of words is for the most part impossible. Consistent with Masataka's findings, Mervis and Bertrand (1997) reported that the two children in their longitudinal study who had not started to produce canonical babble prior to entry into the study began to produce rhythmic hand banging and canonical babble in the same month.

Velleman et al. (2006) provided further evidence that the phonological development of very young children with WS was delayed relative to chronological-age (CA) expectations. The performance of six 18-month-olds with WS was compared with that of same-CA samples of children with DS and TD children. The children with WS or DS produced more immature babble patterns than did the TD children, including a higher proportion of vowel-only syllables, fewer syllables per babble, fewer true consonants per babble and a lower mean babble level (as defined by Stoel-Gammon, 1989). The babble histories of the two children with WS with the most rapid language development were the most similar to those of the TD children, and the child with WS who had the most serious language delay had not met the criterion for canonical babble at age 36 months (Mervis & Becerra, 2007). There have been no systematic studies of the phonologies of older children with WS. However, in their discussion of the literature, Udwin and Yule (1990, p.108) summarised the language of older children and adults as 'fluent and articulate', suggesting that at least for most individuals with WS, the initial phonological delays are eventually resolved. Phonological studies of older children and adults are warranted; longitudinal studies beginning in early childhood and continuing through the school years would be particularly valuable.

The second type of ability important for language acquisition for which delays have been hypothesised involves the segmentation of words from fluent speech. The importance of speech segmentation abilities for later language development has been shown in two retrospective studies of a large sample of TD children conducted by Newman et al. (2006). In the first study, Newman et al. (2006) found that children who at age 24 months were in the top 15% of the sample in CDI expressive-vocabulary size were significantly more likely than children who were in the bottom 15% to have successfully segmented words from fluent speech in studies conducted when they were 7.5-12 months old. In the second study, Newman et al. (2006) showed that TD children aged 4-6 years who had been successful at speech segmentation in the infant studies ('segmenters') earned significantly higher standard scores on measures of both semantics and syntax (but not nonverbal reasoning) than did children who had been 'nonsegmenters' in the infant studies, although all children scored in the average or above-average range.

Nazzi et al. (2003) considered the ability of 17 children with WS aged 15-47 months (mean: 33 months) to segment bisyllabic words with either a strong–weak stress pattern (the predominant pattern in English) or a weak–strong stress pattern from fluent speech. This study was modelled on the research of Jusczyk et al. (1999), who used stimuli and procedures similar to those in the speech segmentation component of Newman et al.'s (2006) research. As a group, the children were able to segment the strong–weak words but not the weak–strong words from the speech stream. Nazzi et al. (2003) theorised that this pattern indicated that children with WS predominately relied on prosodic cues (adequate to identify strong–weak words) to segment words from the speech stream and had difficulty using distributional information (needed to identify weak–strong words) for this purpose. More recently, Cashon et al. (2009) considered the speech segmentation skills of ten children with WS who were aged 9-20 months (mean: 14 months) using a statistical learning paradigm in which all the syllables in an artificial language were equally stressed. In this situation, young toddlers with WS were able to use distributional properties to segment words from fluent speech. Unfortunately, the participants in both studies were older than the ages at which TD children typically first evidence the abilities tested, so for the abilities that were demonstrated, it is unclear if they are initially delayed. As Mervis and Becerra (2007) indicated, the impact of delays in segmenting words from fluent speech will vary depending on the type of compensatory strategies used (either consciously or unconsciously) by the children's carers.

Even under the best possible compensatory scenario, however, in which carers consistently implement strategies such as introducing new words in isolation along with their referents, children who are delayed in acquiring the ability to segment words from fluent speech are probably at a considerable disadvantage in vocabulary acquisition (Newman et al., 2006). Difficulties with segmentation of fluent speech would also be expected to have a negative impact on syntactic development because acquisition of function words and bound morphemes is dependent on segmentation abilities. Longitudinal studies addressing the relations between early speech segmentation abilities and later linguistic abilities for individuals with WS are needed.

The third type of prelinguistic ability for which delays have been reported involves comprehension and production of pointing gestures and engagement in triadic joint attention. These are abilities that have been shown repeatedly to emerge prior to the onset of referential language acquisition not only for TD children (Adamson, 1995) but also for children with DS and children with severe developmental delay of unknown aetiology (Mervis & Bertrand, 1997). This sequential ordering probably occurs because pointing (the cognitive manifestation of reference) provides a particularly useful way for the child to determine the referent of a word. Adults routinely use pointing to indicate the referent of a word, and prelinguistic TD children, prelinguistic children with DS and prelinguistic children with severe developmental delay use pointing gestures to indicate and/or request interesting objects; these gestures are likely to elicit the object name from the child's carer. These situations typically lead to triadic joint attention, with the child and adult jointly attending to the same object or event.

The pattern for children with WS is strikingly different. Mervis and Bertrand (1997) reported that for 9 of 10 children in their longitudinal study, the onset of referential language preceded the onset of referential pointing—by an average of 6 months. Although the triadic joint attention abilities of children with WS have not been systematically studied during the prelinguistic period, the absence of spontaneous triadic joint attention is routinely raised as a concern by parents of young children with WS. Brown et al. (2003) reported that toddlers with WS (mean CA: 29 months) had significantly more difficulty planning visual saccades than did either CA- and MA-matched children with DS or younger MA-matched TD toddlers, and Karmiloff-Smith (2007) has argued that this type of difficulty may lead to difficulties in triadic interactions, including triadic joint attention (see also Chapter 14 for discussion of the relation between attention to faces and the development of triadic joint attention). As joint attention to the referent is necessary for a child to acquire labels, alternative methods of establishing joint attention must be used. Several of these have been documented by Mervis and Bertrand (1993, 1997), all of which also are used occasionally by parents of TD children and children with DS. Nevertheless, the inability of very young children with WS to comprehend and produce pointing gestures, to follow another person's eye gaze and to engage in spontaneous triadic joint attention severely limits their opportunities to acquire new words and almost certainly leads to a reduction in the rate of vocabulary acquisition (Karmiloff-Smith, 2007; Mervis & Becerra, 2007). These difficulties with nonverbal communication presage significant difficulties with pragmatics in both childhood and adulthood.

Lexical development

The modal focus of studies of the language acquisition of toddlers, preschool children and early-primary-school children with WS has been lexical development. In this section, we consider three topics: the conceptual basis for early vocabulary and principles underlying the acquisition of early vocabulary, vocabulary size comparisons with children with DS and the relation between concrete and relational vocabulary for children with WS aged 5-7 years.

Conceptual basis for object words

Studies of TD children and children with DS have identified several links between early cognitive development and early lexical development. As indicated in the previous section, one such link—between the onset of referential pointing and the onset of referential language—does not hold for children with WS. However, two other links do hold. Data from the longitudinal study by Mervis and Bertrand (1993, 1997) mentioned previously indicated that the extensions of the early object labels of all ten children with WS, whether measured by comprehension or by production, corresponded to the children's play patterns with the objects, and both were at the child-basic level. For example, the children rolled a variety of spherical objects whether or not they were balls; they also comprehended and produced 'ball' in relation to these objects even when their mothers attempted to correct them. Nine of the ten children also began to be able to fast-map (identify the referent of a novel label even though the person who used the label did not explicitly indicate its referent) new object names at about the same time as they began to spontaneously sort objects by category; the remaining child began to fast-map new object labels about 2 weeks before she began to sort objects exhaustively by category. Gopnik and Meltzoff (1987, 1992) had argued that the onsets of these abilities should be at about the same time because they represent parallel insights: that all objects belong to some category (cognitive insight) and that all objects have a name (linguistic insight).

Objects in basic-level categories share shape–function correlations (e.g. spherical–roll), and most of the early object labels learnt by very young children are names for basic-level categories. However, categories may also be formed of highly dissimilar objects simply because they have been assigned the same label. Nazzi and his colleagues have addressed the ability of young children with WS to form such categories. In the first study, Nazzi and Karmiloff-Smith (2002) showed 12 children with WS (mean CA: 4.65 years) three highly dissimilar objects and told them a name for each object; two objects were assigned the same name and the third a different name. On the test trial, the researcher held one object out and asked the child to give him 'the object that goes with this one'. The WS group performed at chance. On trials in which two of the three objects were identical and the researcher did not provide a name, however, the children with WS performed significantly above chance. On this basis, the authors argued that children with WS could categorise based on physical appearance but not based on label alone. They further noted that this pattern differed from that found by Nazzi and Gopnik (2001) for a group of TD 20-month-olds, who selected the correct item in the label-alone condition at a rate slightly but significantly above chance. Nazzi et al. (2005) found that a slightly older group of eight children with WS (mean CA: 6.08 years) performed significantly above chance on the label trials but significantly below TD children matched for CA.

Havy et al. (2010) compared the performance of 12 children with WS (mean CA: 5.25 years) with that of three groups of TD children (one matched for CA, one for verbal MA and one for nonverbal MA) using the same type of stimuli as in the label trials in the previous studies. The two labels in each trial were highly similar, differing only by either one consonant or one vowel. The performance of the WS group was above chance and comparable with that of the two MA-matched groups; all three groups performed significantly better on the consonant contrast pairs than on the vowel contrast pairs. Thus, by age 5 years, most children with WS are able to form name-based categories even if there is no physical-appearance support for these categories and the category names differ by only a single phoneme.

Vocabulary size comparisons: young children with Williams syndrome or Down syndrome

When matched for CA, older children and adolescents with WS have significantly larger vocabularies than do children with DS (e.g. Bellugi et al., 2000). This same pattern is present by age 2 years; Mervis and Robinson (2000) reported a mean expressive-vocabulary size, as measured by the CDI: Words and Sentences, of 55.08 words (range: 5-120 words) for children with WS and 19.67 words (range: 0-70 words) for children with DS at age 2.16 years. Two outliers with WS who had expressive vocabularies of more than 400 words were excluded. These children were at the 75th percentile on the CDI norms. However, the remaining children with WS were relatively delayed; 67% were below the 5th percentile (the lowest percentile included in the norms). The wide range for the children in this study presages the considerable variability found for older children on the PPVT-4 and the second edition of the Expressive Vocabulary Test (EVT-2; Williams, 2007) (see Mervis & John, 2010a).

Vicari and colleagues (2002) compared a group of toddlers and preschool children with WS (mean CA: 4.85 years; mean MA: 2.83 years) with a slightly older but MA-matched group of children with DS and a younger MA-matched group of TD children. The mean expressive-vocabulary size as measured by the Italian version of the CDI was highly similar for the three groups (WS: 452 words, DS: 457 words, TD: 488 words). This finding indicates that at least during the preschool period, matching children with WS and DS for MA eliminates the expressive-vocabulary difference found by Mervis and Robinson (2000) for CA-matched groups.

Relation between concrete- and relational/conceptual-vocabulary ability

As mentioned in the Introduction, concrete vocabulary is the area of greatest strength for adolescents and adults with WS. Concrete vocabulary is also the area of greatest strength for young children with WS (Mervis & John, 2010a), with a mean level of performance in the low average range for the general population on both the PPVT-4 (mean: 81.84, range: 20-124) and the EVT-2 (mean: 79.43, range: 20-120). Vocabulary is not monolithic, however. In striking contrast to their performance on concrete-vocabulary measures, children with WS have considerable difficulty with relational/conceptual vocabulary. Mervis and John (2008) compared the concrete- and relational/conceptual-vocabulary abilities of 92 children with WS who were 5-7 years old. Although the mean PPVT-III standard score was 86.73, the mean standard score on the Test of Relational Concepts (TRC; Edmonston & Litchfield Thane, 1988), which measures simple spatial, temporal, quantitative and dimensional concepts, was 55.79. Performance on the TRC was almost as low as performance on the DAS Pattern Construction subtest, the signature weakness for individuals with WS, and performance on these two measures was strongly correlated. The finding that children with WS had difficulty with all types of relational concepts is consistent with Walsh's (2003) argument that a common magnitude system located in the inferior parietal cortex controls spatial, temporal and quantitative processing. This is the same area that Meyer-Lindenberg et al. (2004, 2006) identified as a region of reduced grey matter that served as a roadblock to dorsal-stream information flow in individuals with WS (see also Chapters 12 and 13 for discussion of dorsal-stream processing), suggesting a possible common basis for the findings of extreme difficulty in both visuospatial construction and relational language for individuals with WS.

Early grammatical development

Although a large proportion of the studies addressing the language abilities of adolescents and adults with WS has focused on grammatical abilities (see Chapter 11), there have been very few studies of early grammatical development. Mervis et al. (2003) considered the grammatical abilities of 22 young children with WS who were followed longitudinally from the onset of language acquisition. At age 30 months, only four (18%) children had earned a CDI Sentence Complexity score of at least 1 (10th percentile, the lowest percentile reported). Thus, the onset of grammatical development was considerably delayed for most children with WS. However, grammatical ability was both strongly correlated with expressive-vocabulary size and at the level predicted for expressive-vocabulary size based on the CDI norms. Similar findings were reported for smaller samples of Italian children based on the norms for the Italian CDI (Vicari et al., 2002; Volterra et al., 2003). This finding of strong correlations between expressive-vocabulary size and grammatical ability for young children with WS is consistent with the results of several large-sample studies of TD toddlers and preschool children that used the CDI or CDI-III to measure language abilities (e.g. Bates & Goodman, 1997; Dale et al., 2000; Fenson et al., 1994). Longitudinal studies of TD children have further indicated that language abilities at ages 2-4 years (as measured by the CDI, CDI-III and a related instrument developed for the Twins Early Development Study, Kings College London, UK) are strongly related to reading abilities at ages 7-10 years and that the relation is likely to be causal (Harlaar et al., 2008). Longitudinal studies examining the relations between early language abilities and school-age reading abilities for children with WS are needed.

To further study grammatical development, Vicari et al. (2002) and Volterra et al. (2003) also administered a sentence repetition task to MA-matched WS, DS and TD groups. Although the three groups were well-matched for expressive-vocabulary size, the WS group had a significantly longer mean length of utterance than did the DS group. On the sentence repetition task, the WS and TD groups repeated significantly more sentences accurately than did the DS group. For all three groups, the expressive-vocabulary size was strongly correlated with the percentage of correctly repeated sentences. An error analysis indicated that the most common error was omission. For the WS and DS groups, a significant proportion of errors involved bound morphology; such errors were very rare for the TD group. All three groups produced word order errors. For the TD group, the resulting sentences were still grammatical. By contrast, although the WS and DS groups produced fewer word order errors, many of their word order errors resulted in ungrammatical sentences of types that were rarely produced by even very young TD children, indicating that these errors were probably associated with intellectual disability.

John et al. (2008) studied the language abilities of 39 young 4-year-olds with WS (CA range: 4.00-4.33 years). Seven of these children also had been diagnosed with a comorbid autism spectrum disorder (ASD). Fifteen children (including six with ASD) had a CDI Sentence Complexity score of 0, indicating considerable delay in the onset of grammar. Six children (five with ASD) had a mean length of utterance of 1.00 based on a 30-minute play session with a parent. Fourteen children (two with ASD) were in Brown's (1973) stage 1 of grammatical development, with the remaining 19 children evenly divided among stages 2, 3 and 4. Eight children (five with ASD) did not produce any bound morphemes during the play session. Correlations among CDI-based and play-session-based language measures indicated strong relations between expressive vocabulary and grammatical ability; a further set of correlations indicated strong relations between language abilities and DAS Preschool Verbal cluster, Nonverbal cluster and Recall of Digits standard scores.

Early pragmatics

The ability to coordinate one's attention between a social partner and objects or events of mutual interest (triadic joint attention) facilitates social learning (e.g. Baldwin, 1995; Mundy & Neal, 2001) in that it is fundamental to the development of the ability to understand the intentions, feelings and thoughts of others (e.g. Bretherton, 1991; Tomasello, 1995). Thus, triadic joint attention underlies the development of pragmatics.

As described earlier in this chapter, the emergence of referential pointing, which is important for triadic joint attention, is extremely delayed for most children with WS and almost always occurs after the onset of referential language. Even after children with WS begin to evidence referential pointing and triadic joint attention, their pragmatic abilities remain more limited than expected for their developmental level. Older toddlers and preschool children with WS were significantly less likely to engage in triadic joint attention or to produce referential gestures than were either MA-matched TD children with smaller expressive-vocabulary sizes (Laing et al., 2002) or children with DS individually matched on CA, MSEL ELC score and expressive-vocabulary size (Rowe et al., 2005). In addition, John and Mervis (2010) demonstrated that despite having significantly higher MSEL ELC scores, preschool children with WS were significantly less likely than CA-matched preschool children with DS to infer the communicative intent behind pointing gestures and eye gaze directed at a box in which a toy was hidden; 60% of the children with DS but only 27% of the children with WS found the hidden toy at a rate significantly above that expected by chance. Difficulties in interpreting the social meaning of eye gaze have been reported for adults with WS as well (Tsirempolou et al., 2006; Chapter 14).

These types of findings provided the initial basis for questioning the accuracy of the characterisation of WS as the 'opposite' of autism. The overlap between the phenotypes associated with WS and ASD has been addressed in three studies of older toddlers and preschool children (Klein-Tasman et al., 2007; Klein-Tasman et al., 2009; Lincoln et al., 2007). All of these studies considered performance on the Autism Diagnostic Observation Schedule–Generic (ADOS-G; Lord et al., 2000) Module 1, a semistructured play-based interaction designed to press for behaviours central to the diagnosis of ASD in children who have limited or no expressive language. The results indicated that a large proportion of young children with WS demonstrated behaviours considered to be characteristic of children with ASD. For example, approximately 50% of the participants with WS did not clearly integrate eye contact with their communicative partner in order to reference a desired object that was out of reach, almost 75% did not integrate eye contact or vocalisations with acts of showing objects, and less than 10% spontaneously used a doll or other object as an independent agent or used objects to represent other objects. These difficulties were numerous enough that many children were classified on the ADOS-G algorithm as 'autism spectrum disorder' or 'autism' (47-50% in the Klein-Tasman et al., 2007, 2009, studies and 10% in the study by Lincoln et al., 2007). However, differences between the behavioural phenotypes associated with WS and ASD were also found, suggesting that most children with WS who were classified as 'autism spectrum disorder' on the ADOS-G would not meet the clinical-judgement criterion for a diagnosis of ASD. For example, few children with WS evidenced difficulty in directing vocalisations or facial expressions to other people or sharing affect, and the quality of their social overtures was generally good.

Early language abilities as predictors of later language and cognitive abilities

Most studies of the language abilities of children with WS have been cross-sectional. However, three studies in which the relations between early language abilities and later language and/or cognitive abilities were considered have been reported. Becerra et al. (2010) considered the predictability of the age of attainment of early language milestones for intellectual abilities at age 4 years for the 22 children with WS whose early language development was discussed in Mervis et al. (2003). The ages at attainment of 10-word, 50-word and 100-word expressive vocabularies and first novel word combinations were all strongly related to DAS GCA, Verbal cluster standard score and Nonverbal cluster standard score at 4 years of age (all r values $\geq$ .65). The age of attainment of a 10-word expressive vocabulary (the first language milestone) was very strongly related to the other early language milestones (all r values $\geq$ .88).

To consider the relation between early relational language ability and later relational language ability, Mervis and John (2008) administered the Clinical Evaluation of Language Fundamentals Fourth Edition (CELF-IV; Semel et al., 2003) Formulated Sentences subtest, which includes several advanced relational concepts, to ten children (mean CA: 11.33 years) who had completed the TRC an average of 4.33 years earlier. The children evidenced considerable difficulty with the more advanced relational concepts included on the CELF-IV Formulated Sentences subtest. Furthermore, performance on that subtest was strongly correlated with prior performance on the TRC (r = .87).

Early pragmatic language abilities have recently been shown to predict later pragmatic abilities. John et al. (2010) considered the pragmatic language abilities of 12 children with WS at two time points: first, as 4-year-olds during a 30-minute play session with their mothers, and second, an average of 6.18 years later (mean CA: 10.35 years) during a one-on-one conversation with a familiar researcher. At both time points, there was considerable variability in the proportion of questions that was pragmatically appropriate. At age 10 years, the children's proficiency at asking pragmatically appropriate questions, their DAS-II Verbal, Nonverbal Reasoning and Spatial cluster standard scores and their adaptive behaviour performance were all strongly correlated with the proportion of pragmatically appropriate questions asked at age 4 years (all r values $\geq$ .68).

Conclusion

Considerable progress has been made in our understanding of WS over the past 15-20 years. Perhaps the most important change has been a shift from focusing on the 'end state' of WS and the apparent similarities of adolescents and adults with WS to adults with right-hemisphere brain damage (e.g. Bellugi et al., 1994), characterised by 'linguistic preservation and marked spatial-cognitive deficit' (p.44), to focusing on WS as a neurodevelopmental disorder in which the adult state is determined by the impact of the deleted genes, in transaction with the environment, on the development of brain structure and function and the development of behaviour. The developmental trajectory approach (see Chapter 1) has not specifically been applied in studies of either early language development or its precursors. However, these areas have been well-studied for TD children by multiple research groups, with converging findings, thus providing a solid basis of comparison for studies of children with WS. As described in this chapter, although the onset of language development is delayed for children with WS, the relations among many aspects of language development are similar for children with WS and TD children (e.g. relations between expressive-vocabulary size and grammatical development). At the same time, other relations (e.g. the relation between referential pointing gestures/triadic joint attention and the onset of referential expressive language) are clearly different not only from those shown for TD children but also from those of children with DS or children with severe developmental delay. There is clear developmental continuity both in areas of language that are relative strengths for children with WS (e.g. expressive-vocabulary acquisition) and in areas that are particularly challenging for children with WS (e.g. relational vocabulary, pragmatics). Longitudinal studies of large groups of children with WS are needed to provide a more complete perspective on variability in early language development and its precursors, the factors affecting that variability, and the impact of early variability on variability in later development, both linguistic and nonlinguistic.

Targeted studies using the developmental trajectory method will provide further information regarding relations among different language and cognitive abilities and their similarities or differences to those found for TD children or children with other genetic disorders. When interpreting these studies, it will be important to remember that because children with WS will almost certainly have below-average abilities on the matching variable, one cannot automatically assume that they should evidence the same levels of ability on the target variable as do younger TD children with the same level of ability on the matching variable (see Mervis & Robinson, 2005, Figure 1). This problem is further exacerbated when the TD group has above-average intellectual ability; it is important that the TD children be tested for intellectual ability on the same measure as is being used for the WS group and that the mean for the TD group be very close to 100. Only one neuroimaging study of very young children with WS has been published (Jones et al., 2002); this report was based on structural magnetic resonance imaging (MRI) scans obtained for clinical rather than research purposes. Structural MRI, functional MRI and diffusion tensor imaging studies of very young children with WS who have intellectual abilities in the average range for the general population and CA-matched groups of TD children with similar levels of intellectual abilities will be crucial to understanding brain similarities and differences that underlie the pattern of language strengths and weaknesses found for children with WS. Studies of the rare children with carefully characterised shorter deletions will be critical for beginning to determine the roles of specific deleted genes (or sets of deleted genes) in the course and pattern of language development of children with WS who have classic deletions. Finally, although particularly difficult to accomplish given the rarity of WS, the roles of environmental factors such as the educational levels of the parents, the amount and quality of language directed to the child, and the intensity of early speech/language therapy should be studied, along with the roles of the child's temperament and mastery motivation as language development depends not only on genetics but also on the child's environment and his or her temperament and willingness to persevere.

Editor commentary (Emily K. Farran & Annette Karmiloff-Smith)

In typical development, children can produce 100 words by approximately 18 months. In WS, however, this level often is not achieved until children are 3 years old. To determine the developmental start-point of linguistic delay, the authors considered typical precursors to language acquisition and the longitudinal impact of early language impairments in WS on later development.

Taking the neuroconstructivist stance, the chapter reported that some cross-domain interacting systems that emerge in the first years of life show a typical developmental association, but nonetheless emerge late in WS. By contrast, other systems, such as the relation between referential pointing (triadic joint attention) and referential language are atypical in WS; whereas pointing precedes language onset in typical development, the opposite pattern is observed in WS.

Although the chapter at times pointed to the possibility of similar profiles in infancy and adulthood, the impact of early language differences on later development was shown to be far-reaching. For example, triadic joint attention was compared between WS and autism together with the effects that this has on the development of pragmatics (discussed further in Chapter 11). Crucially, the authors provided an example of how delayed early development in one domain (the verbal domain) has cascading effects across multiple domains (verbal and nonverbal development). This highlights the importance of exploring profiles of abilities at the infant start state in any neurodevelopmental disorder because both delay and deviance in early milestones are crucial to our understanding of later cognitive profiles.

References

Adamson, L.B. (1995). *Communication Development during Infancy*. Madison, WI: Brown and Benchmark.

von Arnim, G., & Engel, P. (1964). Mental retardation related to hypercalcaemia. *Developmental Medicine and Child Neurology*, **6**, 366–77.

Baldwin, D.A. (Ed.). (1995). *Understanding the Link Between Joint Attention and Language*. Hillsdale, NJ: Lawrence Erlbaum.

Bates, E., & Goodman, J.C. (1997). On the inseparability of grammar and the lexicon: evidence from acquisition, aphasia, and real-time processing. *Language and Cognitive Processes*, **12**, 507–84.

Becerra, A.M., Henderson, D.R., John, A.E., & Mervis, C.B. (June 2010). *Relations between Early Linguistic Milestones and Intellectual Abilities at Age 4 Years for Children with Williams Syndrome.* Presented at the Symposium on Research in Child Language Disorders, Madison, WI.

Beilin, H. (1975). *Studies in the Cognitive Basis of Language Development.* New York, NY: Academic Press.

Bellugi, U., Marks, S., Bihrle, A., & Sabo, H. (1988). Dissociation between language and cognitive functions in Williams syndrome. In D. Bishop & K. Mogford (Eds), *Language Development in Exceptional Circumstances* (pp. 177–89). London: Churchill Livingstone.

Bellugi, U., Lichtenberger, L., Jones, W., Lai, Z., & St. George, M. (2000). The neurocognitive profile of Williams syndrome: a complex pattern of strengths and weaknesses. *Journal of Cognitive Neuroscience,* **12 Supplement 1**, 7–29.

Bellugi, U., Wang, P., & Jernigan, T.L. (1994). Williams syndrome: an unusual neuropsychological profile. In S.H. Broman & J. Grafman (Eds), *Atypical Cognitive Deficits in Developmental Disorders: Implications for Brain Function* (pp. 23–56). Hillsdale, NJ: Lawrence Erlbaum.

Bishop, D.V.M. (1998). Development of the Children's Communication Checklist (CCC): a method for assessing the qualitative aspects of communication impairment in children. *Journal of Child Psychology and Psychiatry,* **39**, 879–91.

Bretherton, I. (Ed.). (1991). *Intentional Communication and the Development of an Understanding of Mind.* Hillsdale, NJ: Lawrence Erlbaum.

Brock, J., Jarrold, C., Farran, E.K., Laws, G., & Riby, D.M. (2007). Do children with Williams syndrome really have good vocabulary knowledge? Methods for comparing cognitive and linguistic abilities in developmental disorders. *Clinical Linguistics and Phonetics,* **21**, 673–88.

Brown, J.H., Johnson, M.H., Paterson, S.J., Gilmore, R., Longhi, E., & Karmiloff-Smith, A. (2003). Spatial representation and attention in toddlers with Williams syndrome and Down syndrome. *Neuropsychologia,* **41**, 1037–46.

Brown, R. (1973). A first language: the early stages. Cambridge, MA: Harvard University Press.

Cashon, C.H., Ha, O.R., Allen, C.L., Graf, K.M., Saffran, J.R., & Mervis, C.B. (2009). *9- to 20-Month-Olds with Williams Syndrome are Linguistic Statistical Learners.* Denver, CO: Society for Research in Child Development.

Cowley, G. (18 September 2003). Girls, boys and autism. *Newsweek,* 42–50.

Dale, P.S., Dionne, G., Eley, T., & Plomin, R. (2000). Lexical and grammatical development: a behavioral genetic perspective. *Journal of Child Language,* **27**, 619–42.

Dobbs, D. (8 July 2007). The gregarious brain. *The New York Times.* <http://www.nytimes.com/2007/07/08/magazine/08sociability-t.html> accessed 7 Jul 2011.

Dunn, L.M., & Dunn, L.M. (1981). *Peabody Picture Vocabulary Test—Revised.* Circle Pines, MN: American Guidance Service.

Dunn, L.M., & Dunn, L.M. (1997). *Peabody Picture Vocabulary Test—Third Edition.* Circle Pines, MN: American Guidance Service.

Dunn, L.M., & Dunn, D.M. (2007). *Peabody Picture Vocabulary Test—Fourth Edition.* Minneapolis, MN: Pearson Assessments.

Dunn, L.M., Dunn, L.M., Whetton, C., & Burley, J. (1997). *British Picture Vocabulary Scale—Second Edition.* Windsor: NFER-Nelson.

Edmonston, N.K., & Litchfield Thane, N. (1988). *TRC: Test of Relational Concepts.* Austin, TX: Pro-Ed.

Eilers, R.E., Oller, D.K., Levine, S., Basinger, D., Lynch, M.P., & Urbano, R. (1993). The role of prematurity and socioeconomic status in the onset of canonical babbling in infants. *Infant Behavior and Development,* **16**, 297–315.

Elliott, C.D. (1990). *Differential Ability Scales.* San Antonio, TX: Psychological Corporation.

Elliott, C.D. (2007). *Differential Ability Scales—Second Edition.* San Antonio, TX: Psychological Corporation.

Fenson, L., Dale, P.S., Bates, E., Reznick, J.S., Thal, D.J., & Pethick, S.J. (1994). *Variability in Early Communicative Development*. Monographs of the Society for Research in Child Development, serial no. 242, vol 59, no. 5. Chicago, IL: University of Chicago Press.

Fenson, L., Dale, P.S., Reznick, J.S., Thal, D., Bates, E., Hartung, J.P., et al. (1993). *MacArthur Communicative Development Inventories: User's Guide and Technical Manual*. San Diego, CA: Singular Publishing Group.

Fenson, L., Marchman, V.A., Thal, D.J., Dale, P.S., Reznick, J.S., & Bates, E. (2007). *MacArthur-Bates Communicative Development Inventories: User's Guide and Technical Manual*, 2nd edn. Baltimore, MD: Brookes.

Finn, R. (June 1991). Different minds. *Discover*, 55–58.

Glenn, S., & Cunningham, C. (2005). Performance of young people with Down syndrome on the Leiter-R and British Picture Vocabulary Scales. *Journal of Intellectual Disability Research*, **49**, 239–44.

Gopnik, A. & Meltzoff, A. (1987). The development of categorization in the second year and its relation to other cognitive and linguistic developments. *Child Development*, **58**, 1523–31.

Gopnik, A. & Meltzoff, A. (1992). Categorization and naming: basic-level sorting in eighteen-month-olds and its relation to language. *Child Development*, **63**, 1091–1103.

Harlaar, N., Hayiou-Thomas, M.E., Dale, P.S., & Plomin, R. (2008). Why do preschool language abilities correlate with later reading? A twin study. *Journal of Speech, Language, and Hearing Research*, **51**, 688–705.

Havy, M., Moukawane, S., & Nazzi, T. (2010). Are 3- to 8-year-old children with Williams syndrome good word-learners? *NeuroReport*, **21**, 882–86.

Howlin, P., Davies, M., & Udwin, O. (1998). Cognitive functioning in adults with Williams syndrome. *Journal of Child Psychology and Psychiatry*, **39**, 183–89.

Howlin, P., Elison, S., Udwin, O., & Stinton, C. (2010). Cognitive, linguistic and adaptive functioning in Williams syndrome: trajectories from early to middle adulthood. *Journal of Applied Research in Intellectual Disabilities*, **23**, 322–36.

Jackendoff, R. (1994). *Patterns in the Mind: Language and Human Nature*. New York, NY: Basic Books.

John, A.E., Becerra, A.M., Peregrine, E., & Mervis, C.B. (July 2008). *Variability of Language Abilities of Young 4-Year-Olds who have Williams Syndrome*. Presented at the 12th International Professional Conference on Williams Syndrome, Anaheim, CA.

John, A.E., & Mervis, C.B. (2010). Comprehension of the communicative intent behind pointing and gazing gestures by young children with Williams syndrome or Down syndrome. *Journal of Speech, Language, and Hearing Research*, **53**, 950–60.

John, A.E., Thomas, L.E., Dobson, L.A., & Mervis, C.B. (2010, June). *Preschool Pragmatic Abilities Predict School-Age Pragmatic Abilities of Children with Williams Syndrome*. Madison, WI: Symposium on Research in Child Language Disorders.

Jones, W., Hesselink, J., Courchesne, E., Duncan, T., Matsuda, K., & Bellugi, U. (2002). Cerebellar abnormalities in infants and toddlers with Williams syndrome. *Developmental Medicine & Child Neurology*, **44**, 688–94.

Jusczyk, P.W., Houston, D.M., & Newsome, M. (1999). The beginnings of word segmentation in English-learning infants. *Cognitive Psychology*, **39**, 159–207.

Karmiloff-Smith, A. (2007). Atypical epigenesis. *Developmental Science*, **10**, 84–88.

Klein-Tasman, B.P., Mervis, C.B., Lord, C.E., & Phillips, K.D. (2007). Socio-communicative deficits in young children with Williams syndrome: performance on the Autism Diagnostic Observation Schedule. *Child Neuropsychology*, **13**, 444–67.

Klein-Tasman, B.P., Phillips, K.D., Lord, C., Mervis, C.B., & Gallo, F. (2009). Socio-communicative deficits in young children with Williams syndrome: comparisons to children with autism, pervasive developmental disorders, or other developmental disabilities. *Journal of Developmental and Behavioral Pediatrics*, **30**, 289–99.

Laing, E., Butterworth, G., Ansari, D., Gsödl, M., Longhi, E., Panagiotaki, G., et al. (2002). Atypical development of language and social communication in toddlers with Williams syndrome. *Developmental Science*, 5, 233–46.

Laws, G., & Bishop, D.V.M. (2004). Pragmatic language impairment and social impairment in Williams syndrome: a comparison with Down's syndrome and specific language impairment. *International Journal of Language and Communication Disorders*, 39, 45–64.

Lincoln, A.J., Searcy, Y.M., Jones, W., & Lord, C. (2007). Social interaction behaviors discriminate young children with autism and Williams syndrome. *Journal of the American Academy of Child and Adolescent Psychiatry*, 46, 323–31.

Lord, C., Risi, S., Lambrecht, L., Cook, E.H., Jr., Leventhal, B.L., DiLavore, P.C., et al. (2000). The Autism Diagnostic Observation Schedule-Generic: a standard measure of social and communication deficits associated with the spectrum of autism. *Journal of Autism and Developmental Disorders*, 30, 205–23.

Masataka, N. (2001). Why early linguistic milestones are delayed in children with Williams syndrome: late onset of hand banging as a possible rate-limiting constraint on the emergence of canonical babbling. *Developmental Science*, 4, 158–64.

Mervis, C.B. (1999). The Williams syndrome cognitive profile: strengths, weaknesses, and interrelations among auditory short term memory, language, and visuospatial constructive cognition. In E. Winograd, R. Fivush, & W. Hirst (Eds), *Ecological Approaches to Cognition: Essays in Honor of Ulric Neisser* (pp. 193–227). Mahwah, NJ: Lawrence Erlbaum.

Mervis, C.B. (2006). Language abilities in Williams-Beuren syndrome. In C.A. Morris, H.M. Lenhoff, & P.P. Wang (Eds), *Williams-Beuren Syndrome: Research, Evaluation, and Treatment* (pp. 159–206). Baltimore, MD: Johns Hopkins University Press.

Mervis, C.B., & Becerra, A.M. (2007). Language and communicative development in Williams syndrome. *Mental Retardation and Developmental Disabilities Research Reviews*, 13, 3–15.

Mervis, C.B., & Bertrand, J. (1993). Acquisition of early object labels: the roles of operating principles and input. In A.P. Kaiser & D.B. Gray (Eds) *Enhancing Children's Communication: Research Foundations for Intervention* (pp. 281–316). Baltimore, MD: Brookes.

Mervis, C.B., & Bertrand, J. (1997). Developmental relations between cognition and language: evidence from Williams syndrome. In L.B. Adamson & M.A. Romski (Eds), *Communication and Language Acquisition: Discoveries from Atypical Development* (pp. 75–106). New York, NY: Brookes.

Mervis, C.B., & John, A.E. (2008). Vocabulary abilities of children with Williams syndrome: strengths, weaknesses, and relation to visuospatial construction ability. *Journal of Speech, Language, and Hearing Research*, 51, 967–82.

Mervis, C.B., & John, A.E. (2010a). Cognitive and behavioral characteristics of children with Williams syndrome: implications for intervention approaches. *American Journal of Medical Genetics Part C: Seminars in Medical Genetics*, 154C, 229–48.

Mervis, C.B., & John, A.E. (2010b). Williams syndrome: psychological characteristics. In B. Shapiro & P. Accardo (Eds), *Neurogenetic Syndromes: Behavioral Issues and Their Treatment* (pp. 81–98). Baltimore, MD: Brookes.

Mervis, C.B., & Robinson, B.F. (2000). Expressive vocabulary of toddlers with Williams syndrome or Down syndrome: a comparison. *Developmental Neuropsychology*, 17, 111–26.

Mervis, C.B., & Robinson, B.F. (2005). Designing measures for profiling and genotype/phenotype studies of individuals with genetic syndromes or developmental language disorders. *Applied Psycholinguistics*, 26, 41–64.

Mervis, C.B., Robinson, B.F., Bertrand, J., Morris, C.A., Klein-Tasman, B.P., & Armstrong, S.C. (2000). The Williams syndrome cognitive profile. *Brain and Cognition*, 44, 604–28.

Mervis, C.B., Robinson, B.F., Rowe, M.L., Becerra, A.M. & Klein-Tasman, B.P. (2003). Language abilities of individuals who have Williams syndrome. *International Review of Research in Mental Retardation*, 27, 35–81.

Meyer-Lindenberg, A., Kohn, P., Mervis, C.B., Kippenhan, J.S., Olsen, R.K., Morris, C.A., et al. (2004). Neural basis of genetically determined visuospatial construction deficit in Williams syndrome. *Neuron*, **43**, 623–31.

Meyer-Lindenberg, A., Mervis, C.B., & Berman, K.F. (2006). Neural mechanisms in Williams syndrome: a unique window to genetic influences on cognition and behavior. *Nature Reviews Neuroscience*, 7, 380–93.

Mullen, E.M. (1995). *Mullen Scales of Early Learning*. Circle Pines, MN: American Guidance Service.

Mundy, P., & Neal, A. (2001). Neural plasticity, joint attention, and a transactional social-orienting model of autism. *International Review of Research in Mental Retardation*, **12**, 139–68.

Nazzi, T., & Gopnik, A. (2001). Linguistic and cognitive abilities in infancy: when does language become a tool for cognition? *Cognition*, 80, B11–20.

Nazzi, T., Gopnik, A., & Karmiloff-Smith, A. (2005). Asynchrony in the cognitive and lexical development of young children with Williams syndrome. *Journal of Child Language*, **32**, 427–38.

Nazzi, T., & Karmiloff-Smith, A. (2002). Early categorization abilities in young children with Williams syndrome. *NeuroReport*, **13**, 1259–62.

Nazzi, T., Paterson, S., & Karmiloff-Smith, A. (2003). Early word segmentation by infants and toddlers with Williams syndrome. *Infancy*, **4**, 251–71.

Newman, R., Bernstein Ratner, N., Jusczyk, A.M., Jusczyk, P.W., & Dow, K.A. (2006). Infants' early ability to segment the conversational speech signal predicts later language development: a retrospective analysis. *Developmental Psychology*, **42**, 643–55.

Piattelli-Palmarini, M. (2001). Speaking of learning: how do we acquire our marvellous facility for expressing ourselves in words? *Nature*, **411**, 887–88.

Pinker, S. (1999). *Words and Rules*. London: Weidenfeld and Nicholson.

Rowe, M.L., Peregrine, E., & Mervis, C.B. (April 2005). *Communicative Development in Toddlers with Williams Syndrome*. Presented at the Biennial Meeting of the Society for Research in Child Development, Atlanta, GA.

Searcy, Y.M., Lincoln, A.J., Rose, F.E., Klima, E.S., & Bavar, N. (2004). The relationship between age and IQ in adults with Williams syndrome. *American Journal on Mental Retardation*, **109**, 231–36.

Semel, E., Wiig, E.H., & Secord, W.A. (2003). *Clinical Evaluation of Language Fundamentals—Fourth Edition*. San Antonio, TX: Harcourt Assessment.

Stoel-Gammon, C. (1989). Prespeech and early speech development of two late talkers. *First Language*, **9**, 207–23.

Tomasello, M. (Ed.). (1995). *Joint Attention as Social Cognition*. Hillsdale, NJ: Lawrence Erlbaum.

Tsirempolou, E., Lawrence, K., Lee, K., Ewing, S., & Karmiloff-Smith, A. (2006). Understanding the social meaning of the eyes: is Williams syndrome so different from autism? *World Journal of Pediatrics*, **2**, 288–96.

Udwin, O. & Yule, W. (1990). Expressive language of children with Williams syndrome. *American Journal of Medical Genetics*, **37**, 108–114.

Velleman, S.L., Currier, A., Caron, T., Curley, A., & Mervis, C.B. (May 2006). *Phonological Development in Williams Syndrome*. Presented at the Annual Meeting of the International Clinical Phonetics and Linguistics Association, Dubrovnik, Croatia.

Vicari, S., Caselli, M.C., Gagliardi, C., Tonucci, F., & Volterra, V. (2002). Language acquisition in special populations: a comparison between Down and Williams syndromes. *Neuropsychologia*, **40**, 2461–60.

Volterra, V., Caselli, M.C., Capirci, O., Tonucci, F., & Vicari, S. (2003). Early linguistic abilities of Italian children with Williams syndrome. *Developmental Neuropsychology*, **23**, 33–59.

Walsh, V. (2003). A theory of magnitude: common cortical metrics of time, space and quantity. *Trends in Cognitive Science*, **7**, 483–88.

Williams, K.T. (2007). *Expressive Vocabulary Test—Second Edition*. Minneapolis, MN: Pearson Assessments.

Chapter 11

Later language

Vesna Stojanovik

Introduction

The focus of this chapter is language abilities in individuals with Williams syndrome (WS) after the age of 5 years. The language abilities of individuals with WS have been noted as special since the first research carried out on this population. One of the earliest studies of the cognitive profile of individuals with WS by von Arnim and Engel (1964) reported that individuals with WS showed a facility for language rarely observed in other populations with the same degree of cognitive impairment. It was not until 1978 that the first attempt was made to systematically quantify the intellectual abilities of individuals with WS. Bennett et al. (1978) administered the McCarthy Scales of Children's Abilities (McCarthy, 1972) to seven children with WS (aged between 4 years 6 months and 8 years 5 months) and reported that all children performed better on measures of verbal ability than on fine motor and gross motor skills. The authors concluded that children with WS showed a relative strength in expressive language.

Until recently, interest in the linguistic skills of individuals with WS has mainly centred on morphosyntactic abilities, with comparably fewer studies investigating other linguistic domains, such as phonological, lexical/semantic and pragmatic abilities. In addition, the focus of research into language abilities in the WS population has mainly been on children and adults rather than on infants (see Chapter 10 for discussion of early language skills), resulting in a rich body of literature on later language skills in this population. This focus on the morphosyntactic domain has stemmed from theoretical interest in the contribution of the WS cognitive profile to the debate on whether language, and in particular morpho-syntax, is a separate neural system or module that develops independently of other cognitive abilities (Bellugi et al., 2001; Gerrans, 2003). This issue was first discussed by Bellugi and colleagues (Bellugi et al., 1988; Bellugi et al., 1992; Bellugi et al., 1994), who argued that WS offered *prima facie* evidence that language develops independently of general intellectual ability and is therefore a module, that is, impenetrable to general knowledge and input from other nonmodular cognitive systems (Fodor, 1983). The claim was based on findings that adolescents and adults with WS have relatively good morphosyntactic and lexical-semantic abilities, particularly when compared with individuals with Down syndrome (DS) of similar chronological and mental ages (CA and MA, respectively), and the 'relatively good' quickly slipped into 'preserved' (for example, Bellugi et al., 1999; Levy & Bechar, 2003; Musolino et al., 2010). Although the original proposal on language modularity by Fodor takes language as a whole to be a modular cognitive system, theoretical linguists often focus on the abstract, computational components of language involved in the genera-tion of rules in syntax and phonology as the 'language module'. The few early studies that investigated other linguistic skills in WS made similar claims regarding these skills, such that prosody was viewed as preserved albeit rich in affect intonation (Trevarthen et al., 1998), and lexical semantics was claimed to be independent of general cognitive abilities, characterised by word knowledge above MA level (Bellugi et al., 2000).

The view of language as a module in the Fodorian sense has been challenged, and of particular relevance for the understanding of neurodevelopmental disorders, including WS, has been the challenge to the innateness of modules (Karmiloff-Smith, 1992). This alternative view, the neuroconstructivist view, does not preclude the existence of modular-ity in the adult brain but proposes that rather than being present from the earliest stages of development, as suggested by innate-modularity accounts, modularity is a product of development (e.g. Karmiloff-Smith, 1992, 1998). Development itself and the protracted period of postnatal growth are seen as playing a crucial role in shaping phenotypical out-comes (Karmiloff-Smith, 1998). Thus, research on the language abilities of individuals with WS couched within the neuroconstructivist view of neurodevelopmental disorders has been particularly informative when specifying the development of different language skills over time in terms of onset and rate of development. This theoretical approach sup-ports developmental analyses of data and the building of developmental trajectories (see Chapter 1). Developmental trajectory analysis uses regression methods to plot a function between age and performance on an experimental task or a standardised test, using groups that typically span a large CA range (Thomas et al., 2009). A developmental trajectory analysis allows investigation of performance on a specific task over time as well as providing a description of performance in terms of typicality or atypicality (e.g. slow rate of development, late onset) for specific tasks as a function of age (Thomas et al., 2009). Ideally, development should be studied longitudinally. However, to date, only a few studies have taken that approach (e.g. Jarrold et al., 2001), and knowledge about how different linguistic skills may develop over time in individuals with WS has come primarily through the examination of cross-sectional developmental trajectories for different linguistic skills.

In addition to having a predominantly 'morphosyntax-centric' focus within the domain of later language development in individuals with WS, most studies have been limited by the consideration of data only from English-speaking individuals with WS. Data on the language abilities of individuals with WS speaking languages other than English have only recently been reported. The few published studies have also reported difficulties with language, especially with morphosyntax.

This chapter provides a review of the literature on linguistic abilities in English-speaking older children, adolescents and adults with WS regarding morphosyntax, phonology, lexical semantics and pragmatics, and in those speaking other languages, where data are available. The evidence for the status of different linguistic skills in individuals with WS will be evaluated with reference to the current theoretical debate about the contribution of neurodevelopmental disorders to the understanding of typical cognitive organisation. It will be shown how the neuroconstructivist approach and the use of developmental trajectories have advanced current knowledge of the linguistic profile in this population.

Links between brain abnormalities and resulting phenotypic outcomes will also be discussed.

Morphosyntactic abilities

The morphosyntactic skills of individuals with WS have been studied extensively, primarily for theoretical reasons, as discussed in the Introduction. Owing to the predominant innate-modularity view of language and, in particular, the focus on morphosyntax in the late 1980s and early 1990s, many of the early studies investigated relative strengths in the language domain, predominantly in older children and adults with WS (Bellugi et al., 1988; Bellugi et al., 1992; Bellugi et al., 1994). These studies promoted the view that syntactic abilities in individuals with WS are 'spared' (Bellugi et al., 1994) or 'preserved' (Bellugi et al., 1999) supporting the idea that there is a dissociation between morphosyntax and general cognitive skills. This view was based on findings showing that adolescents with WS are better at comprehension of reversible passive sentences, negation and conditionals than are age- and IQ-matched individuals with DS (Bellugi et al., 1999). Bellugi and her colleagues also reported that children and adolescents with WS are better at detecting syntactic anomalies and are able to correct ungrammatical sentences (Bellugi et al., 1999; Bellugi et al., 1994). Studies from other research laboratories also reported relatively good morphosyntactic skills in individuals with WS. Thus, Clahsen and Almazan (1998) showed that the ability of individuals with WS to comprehend reversible passives, regular past-tense morphology and reflexive anaphors is intact, compared with children with specific language impairment (SLI). Musolino et al. (2010) reported that individuals with WS aged between 11 and 21 years are able to understand core syntactic and semantic relations (i.e. c-command and scope, respectively) and that they perform similarly to MA-matched controls on most measures, thus arguing that 'knowledge of core, abstract principles of grammar is present and engaged in WS' (p. 53).

However, there is no evidence so far to show that individuals with WS perform above their nonverbal MA on tasks assessing morphosyntax. For example, Karmiloff-Smith et al. (1997) reported that English-speaking adolescents and adults with WS perform below their vocabulary age and CA on a standardised test of grammar. In a sentence repetition task requiring participants to repeat relative clauses, adolescents and adults with WS performed at a level equivalent to that of typically developing (TD) children aged 5 years (Grant et al., 2002). Similarly, Joffe and Varlocosta (2007) reported that children with WS performed significantly worse than MA-matched controls on the repetition of wh-questions. In addition, they performed significantly worse than MA-matched children and similarly to children with DS on the Test for Reception of Grammar (Bishop, 2003b), on comprehension and production of wh-questions and on a task assessing understanding of passive sentences. It should be noted however that there have not been any published studies so far that have adopted the developmental trajectory approach when investigating syntactic skills in WS and this is an area that clearly requires further research.

Research from languages with rich morphological systems has provided very useful insights into the language difficulties experienced by people with WS and has complemented

English-language findings about impaired grammatical skills in this population. For example, Levy and Hermon (2003) reported that although Hebrew-speaking adolescents with WS performed well on the basic consonant root structure of Hebrew words, they were poor compared with MA controls on different morphological paradigms. Furthermore, French-speaking adolescents and young adults with WS have been reported to have difficulty with the assignment of grammatical gender compared with younger TD children (Karmiloff-Smith et al., 1997). In particular, despite the fact that the individuals with WS had a higher MA with regard to vocabulary and morphosyntax compared with the younger controls, they performed poorly on assigning concordant grammatical gender markers especially with nonsense words. Similar difficulties with gender assignment were also reported by Monnery et al. (2002), and gender agreement errors have been documented for Italian (Volterra et al., 1996). Lukács et al. (2004) investigated the production of plural and accusative forms on nouns in Hungarian, another language with a rich and complex morphological system. They found that children with WS performed worse than receptive-vocabulary controls and that they had difficulty with both regular and irregular morpho-logical markers. Preposition errors and ungrammatical substitutions of function words or inflected forms in Spanish- or Italian-speaking children with WS have also been reported (Díez-Itza et al., 1998; Volterra et al., 1996).

The issue of regular versus irregular past-tense marking has attracted a lot of interest and debate. A number of research groups studying different languages have shown that individuals with WS perform better on regular than on irregular morphology (Bromberg et al., 1994; Clahsen et al., 2004; Pléh et al., 2003) and that they may be significantly impaired on irregulars compared with controls, but not on regulars (Clahsen &Almazan, 1998; Penke & Krause, 2004; Zukowski, 2004). However, individuals with WS have never been shown to outperform MA controls, either on regular or irregular inflections. Furthermore, studies that have employed large numbers of participants with WS and have taken a developmental trajectory approach controlling for verbal MA show no inter-action between group and regularity (e.g. Thomas et al., 2001). In other words, they failed to replicate the findings that regular morphology in WS is better than irregular morphology. The developmental trajectory approach also revealed that acquisition of the past tense by individuals with WS may follow an atypical trajectory because the individuals with WS, unlike the typical controls in the study, did not show a frequency effect for irregular past-tense forms (Thomas et al., 2001). Thus, the trajectory approach pushes the researcher to ask a more subtle set of questions and often reveals atypical processes.

Knowledge about morphosyntactic abilities in individuals with WS has also benefited from studies that have compared individuals with WS and other atypical populations known to have language deficits, such as individuals with SLI. Such comparisons have been particularly useful because they have pointed out that individuals with WS may not have as good language skills as it was originally thought. Few studies so far have directly compared the language abilities of individuals with WS with those of individuals with SLI; yet, there have been claims made in the literature that individuals with WS show the opposite language and cognitive profile to those with SLI (Pinker, 1999). In contrast to this position, Stojanovik et al. (2004) showed that a small sample of children with WS did not differ from children with SLI when directly compared on receptive and expressive standardised language tests assessing different aspects of morphosyntax. In addition, the children with WS and those with SLI did not differ on the number of correctly and incorrectly used grammatical markers in a spontaneous speech task. Hence, when only morphosyntactic skills were assessed, the two groups looked almost identical. Because of their radically different cognitive abilities, this strongly suggests that morphosyntactic abilities and the acquisition of grammar in WS and SLI are supported by different cognitive mechanisms that are most likely linked to the different genetic abnormalities in the two populations (although currently WS has a much clearer genetic specification than SLI). Given that both groups of children were of a similar CA, their experience of language and level of language input should be fairly comparable.

Such findings can be taken to support the neuroconstructivist view that specific phenotypes result from a unique interaction between specific genes and the environment. It should be noted that such findings also suggest that there is a minimum level of cognitive ability needed to acquire these morphosyntactic abilities and that both groups have reached that minimum level, that is, a threshold effect such that once the minimum level needed is acquired, then having more of that cognitive ability does not matter for acquisition of the particular morphosyntactic ability. However, if one took a nativist perspective, these findings could also be taken to show that language is independent of general cognitive abilities because despite having general cognitive impairments, children with WS still perform similarly to children with SLI who do not have such impairments. This shows that the same data can be interpreted in opposite ways given a specific theoretical position.

It should be noted that Stavrakaki (2004) compared three Greek-speaking children with WS and a group of children with SLI on their ability to produce referential and nonreferential wh-subject and wh-object questions. Two of the three children with WS reached ceiling performance (which was not the case with the children with SLI), but one participant with WS had difficulties with the production of these structures. The authors interpreted the results as implying that children with WS have similar syntactic abilities to TD children and different syntactic abilities when compared with children with SLI. This interpretation should be treated with caution because the sample size for the WS group was very small and only two of the three children performed at ceiling on the syntactic structures under investigation. Research has shown that the WS population is heterogeneous (Porter & Coltheart, 2005; Stojanovik et al., 2006) and it is difficult to get a full picture of the population's language profile if findings are based on two or three participants.

Lexical abilities

When compared with other populations with cognitive deficits, adolescents and adults with WS usually have rather impressive vocabularies. However, it is still unclear whether vocabulary and semantic processing in individuals with WS is typical, delayed or atypical. Individuals with WS often score better than what would be expected for their MA on standardised measures of receptive vocabulary (Bellugi, et al., 1988; Rossen et al., 1996; Clahsen et al., 2004), but note that it has recently been found that it is concrete vocabulary that is a relative strength in individuals with WS rather than conceptual/relational vocabulary (see Chapter 10; Mervis & John, 2008). Studies based on observations in which context was not controlled have reported that individuals with WS sometimes use unusual, low-frequency and idiosyncratic phrases, such as 'to evacuate the glass' instead of 'to empty the glass' (Bellugi et al., 1992), and that they produce semantic alternatives not appropriate for the context (Rossen et al., 1996). Such reports have been taken as evidence by some that certain aspects of language, such as lexical semantics, are independent of general cognitive abilities (Bellugi et al., 2000). However, when the conversational context was controlled, that is, when individuals with WS were given a wordless picture book and asked to generate a story based on the book, they did not produce a larger number of low-frequency words than did controls matched for language age, nonverbal age or CA (Stojanovik & van Ewijk, 2008).

Yet other reports in the literature suggest that semantic organisation in WS is atypical. For example, Temple et al. (2002) reported that children with WS have difficulties with naming, but they also found that when naming was accurate, it was faster than that of MA-matched controls. This is supported by evidence from a study by Ypsilanti et al. (2005), who showed that older children and adolescents with WS and those with DS produced atypical responses compared with MA-matched controls in a word definitions task. Rossen et al. (1996) found that older children and adolescents with WS had a reduced bias when pairing a homonym with its most likely associate in a task that required them to pair two words that go together. However, no atypicality has been revealed in online language processing. In a study by Tyler and colleagues (1997) who investigated priming effects of category structure and functional relations, adolescents and adults with WS performed no differently from controls, suggesting no atypical semantic organisation. These results indicate that individuals with WS seem to have normal semantic organisation and are able to access semantic information for individual words in the same way as TD individuals. However, their ability to integrate semantic information when processing sentences may be atypical.

Delayed rather than deviant semantic organisation in WS was reported in a study by Scott et al. (1995), who compared children with WS and those with DS with CA- and MA-matched TD controls on a task requiring the children to name as many animals as possible in 60 seconds. The four groups of participants were compared on fluency, representativeness, word frequency and category composition. The children with WS performed as expected for their MA on most measures of semantic fluency apart from knowledge of the most unusual items in a given category, which was in line with their CA. However, the finding is not specific to WS as this also happened in the DS group. These findings have been replicated by Volterra et al., (1996) and Lukács (2005). In a study using developmental trajectory analysis, Thomas et al. (2006) showed that frequency and semantic-category effects in a speeded picture-naming task were in line with receptive-vocabulary skills, arguing that the trajectory of semantic development in WS is delayed rather than atypical. They also argued that the use of unusual words by individuals with WS may be attributable to the specifics of the pragmatic profile of these individuals.

Research into lexical abilities (in particular into the claimed use of unusual exemplars from a given category) in WS has also benefited from cross-syndrome comparisons. Comparisons of individuals with WS and individuals classified with moderate learning difficulties have provided compelling evidence that there is not much unusual about the spontaneous production of vocabulary items in individuals with WS. Jarrold et al. (2000) compared a group of adolescents and adults with WS with a group of individuals with learning disability matched to the WS group on level of receptive vocabulary on a semantic fluency task. Contrary to the results of Bellugi and colleagues (Bellugi et al., 1994), Jarrold and colleagues found that there was little that was unusual about the semantic fluency performance of individuals with WS and that they produced the same number of novel items as the receptive-vocabulary-matched individuals with learning disability. Similar findings were also reported for Hebrew-speaking individuals by Levy and Bechar (2003), who compared individuals with WS with individuals with learning difficulties matched for CA and MA and two groups of TD children, highlighting the fact that findings are more general than just being applicable to English. Not only were there no differences on the semantic fluency task between the WS group and the learning disability group, but there also were no differences between the WS and the two TD groups.

Furthermore, Ypsilanti et al. (2005) showed that when defining vocabulary items, individuals with WS made semantic errors, whereas individuals with DS made morphosyntactic errors; yet, the groups were indistinguishable with regard to their overall expressive-vocabulary scores and MA. This highlights the fact that test results should be taken with caution and analysed qualitatively where possible so that we get a deeper and more accurate understanding of the specific language skills in different atypical populations.

Phonological abilities

Phonological abilities in WS have so far received relatively little interest, possibly because of the fact that individuals with WS do not have difficulties with the production of the sounds of their native language, although they may sometimes find it difficult to produce some polysyllabic words (Semel & Rosner, 2003). In a large-scale study including 43 children and adolescents with WS, Udwin and Yule (1990) reported that 84% of them had fluid intelligible speech. When 20 of the children with WS were compared with age- and verbal-IQ-matched individuals with learning difficulties, the WS group produced a greater proportion of intelligible and complete utterances.

Prosody, on the other hand, which refers to suprasegmental aspects of speech such as intonation, loudness, speech rhythm and syllabic features, has received more attention, though comparably less than other linguistic skills. Using prosody effectively and interpreting the prosodic features of other people's speech enables the listener to participate in the social rituals of his or her community: it is important to know when another speaker is finishing or preparing to speak further as well as signal one's own intention to finish or speak further, to decide where emphasis has been placed and be able to place emphasis, and to understand another speaker's emotional state and express one's own emotional state (see Chapter 15). One of the first studies to investigate the cognitive profile of individuals with WS noted that adolescents with WS had expressive prosody that was over-rich in affect intonation (Reilly et al., 1990). The first published studies to investigate both comprehension and production of prosody in children and adolescents with WS showed that they performed similarly to younger TD children on tasks assessing affective and linguistic prosody (Catterall et al., 2006; Stojanovik et al., 2007; Setter et al., 2007). Children and adolescents with WS have been found to have an abnormally high pitch range, which makes them sound twice as emotionally involved when telling a story as controls matched for language age and CA (Setter et al., 2007).

Using developmental trajectory analysis, Stojanovik (2010) showed that when MA is taken into account, children with WS do not show either a delay in onset or a slowed rate of development in any aspect of linguistic prosody apart from the ability to use prosody to regulate conversational behaviour. Furthermore, although an earlier study by Stojanovik et al. (2007) showed no differences between the WS group and CA-matched controls on the production of questioning versus declarative intonation, the developmental trajectory results showed that this prosodic skill develops at a slower rate in children with WS but eventually develops to a level commensurate with their CA. The developmental trajectory analysis also showed that, relative to CA, children and adolescents with WS have a delayed onset of the ability to use prosody to signal the most important word in an utterance, and delayed rates of development in the ability to perceive and produce prosody to disambiguate complex noun phrases and the ability to use prosody to perceive the most prominent word in an utterance (Stojanovik, 2010).

Some of these findings may not be syndrome-specific, however. Stojanovik and Setter (2011) compared children with WS and those with DS matched on receptive language and nonverbal skills on a number of prosodic tasks, both receptive and expressive. This study used a group-matching design, so did not address possible developmental trajectory differences between the two populations. However, the results showed two rather distinct profiles. Whereas the children with WS and those with DS performed similarly on tasks assessing the perception of the most prominent word in an utterance and were also similar in their ability to use prosody to disambiguate complex noun phrases, there were marked between-group differences with regard to all other aspects of prosody assessed in the study. In particular, the children with DS scored much lower than the children with WS on the ability to perceive and produce the affective and the turn-end functions of prosody. This between-syndrome comparison allows us to discover any syndrome-specific characteristics. What we know so far tells us that in WS, prosodic skills are in line with other cognitive abilities, whereas the prosodic profile in DS is mixed with severe weaknesses evident in some prosodic domains.

Research into the prosodic abilities of individuals with WS speaking languages other than English and cross-linguistic comparisons have highlighted the fact that comprehension and production of prosody is a weakness relative to CA in Spanish-speaking children and adolescents with WS (Martínez-Castilla et al., 2011). This study used a comprehensive battery of tasks from the Profiling Elements of Prosody in Speech Communication test (Peppé et al., 2003) assessing different aspects of prosody form and function. The tasks were identical, but the stimuli were different in the two languages. Furthermore, when English- and French-speaking individuals with WS were compared on their spontaneous use of language and their pitch range was measured, the results for the English and French individuals with WS were similar in that they showed an abnormally high pitch range compared with CA-matched controls in a story generation task (Lacroix et al., 2010b).

Pragmatic abilities

Pragmatics is often defined as the 'study of the way humans use language in communication' (Mey, 2001). However, the scope of pragmatic abilities is wide-ranging and includes the use of both linguistic and nonlinguistic abilities for the purposes of communication (Perkins, 2007). Research into the pragmatic abilities of children, adolescents and adults with WS has so far concentrated on the way in which individuals with WS use their linguistic abilities for the purpose of communication.

Knowledge about the pragmatic abilities of individuals with WS has come from studies that have investigated their conversational abilities, narrative skills and metapragmatic skills, such as understanding and use of idioms, metaphors and metonyms. Early descriptions of the communication skills of adolescents with WS characterised them as being 'highly social' (Reilly et al., 1990) and 'having remarkable social understanding' (Reilly et al., 1990). More recently, Jones et al. (2000) referred to individuals with WS as 'overly social'. This overly social personality has been interpreted by some, such as Rice et al. (2005), to suggest that social communication is not a weakness in children with WS. Based on findings from a series of tasks, Jones and colleagues (2000) reported that individuals with WS included more inferences about the affective state and motivation of story characters than did TD children or children with DS. In addition, individuals with WS provided a greater number of descriptions of affective states and evaluative comments during an interview task and were more likely to ask the interviewer personal questions. The authors interpreted such behaviours as showing that individuals with WS are hypersocial.

However, other research groups have reported that individuals with WS are not sensitive to the needs of their conversational partner (Udwin & Yule, 1991) and that they have difficulties making friends and establishing social relationships (Davies et al., 1998). More recently, Laws and Bishop (2004) compared caregiver or teacher reports of the pragmatic abilities of children and young adults with WS with those of individuals with DS or SLI using the Children's Communication Checklist (Bishop, 1998). Only the WS group differed significantly from younger TD control children on all five subscales that form the Pragmatics composite (Stereotyped Conversation, Use of Context, Rapport, Inappropriate Initiation of Conversation, Coherence). The WS group was also described as using considerably more stereotyped conversation than either the DS or SLI groups, indicating that stereotyped conversation may be a specific feature of the language of individuals with WS when compared with individuals with DS and those with SLI. The WS group also had the lowest score on social relationships when compared with younger TD children, children with SLI and those with DS. However, Philofsky et al. (2007) compared a group of school-aged children with WS with a group of school-aged children with autism using the

Children's Communication Checklist 2 (Bishop, 2003a) and found that the performance of children with WS was significantly better on the Pragmatic composite scale and on the Coherence, Stereotyped Language, Nonverbal Communication and Social Relations subscales than that of the children with autism. Thus, it seems that when compared with children who are known to have difficulties with pragmatic language functioning, such as those with autism spectrum disorders, children with WS do not seem to have quite such severe pragmatic language difficulties. This highlights the importance of cross-syndrome comparisons because we may get a slightly different picture of relative strengths and weaknesses depending on which other clinical population is used as a comparison group to the WS group.

Researchers studying the pragmatic abilities of people with WS have also investigated how individuals with WS understand figurative language (see also Chapter 1). Successful communication skills involve interpreting other people's intended meaning, which is not always the literal meaning of what was said. In typical development, idiom comprehension starts to develop from early childhood and continues to improve into adolescence and through adulthood. The first study of figurative language was with 11 adults with WS (Karmiloff-Smith et al., 1995). The authors reported that half of the participants were unable to explain the meaning of the metaphorical and sarcastic expressions in a story. However, the study lacked a control group and therefore it is difficult to conclude whether adults with WS had real difficulties with figurative language given their MA. A later study by Sullivan et al. (2003) included older children and young adults with WS as well as two comparison groups: CA- and IQ-matched adolescents with Prader–Willi syndrome and CA- and IQ-matched adolescents with nonspecific intellectual disability. The participants listened to stories that ended in either a lie or a joke and they were asked to identify which was which and justify their answers. The study reported that individuals with WS had difficulty distinguishing between lies and ironic jokes, but they did not differ from the other two populations, suggesting that the difficulty is not syndrome-specific. Unfortunately, the analyses of the data did not include any developmental trajectories because the design was one that matched at a group level, which by default does not take development into account. Nevertheless, the results do emphasise the fact that although the three groups of participants did not differ in the number of accurate responses they gave, they seem to be reasoning about their answers differently. The individuals with WS justified their answers by looking at the pictures and referring to what actually happened, whereas the other two groups justified their answers by referring to the mental state of the characters. According to the authors, the pattern of errors of the individuals with WS was similar to that for younger TD children but different from those made by patients with acquired brain damage.

A significant step forward in the understanding of how this aspect of pragmatics, figurative language, develops in individuals with WS was made in a recent study by Annaz et al. (2009), who included children with WS aged between 6 and 10 years. The study investigated comprehension of two types of figurative expressions: metaphors and metonyms. The data were analysed using developmental trajectories. The results showed that while for TD children there is a linear relation between increasing CA and understanding of lexicalised metaphor and metonymy, no such relationship held for the children with WS, although there was a significant relationship with receptive-vocabulary age. Furthermore, metaphor comprehension in the WS group was worse than expected for their level of receptive vocabulary, whereas metonymy comprehension was in line with their receptive vocabulary level. The developmental trajectory approach allowed for a finer account of two pragmatic subskills: both skills are delayed but metaphor comprehension seems to be very delayed, and the authors question whether this ability will ever develop.

Understanding of idiomatic expressions has also been investigated in individuals with WS. Mervis et al. (2003) investigated the understanding of idiomatic expressions in English-speaking adolescents and adults with WS and found that the majority of them had difficulty with the understanding of idiomatic expressions, with ability to comprehend idioms strongly related to performance on Piagetian conservation tasks. A study by Lacroix et al. (2010a) also investigated understanding of idiomatic expressions, but in French-speaking children and adolescents with WS using the developmental trajectory approach. The analyses showed that the children with WS have a slower rate of development regarding the comprehension of idiomatic expressions, but that their understanding of idioms increases with increasing CA. Owing to the slower rate of development, individuals with WS may never reach typical proficiency with regard to idiom comprehension.

General discussion

This chapter presented an overview of the current state of knowledge regarding the phonological, lexical, morphosyntactic and pragmatic abilities of older children, adolescents and adults with WS. The presented evidence strongly suggests that none of these abilities is 'preserved' in individuals with WS and that the language profile of individuals with WS does not support innate modularity. Indeed, as Mervis and Becerra (2007) argue, 'rather than being the paradigm case for the independence of language from cognition, WS provides strong evidence for the interdependence of many aspects of language and cognition'.

A significant contribution to the understanding of how different aspects of language in individuals with WS may be developing over time has been made by advances in theoretical thought and the introduction of the developmental trajectory approach to data analysis and interpretation. Cross-syndrome comparisons have also allowed for the identification of syndrome-specific profiles and data from languages other than English confirm that the language abilities in individuals with WS are not preserved.

Technological advances in the field of cognitive neuroscience have made it possible to investigate brain–behaviour relationships in typical and atypical populations, paving the way towards the bridging of the gap between brain structure and function and phenotypic outcomes related to the language profile of this population. Some evidence comes from magnetic resonance imaging studies. For example, the atypical prosody reported in individuals with WS may be related to increased cortical thickness (Thompson et al., 2005) spanning a broad anatomical area including the perisylvian regions, which, especially in the right hemisphere, are responsible for processing linguistic and musical syntax and prosody (Ross & Mesulam, 1979; Cabeza & Nyberg, 2000; as cited in Thompson et al., 2005). The hypersocial behaviour of individuals with WS may be related to the aberrant morphology of the ventral anterior prefrontal cortex, which is a pivotal contributing factor to the abnormal size and shape of the cerebral cortex (Gothelf et al., 2008). Meyer-Lindenberg et al. (2005) reported abnormal activation and interaction of prefrontal regions linked to the amygdala, which may be associated with the hypersociability and nonsocial anxiety in individuals with WS.

Event-related potential studies have shown that individuals with WS do not develop the hemispheric asymmetries associated with the processing of closed versus open class words by individuals in the general population (Neville et al., 1994), which suggests that the neural organisation of some aspects of language in WS is different from that in the general population. However, these studies are far from definitive and future research is needed to fully uncover the underlying brain structure and function responsible for the WS phenotype. As detailed in Chapter 2, currently we mainly have information about the adult brain in individuals with WS. Future research is important to establish how the language phenotype later on in life is affected by cortical anomalies in infancy and childhood and by any anatomical changes that occur in the WS brain because of the genetic abnormality. Little is also known about which other cognitive processes may underlie the language abilities in WS. Phonological memory ability and verbal working memory ability have been found to be related to vocabulary and grammatical ability for individuals with WS (Grant et al., 1997; Pléh, et al., 2003; Robinson et al., 2003), but there may be other cognitive skills that are important and need to be identified (see Chapter 18 for discussion of the impact of attentional mechanisms on language development). Finally, very little is known about how individuals with WS process language online and future research should close this gap.

Editor commentary (Emily K. Farran & Annette Karmiloff-Smith)

The phenomenon that language skills are stronger than visuospatial and motor abilities is often seen as the hallmark of the adult WS cognitive profile. Following exploration in the previous chapter (Chapter 10) of the emergence of language in WS, this chapter detailed the subsequent development of the WS language profile, with reference to morphosyntax, lexical development, phonology and pragmatics. The chapter included multiple examples that showed that, despite its relative strength in WS, the development of language has proceeded through qualitatively different trajectories. Lexical ability, for example, is the strongest aspect of language in WS, yet individuals with WS and DS with the same overall level of vocabulary show different error patterns. Furthermore, children with WS show an uneven profile of weaker vocabulary for conceptual and relational words than concrete words, which further testifies to atypical developmental trajectories of lexical abilities in WS. The same is true of morphosyntax, where atypical developmental patterns are also described. Accurate perception of prosody, on the other hand, emerges late with a slow rate of development but eventually reaches age-appropriate levels. Indeed, in WS, speech output is very intelligible and this contrasts with many other neurodevelopmental disorders.

Pragmatics, or the use of language in communication (also discussed in Chapter 1), is weaker in WS than in individuals with DS or SLI, but is stronger than in individuals with autism. Cross-syndrome association between the pragmatic abilities of individuals with WS and those with Prader–Willi syndrome further emphasises different cognitive/brain/genetic causes for impairment, despite similar levels of ability.

Just as language is not 'spared' in WS, can language be specifically impaired, leaving other processes 'intact'? Evidence has shown that children with dyslexia, which is described as a specific reading deficit, can also have visual impairments and deficits in motor tapping tasks (Geuze & Kalverboer, 1994), whereas children with SLI revealed postural errors when asked to produce familiar hand positions for, say, brushing their teeth (Hill et al., 1998), as well as deficits in visuospatial short-term memory (Hick et al., 2005). Furthermore, although within the normal range, nonverbal intelligence in children with SLI is significantly lower than that in their siblings (see Botting, 2005) suggesting some more subtle general deficits. This lends credence to the neuroconstructivist view of gradual specialisation. Multilevel developmental interactions are vital to truly understand phenotypic outcome.

References

Annaz, D., Van Herwegen, J., Thomas, M., Fishman, R., Karmiloff-Smith., A., et al. (2009). Comprehension of metaphor and metonymy in children with Williams syndrome. *International Journal of Language and Communication Disorders*, **44**, 962–78.

von Arnim, G., & Engel, P. (1964). Mental retardation related to hypercalcaemia. *Developmental Medicine and Child Neurology*, **6**, 366–77.

Bellugi, U., Bihrle, A., Neville, H., Jernigan, T., & Doherty, S. (1992). Language, cognition, and brain organization in a neurodevelopmental disorder. In M. Gunnar & C. Nelson (Eds), *Developmental Behavioral Neuroscience* (pp. 201–232). Hillsdale, NJ: Lawrence Erlbaum.

Bellugi, U., Korenberg, J.R., & Klima, E.S. (2001). Williams syndrome: an exploration of neurocognitive and genetic features. *Clinical Neuroscience Research*, **1**, 217–29.

Bellugi, U., Lichtenberger, L., Jones, W., Lai, Z., & St. George, M. (2000). The neurocognitive profile of Williams syndrome: a complex pattern of strengths and weaknesses. *Journal of Cognitive Neuroscience,* **12 Supplement 1**, 7–29.

Bellugi, U., Lichtenberger, L., Mills, D., Galaburda, A., & Korenberg, J.R. (1999). Bridging cognition, the brain and modular genetics: evidence from Williams syndrome. *Trends in Neuroscience*, **22**, 197–207.

Bellugi, U., Marks, S., Bihrle, A., & Sabo, H. (1988). Dissociations between language and cognitive functions in Williams syndrome. In D. Bishop & K. Mogford (Eds), *Language Development in Exceptional Circumstances* (pp. 177–89). Edinburgh: Churchill Livingstone.

Bellugi, U., Wang, P.P., & Jernigan, T.L. (1994). Williams syndrome: an unusual neuropsychological profile. In S.H. Broman & J. Grafman (Eds), *Atypical Cognitive Deficits in Developmental Disorders: Implications for Brain Function* (pp. 23–56). Hillsdale, NJ: Lawrence Erlbaum.

Bennett, F.C., La Veck, B., & Sells, C.J. (1978). The Williams elfin faces syndrome: the psychological profile as an aid in syndrome identification. *Pediatrics*, **61**, 303–306.

Bishop, D.M. (1998). *Children's Communication Checklist*. London: The Psychological Corporation.

Bishop, D.M. (2003a). *Children's Communication Checklist Second Edition*. London: The Psychological Corporation.

Bishop, D.M. (2003b). *Test for the Reception of Grammar*. London; Harcourt Assessment.

Botting, N. (2005). Non-verbal cognitive development and language impairment. *Journal of Child Psychology and Psychiatry*, **46**, 317–26.

Bromberg, H.S., Ullman, M., Marcus, G., Kelley, K.B., & Levine, K. (July 1994). *The Dissociation between Lexical Memory and Grammar in Williams Syndrome: Evidence from Inflectional Morphology.* Presented at the Professional Conference on Williams Syndrome, San Diego, CA. Language and Williams syndrome: how intact is "intact"? *Child Development*, **68**, 246–62.

Cabeza, R., & Nyberg, L. (2000). Imaging cognition II: an empirical review of 275 PET and fMRI studies. *Journal of Cognitive Neuroscience*, **12**, 1–47.

Catterall, C., Howard, S., Stojanovik, V., Szczerbinski, M., & Wells, B. (2006). Investigating prosodic ability in Williams syndrome. *Clinical Linguistics and Phonetics*. **20**, 531–38.

Clahsen, H., & Almazan, M. (1998). Syntax and morphology in Williams syndrome. *Cognition*, **68**, 167–98.

Clahsen, H., Ring, M., & C. Temple. (2004). Lexical and morphological skills in English-speaking children with Williams syndrome. In S. Bartke & J. Siegmüller (Eds), *Williams Syndrome across Languages* (pp. 221–44). Amsterdam: John Benjamins.

Davies, M., Udwin, O., & Howlin, P. (1998). Adults with Williams syndrome. Preliminary study of social, emotional and behavioural difficulties. *British Journal of Psychiatry*, **172**, 273–76.

Díez-Itza, E., Antón, A., Fernández-Toral, J., & García-Pérez, M.L. (1998). Language development in Spanish children with Williams syndrome. In A. Aksu Koç, E. Erguvanli Taylan, A. Sumru Özsoy & A. Küntay (Eds), *Perspectives on Language Acquisition. Selected Papers from the VIIth International Congress for the Study of Child Language* (pp. 309–24). Istanbul: Bogazici University Printhouse.

Fodor, J. (1983). *The Modularity of Mind*. Cambridge, MA: MIT Press.

Gerrans, P. (2003). Nativism and neuroconstructivism in the explanation of Williams syndrome. *Biology and Philosophy*, **18**, 41–52.

Geuze, R.H., & Kalverboer, A.F. (1994). Tapping a rhythm: a problem of timing for children who are clumsy and dyslexic? *Adapted Physical Activity Quarterly*, **11**, 203–213.

Gothelf, D., Searcy, Y.M., Reilly, J., Lai, P.T., Lanre-Amos, T., Mills, D., et al., (2008). Association between cerebral shape and social use of language in Williams syndrome. *American Journal of Medical Genetics Part A*, **146A**, 2753–61.

Grant, J., Karmiloff-Smith, A., Gathercole, S.A., Paterson, S., Howlin, P., Davies, M., et al. (1997). Phonological short-term memory and its relationship to language in Williams syndrome. *Cognitive Neuropsychiatry*, **2**, 81–99.

Grant, J., Valian, V., & Karmiloff-Smith, A. (2002). A study of relative pronouns in Williams syndrome. *Journal of Child Language*, **29**, 403–416.

Hick, R., Botting, N., & Conti-Ramsden, G. (2005). Cognitive abilities in children with specific language impairment: consideration of visuo-spatial skills. *International Journal of Language and Communication Disorders*, **40**, 137–49.

Hill, E.L., Bishop, D.V.M., & Nimmo-Smith, I. (1998). Representational gestures in Developmental Coordination Disorder and specific language impairment: error-types and the reliability of ratings. *Human Movement Science*, **17**, 655–78.

Jarrold, C., Baddeley, A.D., Hewes, A.K., & Phillips, C. (2001). A longitudinal assessment of diverging verbal and non-verbal abilities in the Williams syndrome phenotype. *Cortex*, **37**, 423–31.

Jarrold, C., Hartley, S.J., Phillips, C., and Baddeley, A.D. (2000). Word fluency in Williams syndrome: evidence for unusual semantic organisation? *Cognitive Neuropsychology*, **5**, 293–319.

Joffe, V., & Varlocosta, S. (2007). Patterns of syntactic development in children with Williams syndrome and Down's syndrome: evidence from passives and wh-questions. *Clinical Linguistics and Phonetics*, **21**, 705–27.

Jones, W., Bellugi, U., Lai, Z., Chiles, M., Reilly, J., Lincoln, A., et al. (2000). Hypersociability in Williams syndrome. *Journal of Cognitive Neuroscience*, **12**, 30–46.

Karmiloff-Smith, A. (1992). *Beyond Modularity: a Developmental Perspective on Cognitive Science*. Cambridge, MA: MIT Press.

Karmiloff-Smith, A. (1998). Development itself is the key to understanding developmental disorders. *Trends in Cognitive Sciences*, **2**, 389–98.

Karmiloff-Smith, A., Grant, J., Berthoud, I., Davies, M., Howlin, P., & Udwin, O. (1997). How intact is "intact"? *Child Development*, **68**, 274–90.

Karmiloff-Smith, A., Klima, E.S., Bellugi, U., Grant, J., & Baron-Cohen, S. (1995). Is there a social module? Language, face processing, and theory of mind in individuals with Williams syndrome. *Journal of Cognitive Neuroscience* 7, 196–208.

Lacroix, A., Aguert, M., Dardier, V., Stojanovik, V., & Laval, V. (2010a). Idiom comprehension in French-speaking children and adolescents with Williams syndrome. *Research in Developmental Disabilities*, **31**, 608–616.

Lacroix, A., Stojanovik, V., Laval, V., & Dardier, V. (2010b). Prosodie et syndrome de Williams: une étude inter-culturelle. *Enfance*, **3**, 287–300.

Laws, G. & Bishop, D. (2004). Pragmatic language impairment and social deficits in Williams syndrome: a comparison with Down's syndrome and specific language impairment. *International Journal of Language and Communication Disorders*, **39**, 45–64.

Levy, Y., & Bechar, T. (2003). Cognitive, lexical, and morpho-syntactic profiles of Israeli children with Williams syndrome. *Cortex*, **39**, 255–71.

Levy, Y., & Hermon, S. (2003). Morphological abilities of Hebrew speaking adolescents with Williams syndrome. *Developmental Neuropsychology*, **23**, 59–83.

Lukács, A. (2005). *Language Abilities in Williams Syndrome*. Budapest, Hungary: Akadémiai Kiadó.

Lukács, A., Pléh, C., & Racsmány, M. (2004). Language in Hungarian children with Williams syndrome. In S. Bartke & J. Siegmüller (Eds), *Williams Syndrome across Languages* (pp. 187–220). Amsterdam: John Benjamins.

Martínez-Castilla, P., Stojanovik, V., Setter, J., & Sotillo, M. (2011). Prosodic abilities in Spanish and English children with Williams syndrome. *Applied Psycholinguistics* [Epub ahead of print 4 August 2011].

McCarthy, D. (1972). *McCarthy Scales of Children's Abilities*. New York, NY: Psychological Corporation.

Mervis, C.B., & Becerra, A.M. (2007). Language and communicative development in Williams syndrome. *Mental Retardation and Developmental Disabilities Research Reviews*, **13**, 3–15.

Mervis, C.B., & John, A.E. (2008). Vocabulary abilities of children with Williams syndrome: strengths, weaknesses and relation to visuospatial construction ability. *Journal of Speech, Language and Hearing Research*, **51**, 967–82.

Mervis, C.B., Robinson, B.F., Rowe, M.L., Becerra, A.M., & Klein-Tasman, B.P. (2003). Language abilities of individuals with Williams syndrome. *International Review of Research in Mental Retardation*, **27**, 35–81.

Mey, J. (2001). *Pragmatics: An Introduction*. Oxford: Blackwell.

Meyer-Lindenberg, A., Hariri, A.R., Munoz, K.E., Mervis, C.B., Mattay, V.S., Morris, C.A., et al. (2005). Neural correlates of genetically abnormal social cognition in Williams syndrome. *Nature Neuroscience*, **8**, 991–93.

Monnery, S., Seigneuric, A., Zagar, D., & Robichon, F. (2002). A linguistic dissociation in Williams syndrome: good at gender agreement but poor at lexical retrieval. *Reading and Writing*, 15, 589–612.

Musolino, J., Chunyo, G., & Landau, B. (2010). Uncovering knowledge of core syntactic and semantic principles in individuals with Williams syndrome. *Language Learning and Development*, **6**, 126–61.

Neville, H.J., Mills, D.L., & Bellugi, U. (1994). Effects of altered auditory sensitivity and age of language acquisition on the development of language relevant neural systems: preliminary studies of Williams syndrome. In S. Broman., & J. Grafman (Eds). *Atypical Cognitive Deficits in Developmental Disorders: Implications for Brain Function* (pp. 67–83). Hillsdale, NJ: Lawrence Erlbaum.

Penke, M., & Krause, M. (2004). Regular and irregular inflectional morphology in German Williams syndrome. In S. Bartke, & J. Siegmüller, J. (Eds), *Williams Syndrome across Languages* (pp. 245–70). Amsterdam: John Benjamins.

Peppé, S., McCann, J., & Gibbon, F. (2003). *Profiling Elements of Prosody in Speech-Communication (PEPS-C)*. Edinburgh: Queen Margaret University College.

Perkins, M. (2007). *Pragmatic impairment*. Cambridge: Cambridge University Press.

Philofsky, A., Fidler, D.J., & Hepburn, S. (2007). Pragmatic language profiles of school-age children with autism spectrum disorders and Williams syndrome. *American Journal of Speech-Language Pathology*, **16**, 368–80.

Pinker, S. (1999). *Words and Rules*. London: Weidenfield and Nicolson.

Pléh, C., Lukács, A., & Racsmány, M. (2003). Morphological patterns in Hungarian children with Williams syndrome and the rule debates. *Brain and Language*, **86**, 377–83.

Porter, M., & Coltheart, M. (2005). Cognitive heterogeneity in Williams syndrome. *Developmental Neuropsychology*, **27**, 275–306.

Reilly, J., Klima, E.S., & Bellugi, U. (1990). Once more with feeling: affect and language in atypical populations. *Development and Psychopathology*, **2**, 367–91.

Rice, M.L, Warren, S.F, & Betz, S.K. (2005). Language symptoms of developmental language disorders: an overview of autism, Down syndrome, fragile X, specific language impairment, and Williams syndrome. *Applied Psycholinguistics*, **26**, 7–27.

Robinson, B.F., Mervis, C., & Robinson, B.W. (2003). The roles of verbal short-term memory and working memory in the acquisition of grammar by children with Williams syndrome. *Developmental Neuropsychology*, **23**, 13–31.

Ross, E.D., & Mesulam, M.M. (1979). Dominant language functions of the right hemisphere? Prosody and emotional gesturing. *Archives of Neurology*, **36**, 144–48.

Rossen, M., Klima, E.S., Bellugi, U., Bihrle, A., & Jones, W. (1996). Interaction between language and cognition: evidence from Williams syndrome. In J.H. Beitchman, N. Cohen, M. Konstantareas & R. Tannock (Eds), *Language, Learning, and Behavior Disorders: Developmental, Biological, and Clinical Perspectives* (pp. 367–92). New York, NY: Cambridge University Press.

Scott, P., Mervis, C.B., Bertrand, J., Klein, B.P., Armstrong, S.C., & Ford, A.L. (1995). Semantic organization and word fluency in 9-and 10-year-old children with Williams syndrome. *Genetic Counselling*, **6**, 172–73.

Semel, E.M., & Rosner, S.R. (2003). *Understanding Williams Syndrome: Behavioural Patterns and Interventions*. Mahwah, NJ: Lawrence Erlbaum.

Setter, J.E., Stojanovik, V., van Ewijk, L., & Moreland, M. (2007). Affective prosody in children with Williams syndrome. *Clinical Linguistics and Phonetics*, **21**, 9, 659–72.

Stavrakaki, S. (2004). Wh-questions in Greek children with Williams syndrome: a comparison with SLI and normal development. In S. Bartke & J. Siegmüller (Eds), *Williams Syndrome across Languages* (pp. 295–312). Amsterdam: John Benjamins.

Stojanovik, V. (2010). Understanding and production of prosody in children with Williams syndrome: a developmental trajectory approach. *Journal of Neurolinguistics*, **23**, 112–26.

Stojanovik, V, & van Ewijk, L. (2008). Do children with Williams syndrome have unusual vocabularies? *Journal of Neurolinguistics*, **21**, 18–34.

Stojanovik, V., Perkins, M., & Howard, S. (2004). Williams syndrome and specific language impairment do not support claims for developmental double dissociations and innate modularity. *Journal of Neurolinguistics*, **17**, 403–24.

Stojanovik, V., Perkins, M., & Howard, S. (2006). Linguistic heterogeneity in Williams syndrome. *Clinical Linguistics and Phonetics*, **20**, 547–52.

Stojanovik, V., Setter, J., & van Ewijk, L. (2007). Intonation abilities in children with Williams syndrome: a preliminary investigation. *Journal of Speech, Language and Hearing Research*, **50**, 1610–17.

Stojanovik, V., & Setter, J. (2011). Prosody in two genetic disorders: Williams and Down's syndrome. In V. Stojanovik & J. Setter (Eds), *Prosody in Atypical Populations* (pp. 25–44). Guildford: J&R Press.

Sullivan, K., Winner, E., & Tager-Flusberg, H. (2003). Can adolescents with Williams syndrome tell the difference between lies and jokes? *Developmental Neuropsychology*, **23**, 85–103.

Temple, C.M., Almazan, M., & Sherwood. (2002). Lexical skills in Williams syndrome: a cognitive neuropsychological analysis. *Journal of Neurolinguistics*, **15**, 463–59.

Thomas, M.S.C., Annaz, D., Ansari, D., Scerif, G., Jarrold, C., & Karmiloff-Smith, A. (2009). Using developmental trajectories to understand genetic disorders. *Journal of Speech, Language, and Hearing Research*, **52**, 336–58.

Thomas, M.S., Dockrell, J.E., Messer, D., Parmigiani, C., Ansari, D., & Karmiloff-Smith, A. (2006). Speeded naming, frequency and the development of the lexicon in Williams syndrome. *Language and Cognitive Processes*, **21**, 721–59.

Thomas, M.S.C., Grant, J., Barham, Z., Gsödl, M., Laing, E., & Lakusta, L. (2001). Past tense formation in Williams syndrome. *Language and Cognitive Processes*, **16**, 143–76.

Thompson, P.M., Lee, A.D., Dutton, R.A., Geaga, J.A., Hayashi, K.M., Eckert, M.A., et al. (2005). Abnormal cortical complexity and thickness profiles mapped in Williams syndrome. *Journal of Neuroscience*, **25**, 4146–58.

Trevarthen, C., Aitken, K., Papoudi, D., & Robarts, J. (1998). *Children with Autism: Diagnosis and Intervention to Meet their Needs*, 2nd edn. London: Jessica Kingsley.

Tyler, L.K., Karmiloff-Smith, A., Voice, J.K., Stevens, T., Grant, J., Udwin, O., et al. (1997). Do individuals with Williams syndrome have bizarre semantics? Evidence for lexical organization using an on-line task. *Cortex*, **33**, 515–27.

Udwin, O., & Yule, W. (1990). Expressive language of children with Williams syndrome. *American Journal of Medical Genetics Supplement*, **6**, 108–114.

Udwin, O., & Yule, W. (1991). A cognitive and behavioural phenotype in Williams syndrome. *Journal of Clinical and Experimental Neuropsychology*, **13**, 232–44.

Volterra, V., Capirci, O., Pezzini, G., Sabbadini, L., & Vicari, S. (1996). Linguistic abilities in Italian children with Williams syndrome. *Cortex*, **32**, 663–77.

Ypsilanti, A., Grouios, G., Alevriadou, A., & Tsapkini, K. (2005). Expressive and receptive vocabulary in children with Williams and Down syndromes. *Journal of Intellectual Disability Research*, **49**, 353–64.

Zukowski, A. (2004). Investigating knowledge of complex syntax: insights from experimental studies of Williams syndrome. In M. Rice & S. Warren (Eds), *Developmental Language Disorders: From Phenotypes to Etiologies* (pp. 99–119). Mahwah, NJ: Lawrence Erlbaum.

Visual Domain

Chapter 12

Visual perception and visuospatial cognition

Emily K. Farran and Susan C. Formby

Introduction

One of the core cognitive characteristics of Williams syndrome (WS) is the marked contrast between poor levels of visuospatial ability relative to stronger verbal abilities. Visuospatial cognition enables us to perceive and interact with our visual world. It includes everyday skills such as the ability to reach for and grasp our knife and fork and to recognise the food on the plate, the visual search skills required to locate our favourite cereal on a supermarket shelf or our coat on a coat rack, the processes that enable us to individuate objects in order to count them, to draw pictures, to write and recognise words and to complete puzzles, and even the ability to know which bus stop to get off at when travelling. In WS, many of these visuospatial skills do not develop beyond the level of a typically developing (TD) 6-year-old. However, there is considerable variation across levels of ability within this domain, as illustrated in Figure 12.1. It is also important to note that, despite a high prevalence of sensory visual problems such as strabismus in WS, sensory status does not correlate with visuospatial cognition (Atkinson et al., 2001; Van der Geest & Frens, 2005). In this chapter, we outline the characteristic profile of visuospatial abilities in WS within the context of developmental interactions between genes, brain, the environment and behaviour.

Visuospatial construction

Poor visuospatial-construction ability is considered a hallmark of the WS cognitive phenotype as it represents one of the poorest abilities within the visuospatial domain in WS, with performance in children and adults with WS at the level of a typical 4-year-old (Atkinson et al., 2001; Farran et al., 1999). Evidence is based on studies that have employed standardised visuospatial-construction tasks such as the Block Design task (e.g. Wechsler Intelligence Scale for Children; Wechsler, 2004) or the Pattern Construction task (Differential Ability Scales; Elliot, 1990). These tasks require the participant to arrange the upper faces of three-dimensional blocks to resemble a two-dimensional model image. Longitudinal assessment by Jarrold et al. (2001) demonstrated that pattern construction mental age (MA) increased linearly in children and adults with WS (range: 7-28 years) by approximately 10 months over a 40-month period, one-quarter the rate of increase in chronological age. This compared with an increase in MA of approximately 24 months for the development of receptive vocabulary, a relative strength in WS. This demonstrates not only that visuospatial-construction ability develops extremely slowly in WS, but also that the WS cognitive profile is an emergent product of development with verbal and visuospatial domains diverging as an individual matures.

Visuospatial-construction performance in WS is characterised by solutions that lack global cohesion such that the blocks are not organised into the correct spatial arrangements. This led researchers to hypothesise that visuospatial cognition in WS reflects a local processing bias (e.g. Bellugi et al., 1988a). However, comparison with the autism literature demonstrates that a local bias in perception on this task benefits rather than impairs performance because participants who process locally are better able to perceptually segment the model image into the component parts, that is, the individual block faces (Shah & Frith, 1993). Furthermore, Farran et al. (2001), used the Children's Embedded Figures Task (Witkin et al., 1971) and a segmented version of a block construction task to present evidence against a local bias in perception in children and adults with WS (range: 10-39 years), concluding that the lack of global cohesion relates to the production demands of the task and not to its perception demands.

A number of visuospatial factors have been identified to explain how the above characteristic pattern is produced. Farran and Jarrold (2005) demonstrated that the encoding of the spatial relationships between local elements is atypical in children and adults with WS (range: 11-33 years). This is thought to negatively impact on the ability to recreate the spatial relationships perceived in the visual array, leading to configural errors in production. Related to this, in studies of children with WS (range: 7-14 years) and a group of children and adults with WS (range: 10-39 years), participants also confused mirror-imaged block faces, such as confusing a block face with white above red with the opposite arrangement of red above white. This indicates that they also have a weak representation of the spatial relationships of the parts within a block face (Farran & Jarrold, 2004; Hoffman et al., 2003). In addition, the strategies used by individuals with WS are suboptimal. TD children employ mental imagery to imagine the blocks at different rotations and configurations before manually moving a block into place. By contrast, children and adults with WS rely on manually manipulating the blocks throughout to reach a solution, which slows down completion time (Farran et al., 2001; Stinton et al., 2008).

The above visuospatial impairments are also likely to interact with the attention, executive function and working memory requirements of the task (see Chapters 6, 8 & 9). For example, in both block construction and drawing tasks, children and adults with WS show evidence of typical executive planning abilities for simple puzzles (WS age range: 7-14 years) and drawings (WS age range: 9-43 years), whereas complex puzzles and drawings are completed using atypical strategies (Hoffman et al., 2003; Hudson & Farran, 2011). This indicates that the ability to use executive functions is dictated by the limits of visuospatial perceptual abilities in WS. Analytic investigation has therefore unravelled the multifactorial nature of the visuospatial-construction deficit in WS. This level of understanding is necessary if we are to understand how behavioural deficits relate to genetic expression, environmental influence and brain development.

The dorsal visual stream and developmental vulnerability

Two visual streams are hypothesised in the typical brain, the dorsal and the ventral visual streams (see also Chapter 13). The dorsal stream runs from the occipital lobe to the parietal lobe and is thought to be responsible for the visual control and guidance of action. The ventral stream runs from the occipital lobe to the inferior temporal lobe and is thought to be responsible for perception (Milner & Goodale, 1995, 2008). Atkinson et al. (1997) report that individuals with WS display impairments on tasks that activate the dorsal visual stream and thus put forward the dorsal-stream-vulnerability hypothesis. In support of this, many of the factors involved in visuospatial construction are functions of the dorsal visual stream (e.g. mental rotation: Alivisatos & Petrides, 1997; coding spatial relations: Goldenberg, 2009; location processing and visuomotor action: Milner & Goodale, 1995).

There are three considerations to take into account in relation to the dorsal-stream-vulnerability hypothesis. First, as Braddick et al. (2003) point out, a dorsal-stream deficit might not be syndrome-specific and has been observed across a number of neurodevelopmental disorders, such as dyslexia, autism and specific language impairment (Eden et al., 1996; Lovegrove et al., 1990; Spencer et al., 2000). This cross-syndrome vulnerability has been related to the later emergence or to relatively long developmental trajectories of dorsal-stream functions in typical children and thus greater susceptibility to genetic and environmental influences than ventral-stream functions.

Second, because competency in a skill is the product of coordination of multiple brain areas, one must consider the network-focused approach to neural activation: although ventral and dorsal pathways are functionally separate, there are many structural connections and functional interactions between them (Van Essen et al., 1992), and thus a deficit unique to one visual stream is unlikely (see McIntosh & Schenk, 2009) and, more broadly, dorsal-stream activation must be considered within the context of correlated activity with domain-general (and other domain-specific) processes, as discussed in Chapter 13.

Finally, owing to brain plasticity, functions typically attributed to the dorsal stream might develop via alternative neural pathways in groups with neurodevelopmental disorders. These considerations are taken into account in our discussion of dorsal-stream vulnerability in WS.

Children with WS show impairment on a 'dorsal stream' postbox task in which the individual posts a card into a slot, relative to a 'ventral stream' postbox task in which the participant matches the orientation of a card to that of the posting slot (Atkinson et al., 1997; Dilks et al., 2008). Dilks et al. (2008) demonstrated that this pattern of performance in their group of children with WS (range: 8-16 years) was akin to the pattern observed in TD 4-year-olds, and that by 6 years TD children no longer showed this disparity because

performance on the dorsal task had 'caught up' with that on the ventral task. The disparity observed in WS, however, does not reflect a simple delay because Atkinson et al.
(1997) report atypical errors in hand posture in WS children (range: 4-14 years) on this
task, indicative of atypical completion strategies. Performance on multiple object-track-
ing tasks shows a similar pattern. O'Hearn et al. (2005) presented participants with a
computer display of eight square cards that flipped over to reveal 1-4 targets (e.g. a cat).
The cards then flipped back to hide the target cards and either remained static (ventral-
stream task) or were dynamic (dorsal-stream task) for 6 seconds, after which the participant was required to click on the cards that they thought were the target cards. Individuals
with WS (range: 10-38 years) performed at the level of TD 5-year-olds on the ventral-
stream task, but at the level of TD 4-year-olds on the dorsal-stream task. Analysis of error
types demonstrated that when targets were dynamic, both groups made errors that
reflected that they had chosen a distracter object that was near to the target position.
However, the WS group made many more random errors than TD children of the same
mental age, indicative of guessing. Investigation of how a task is completed, therefore, is
extremely fruitful to better understand why behaviour might be impaired in an atypical
group. Furthermore, although a dorsal-stream deficit might be observed across many
neurodevelopmental disorders, analysis of completion strategies can differentiate syndrome-specific characteristics.

Atkinson et al. (1997, 2003, 2006) explored WS performance on a dorsal-stream motion
coherence segmentation task (a task that involves detecting a rectangle of coherent motion
that opposes the coherent motion of the background) and a ventral-stream form coherence task (a task that involves discriminating a set of elements that can be grouped into a
coherent form from randomly oriented elements). They report a relative deficit in motion
coherence segmentation compared with form coherence in both children with WS (range:
4-14 years) and adults with WS (range: 16-47 years) that did not change with increasing
chronological age; however, this was not universally observed across all WS participants.
They also observed poorer motion than form coherence in TD children aged 4-5 years. As
such, when coupled with evidence that poorer motion than form coherence is observed
in other neurodevelopmental disorders (e.g. autism: Koldewyn et al., 2010; preterm children: Taylor et al., 2009; dyslexia: Hansen et al., 2001), comparison of performance
between these two tasks has weak sensitivity and specificity to differentiate any one of
these neurodevelopmental disorders from another. Finally, it is also possible that these
tasks can be completed via alternative neural pathways. Indeed, Atkinson and colleagues
(Atkinson et al., 2003, 2006) demonstrated that individuals with WS who showed motion
coherence segmentation thresholds in the normal range were not exempt from showing
visuospatial deficits.

Contrary to predictions of a dorsal-stream deficit, children with WS (range: 9-18 years
and 11-16 years) and adults with WS (range: 20-40 years) are able to detect biological
motion, such as walking, from point-light displays of walkers (biological figures represented by light dots that are positioned at each joint) to the same level as TD adults and
to a significantly higher level than TD MA-matched controls (Jordan et al., 2002; Reiss

et al., 2005). This cannot be accounted for by differences in developmental vulnerability of the dorsal stream because TD children show a similar rate of development for biological motion tasks and motion coherence segmentation tasks (Reiss et al., 2005). Equally, other groups who are purported to show a dorsal-stream deficit and who show a motion coherence deficit, such as those with autism and preterm children, do show impairment on biological motion tasks (Koldewyn et al., 2010; Taylor et al., 2009). In light of this, it is useful to consider the possibility that this cross-syndrome difference reflects an environmental impact on cortical development.

Individuals with WS spend a lot of time fixating on faces (Elgar & Campbell, 2001) with an associated positive impact on face-processing abilities (see Chapter 14). The same could be true of biological motion. Indeed, evidence from TD 12-month-old infants of a developmental interaction between biological motion perception and social cognition (Yoon & Johnson, 2009) corroborates this suggestion. Thus, an environmental preference to observe people could support the maturation of this ability in WS. Consistent with this, Meyer-Lindenberg et al. (2004) and Sarpal et al. (2008) suggest alternative cortical pathways that could process biological motion in WS. Recent evidence, however, has shown typical activation of the superior temporal sulcus in an adult with WS while viewing biological motion (Hirai et al., 2009), which indicates that at least some of the cortical network involved in processing biological motion is typical in WS.

An opposite argument could be made for individuals with autism in that an aversion to observe people might elicit a qualitatively different impairment in biological motion, relative to other groups who show evidence of dorsal-stream vulnerability. Future research could explore this using cross-syndrome methodology.

In summary, although the WS profile of visuospatial cognition is heavily influenced by vulnerability of the dorsal stream, it is not characterised by a universal impairment in functions attributed to dorsal-stream activation, and we discuss later in this chapter that the visuospatial phenotype in WS also includes impairment in cognitive functions that are not typically associated with dorsal-stream activation (see Figure 12.1). To date, research has given little attention to exploring cross-domain interactions with dorsal-stream functions. However, one possibility is that dorsal-stream function is multifaceted, with dorsal-stream networks overlapping heavily with top-down attentional networks involved in executive-function tasks. This convincing argument, which is beyond the scope of this chapter, is fully explored in Chapter 13. Clearly, exploration of dorsal-stream functions and other developmentally vulnerable functions, such as those overlapping with networks for executive control, is fruitful when considered in the context of syndrome-specific genetic expression, environmental influence and brain development. Future research should also aim to characterise typical developmental trajectories because the time point at which a function emerges and the rate of development of an ability can provide clues to help us to understand the profiles of abilities in atypical groups. Research should also identify deficits in atypical groups that seem to be similar across syndromes, as well as those that are different, to determine which of these deficits might be driven by syndrome-specific mechanisms.

Orientation coding and task complexity

Orientation coding is posited as a specific deficit in WS, based on performance on the Benton Judgement of Line Orientation Test (JLOT; Benton et al., 1978), which is often at 'floor' in children and adults with WS (Bellugi et al., 1988b; Rossen et al., 1996; Wang et al., 1995). This task requires participants to match the orientation of a target line to 1 of 11 lines. However, it has been shown to activate brain areas associated with both visuospatial ability and executive planning (Kesler et al., 2004), which makes it difficult to determine the source of impairment in WS. In addition, evidence from the typical population has demonstrated that different orientation-coding tasks elicit task-dependent developmental trajectories (Lewis et al., 2007; Palomares et al., 2009a) and patterns of brain activation (Dupont et al., 1998; Faillenot et al., 2001; Kitada et al., 2006). This indicates that 'orientation coding' refers to a collection of discrete mechanisms and that the claim for impaired orientation coding in WS is simplistic. In support of this, evidence has shown relative deficits on complex but not simple orientation-coding tasks in both children with Turner syndrome (range: 7-18 years) and children and adults with autism (range: 11-31 years), compared with TD controls (Bertone et al., 2005; Kesler et al., 2004).

In children and adults with autism, effects of complexity have been attributed to atypical cortical connections between early and higher visual areas (Bertone et al., 2005). However, as with dorsal-stream vulnerability, effects of complexity might not be syndrome-specific. One might argue that effects of complexity on orientation coding are also observed in children and adults with WS and in TD children. Farran (2006) compared WS performance on a modified version of the JLOT to performance on an orientation discrimination task (in which participants determined whether two lines had the same or a different orientation). For both tasks, the WS group (range: 8-41 years) performed at the same level as TD children aged 5-6 years who were matched on nonverbal ability. However, both groups showed stronger orientation sensitivity on the orientation discrimination task than on the modified JLOT. This indicates that the difficulties experienced by individuals with WS on the Benton JLOT (e.g. Wang et al., 1995) are a reflexion of the complexity of the task and, importantly, that a relative impairment on this type of task over a simple orientation discrimination task is not atypical.

A second effect of task complexity in WS, however, does deviate from typical development. In children and adults with WS, performance on mental image transformation tasks and orientation-coding tasks, when investigated in isolation, was at the level of TD children aged 5-years who were matched on nonverbal ability (Farran & Jarrold, 2004; Farran, 2006). However, when investigated in combination in a mental rotation task, performance of children and adults with WS from the same group as that studied previously was below the level of TD 5- to 6-year-olds (Farran et al., 2001). This is indicative of an atypical effect of task complexity in WS.

For some, but not all, aspects of orientation coding, WS performance is vulnerable to task complexity in a manner that is not observed in typical development. Thus, although one must be cautious in assuming similar definitions of the term 'complexity', one can tentatively argue that atypical effects of task complexity are observed in WS, as well as in

Turner syndrome and autism, which in turn questions the specificity of a complexity hypothesis in autism research.

Palomares et al. (2009a) report that performance on a task that involved matching the orientation of a target to one of four choice stimuli reached adult levels at 7-9 years in typical development, but orthogonal errors (the oblique effect) in matching were observed through to adulthood. They also showed that when participants were asked to detect a linear contour of similarly oriented lines among randomly oriented distracter lines (orientation integration), performance reached adult levels at 5-6 years. In their WS group (range: 12-24 years), thresholds for orientation matching were most similar to those in children aged 3-4 years, and orthogonal errors were made significantly more frequently than among the 3- to 4-year-olds. By contrast, orientation integration performance in WS did not differ from typical adults. This profile supports the notion, put forward with reference to the dorsal visual stream, that functions that show long developmental trajectories in typical development are more susceptible to atypical development. However, differences in the rate of development of developmental trajectories do not seem to neatly dissociate in terms of whether or not they are associated with activation of the dorsal stream. Perhaps, then, we should consider developmental vulnerability more broadly, rather than only in terms of dorsal-stream developmental vulnerability.

In conclusion, studies that have interpreted patterns of performance as relating to task complexity should not assume that the effects are syndrome-specific. In addition, it seems that the characteristics of developmental trajectories in the typical population should also be taken into account when exploring atypical development. Cross-syndrome comparison of orientation-coding performance will advance our knowledge of syndrome-specific gene–brain–environment interactions on development in relation to both developmental vulnerability and task complexity hypotheses.

Visuospatial perception

Research into visuospatial cognition in WS has primarily focused on relatively weaker areas, as outlined earlier in this chapter. Perceptual measures are therefore often employed as a benchmark ability to demonstrate these relative impairments and it is assumed that perception is delayed rather than atypical. The majority of studies of perception in WS are aimed to determine whether there is a local processing bias at the level of perception in WS. Results consistently provide evidence against a local bias and indicate that this group perceive local and global information in a typical manner (e.g. Deruelle et al., 2006; Farran et al., 2001, 2003; Farran & Jarrold, 2003; Hoffman et al., 2003; Mervis et al., 1999; Pani et al., 1999; Rondan et al., 2008; however, see Porter & Coltheart, 2006, for discussion of a fractionation between perception and attention in WS). Further probing of perceptual processes has focused on the fine-grain perceptual properties of gestalt perception (the integration and segmentation of local elements on the basis of shared properties, e.g. shape, luminance, proximity) and on detailed investigation of task completion strategies and error analysis.

Farran et al. (2007) explored perceptual integration, an index of gestalt processing, in infants and toddlers with WS aged 14-36 months. Infants and toddlers with WS perceived a matrix of circles as perceptually integrated into rows or columns on the basis of shared luminance (alternating rows or columns of black-and-white circles), an ability that had not been evident in an assessment 8 months earlier, but they did not perceptually integrate stimuli that were grouped onto rows or columns on the basis of proximity (e.g. circles were more proximal horizontally than vertically, and so could be perceived as rows). This resembles typical development, where integration by luminance is evident at birth (e.g. Farroni et al., 2000), whereas integration by proximity is not evident until 8 months (Farran et al., 2007). By comparison, when presented with a similar matrix of elements, older children and adults with WS (range: 8-39 years) showed a discrepancy with TD individuals aged 5-6 years in terms of their perceptual integration abilities: integration by luminance, closure (alternating rows or columns of closed and open shapes) and alignment (e.g. objects are linearly aligned vertically but misaligned horizontally) was at the level of the TD children, whereas perceptual grouping by shape similarity (alternating rows or columns of circles and squares), orientation similarity (alternating rows or columns of 0° and 30° orientated lines) and proximity was much poorer (Farran, 2005). Indeed, unpublished data from this study demonstrated that performance on these three grouping types was below the level of TD 4-year-olds. This comparison between infancy and later stages of development is in line with a developmental vulnerability account, that is, integration by luminance, which emerges earlier, has a better developmental outcome than integration by proximity in WS, which emerges later. Interestingly, perceptual integration observed on these tasks in children with autism (range: 9-15 years) is relatively weak for integration by shape only (Farran & Brosnan, 2011), highlighting potential avenues for future investigation of syndrome-specific genetic and environmental influences on development.

Gestalt processing does not always show an atypical profile in WS; perceptual segmentation (e.g. segmenting an image from a background texture; Farran & Wilmut, 2007) and implicit perceptual integration using visual illusions (Farran & Cole, 2008; Palomares et al., 2009b) show relatively typical behavioural patterns in children and adults with WS. Farran & Cole (2008) demonstrated typical illusory biases in WS participants (range: 14-41 years) who were asked to judge the distance between pairs of elements that were grouped on the basis of proximity, shape, luminance or orientation similarity. The study showed that distances between elements that were displayed as part of the same perceptual group (e.g. two black circles) were underestimated, whereas distances between elements that belonged to different perceptual groups (e.g. a black circle and a white circle) were overestimated, as in typical development.

In support of this, Palomares et al. (2009b) demonstrated typical susceptibility to visual illusions (Ponzo, Kanizsa occlusion, Müller–Lyer and Ebbinghaus illusions) in WS (range: 10-41 years), all of which rely on the integration of a local element within the surrounding elements. The authors also note no developmental differences in performance between participants with WS who were under 18 years of age and adult WS participants. However, Grice et al. (2003) report that although participants with WS (range: 10-50 years) seemed to perceive illusory contours in a typical manner (when presented with the Kanizsa square), as indicated by their behaviour, their neural responses were not typical. This indicates that individuals with WS were completing the task using an atypical neural pathway and exemplifies that behavioural competence cannot always be attributed to typical neural activation.

Subtle behavioural differences in WS were uncovered by Palomares et al. (2008). Participants were asked to determine whether two central parallel lines were vertically aligned with two squares (control condition) or two notched circles (visuospatial inter-polation condition), thus creating illusory contours of a rectangle on top of two circles. Palomares et al. (2008) demonstrated an apparently typical facilitation effect of illusory contours in participants with WS (range: 11-24 years) in the visuospatial interpolation condition. However, when the illusion was progressively weakened by spacing the notched circles further apart, the WS group was affected to the same extent as TD children aged 4-6 years and to a greater extent than TD children aged 7-9 years. Coupled with evidence for atypical neural processing, this indicates that implicit perceptual integration is not entirely typical in WS.

Palomares et al. (2008) suggest that the contrast between stronger implicit than explicit perceptual integration relates to the early emergence (at 2 months in typical development) of implicit perceptual grouping abilities (Curran et al., 1999), which seems to support a developmental vulnerability account. However, the fact that implicit perceptual integration is supported by atypical neural processing (Grice et al., 2003) provides evidence that development of this ability has proceeded atypically despite being an early emerging skill in the typical population. This has implications for relying on behavioural measures alone to characterise abilities because it is raises the possibility that many of the 'typical' functions discussed in previous sections are driven by atypical neural activation.

Exploration of the strategies employed to support perceptual processing provides an additional window into the mechanisms that drive behaviour. It is important to determine such mechanisms not only for areas of relative weakness but also areas of relative strength. Visual search tasks, which involve the ability to search for a prespecified target among a number of distracter elements, are ideal tasks to explore strategy use.

Scerif et al. (2004) report that toddlers with WS made more errors than MA-matched TD children on a visual search task because they were more likely to confuse targets with distracters (targets and distracters were differentiated by size), but they showed typical search paths and search times. This indicates a perceptual discrimination deficit, rather than a procedural or attentional difficulty, in toddlers with WS. By contrast, toddlers with fragile X syndrome showed the same number of errors as the WS group but had procedural difficulties owing to repetitive touching of the same targets, which emphasises the existence of syndrome-specific patterns of impairment in these two groups. Formby and Farran (2010) demonstrated that the ability to complete visual search tasks in a typical manner is also observed later in development in WS. Older children and adults with WS (range: 9-43 years) showed patterns of performance akin to those of TD children aged 5-6 years and matched for nonverbal ability; repeated mouse clicks on targets, clicks on distracters and clicks on locations that did not contain a stimulus were observed to a similar extent in WS and TD groups. Visual search performance, however, has a long developmental trajectory in the typical population, and search behaviour in children and adults with WS (range: 8-41 years) showed many differences to TD adult performance, as demonstrated on both small-scale (Montfoort et al., 2007) and large-scale (Smith et al., 2009) environments in which WS adult participants were situated egocentrically within the search space. Visual search performance, therefore, resembles that observed in typical development at 6 years, and although performance does not proceed beyond this level, it represents a relative strength within the visuospatial domain in WS. However, in light of the findings by Grice et al. (2003), investigation of associated cortical activation is required to fully support the notion that visual search performance is simply delayed in WS.

Visuospatial cognition in large-scale space

Visuospatial cognition is not restricted to performance on small-scale tasks; yet, WS performance in large-scale space has only been addressed by a handful of studies: the large-scale visual search task discussed earlier and investigation of route learning ability and spatial reorientation. With reference to route learning, Farran et al. (2010) demonstrated that individuals with WS (range: 8-25 years) were able to learn the sequence of landmarks and turns (route knowledge) of a novel route through a university campus but showed little understanding of the spatial relations between landmarks (relational knowledge). In a subsequent study, when individuals with WS (range: 11-41 years) learnt a route through a virtual environment, error pattern analysis revealed subtle deficits in route knowledge that seemed to reflect poor inhibitory processes in WS (Farran et al., submitted) (see Chapters 6 and 9 for discussion of inhibition in WS). Indeed, Farran et al. (submitted) report that the level of nonverbal ability was related to the knowledge of landmarks along a route in children and adults with WS, but not in TD children with the same range of nonverbal abilities. These findings indicate that route knowledge is supported by qualitatively different mechanisms in WS than in typical development.

Route knowledge and relational knowledge tap into egocentric (viewpoint-dependent) and allocentric (viewpoint-independent) frames of reference, respectively. In typical development, young children rely on viewpoint-dependent representations and do not spontaneously use viewpoint-independent representations until the school-age years (e.g. Bullens et al., 2010), and so it is unsurprising that individuals with WS do not seem to exhibit relational knowledge. In typical development, relational knowledge activates the hippocampus (Doeller et al., 2008), an area that shows reduced metabolism in WS (Meyer-Lindenberg et al., 2005). This is indicative of atypical brain–behaviour associations in WS. Impairments in viewpoint-independent representations have also been reported in small-scale environments in children and adults with WS (Nardini et al., 2008). Furthermore, although the authors demonstrated developmental progression between the ages of 5 and 42 years in WS, it was only equivalent to that observed between the ages of 3 and 4 years in TD children.

The hippocampus has also been implicated in spatial reorientation (see Landau & Lakusta, 2009). In a spatial reorientation task employed by Lakusta et al. (2010), individuals with WS (range: 10-28 years) did not benefit from the geometry of the room to reorient themselves, an ability that is present at 18-24 months in typical development (Hermer & Spelke, 1996); however, reorientation in WS was facilitated in a condition that included a single blue wall as a landmark. This supports the previously mentioned findings that individuals with WS are able to use landmarks to orient themselves within their environment and that functions typically attributed to the hippocampus are relatively impaired in WS. This possibility is discussed further in Chapter 13, with reference to dorsal-stream connections to the hippocampus.

Cross-domain interactions

Optimum development involves extensive interaction across domains. Thus, although this chapter focuses on a single domain, it is important to touch on the integration of visuospatial cognition with other domains. Earlier in this chapter, we referred to interactions between visuospatial cognition, executive function and memory, as well as the effects of task complexity. Here, we discuss integration across areas of strength and weakness of the WS cognitive profile.

Areas of strength can be exploited to augment areas of weakness. This has proved beneficial in large-scale navigation tasks, where a new route is learnt better in WS if the landmarks are verbally labelled along the route (Farran et al., 2010). Furthermore, across the Performance subtests of the Wechsler Intelligence Scale for Children (Wechsler, 1992), verbal ability correlates with performance on subtests that represent relatively higher levels of visuospatial ability in WS (range: 9-38 years), which is indicative of a spontaneous verbal mediation strategy (Farran et al., 1999). Comparisons with other syndromes where the opposite pattern of weaker verbal than visuospatial ability is observed (e.g. Down syndrome: Laws, 2002; autism: Williams et al., 2008) show that verbal coding of visuospatial stimuli does not take place spontaneously in these groups, despite its appearance from as young an age as 6 years in typical development.

Cross-domain interactions can also impair performance in an otherwise strong area of ability. For example, comprehension of spatial language terms, such as 'in front of', 'above', 'in' and 'on', represents a relative weakness within the verbal domain in children and adults with WS (Laing & Jarrold, 2007; Phillips et al., 2004). Consistently, young children with WS (range: 5-7 years), demonstrate impaired relational vocabulary relative to concrete vocabulary (Mervis & John, 2008; also discussed in Chapter 10).

Landau and Hoffman (2005) showed that children with WS (range: 8-14 years), but not adults with WS (range: 14-30 years), make directional errors between above and below (as observed by Clark, 1973, in 3-year-old TD children), and both children and adults with WS confuse left and right, a skill typically accomplished by 12 years of age (Landau & Hoffman, 2005). They note that this developmental sequence mirrored that observed in typical development, but that development is limited, that is, even adults with WS did not differ in performance from a group of 5-year-old TD children.

Interestingly, spatial language comprehension is also poor in Down syndrome (Laws & Lawrence, 2001). Given the cognitive profile of poorer verbal than visuospatial ability in Down syndrome, this indicates that visuospatial scaffolding does not take place in this group. It would be interesting to note the relative relationships between spatial representations and spatial language in autism, Down syndrome and WS. This might not only inform us about development in these groups, but might also inform larger debates regarding perception and language (see Levinson et al., 2002; Li & Gleitman, 2002).

Visuospatial cognition and the brain

Many areas of the brain that are associated with visuospatial processing are structurally atypical in WS (see also Chapter 2), with the most consistent evidence for the occipital cortex (including low-level visual processing in V1) and dorsal visual areas (parietal cortex, intraparietal cortex; Mercuri et al., 1997; Eckert et al., 2005; Galaburda et al., 2002; Meyer-Lindenberg et al., 2004; Reiss et al., 2004; Schmitt et al., 2002). Although we must take brain plasticity into account in neurodevelopmental disorders, these structural differences can inform cognitive and genetic theories of visuospatial cognition in WS.

A small number of studies have explored functional brain activation for visuospatial processes in adolescents and adults with WS. Mobbs et al. (2007) employed Navon-type hierarchical stimuli (Navon, 1977), in which a large shape is made up of smaller shapes (e.g. a square is made up of triangles). Contrary to previous findings (e.g. Farran et al., 2001; Deruelle et al., 2006), Mobbs et al. (2007) demonstrated an impairment in processing the global-level shape in their WS sample (range: 15-48 years). They report reduced activation in the occipital and parietal cortex (dorsal visual stream), with typical activation of the occipitotemporal cortex (ventral visual stream). Mobbs et al. (2007) also report increased activation in thalamic areas that are connected to both dorsal and ventral streams and suggest that this could indicate atypical functioning in WS in pathways that feed into (and receive feedback from) ventral and dorsal visual streams.

Meyer-Lindenberg et al. (2004) explored visuospatial matching and construction (participants mentally manipulated two shape parts to form a single shape), and location versus content processing. Their sample of adults with WS was selected because they had IQs within the normal range, which is unusual in WS (see Chapter 5). Despite this, the patterns of activation were consistent with those reported by Mobbs et al. (2007); the participants with WS showed typical ventral-stream activation but reduced dorsal-stream activation relative to controls. Coupled with their findings of structural atypicalities, this provides support for impaired dorsal-stream functioning in WS. As discussed earlier, Meyer-Lindenberg et al. (2004) also highlight the possibility that cross-talk between ventral and dorsal visual streams might enable individuals with WS to process motion via an alternative pathway, such that some aspects of motion perception activate visual area MT in the temporal lobe, that is, via the ventral stream, rather than via the intraparietal sulcus of the dorsal stream.

Although the studies so far report typical brain–behaviour relations for occipitotemporal (ventral-stream) functioning in WS, evidence from event-related potentials data, discussed earlier, demonstrated atypical neural activation to illusory contours in occipitotemporal areas (ventral stream) in children and adults with WS (Grice et al., 2003). Furthermore, in the only study to apply functional connectivity analysis (see Chapter 2 for a discussion of structural connectivity) to explore visuospatial cognition in WS, Sarpal et al. (2008), who used the same high-functioning adult WS sample as Meyer-Lindenberg et al. (2004), report reduced connectivity in WS in circuits that involved both ventral and dorsal regions. For example, both the fusiform face area, an area related to face processing (ventral stream), and the parahippocampal place area, an area that is crucial for spatial navigation, showed reduced connections to the intraparietal sulcus, which is part of the dorsal visual stream. Sarpal et al. (2008) also showed areas of increased connectivity in WS, which they hypothesise relates to compensatory functional reorganisation during development. They suggest that increased connectivity between the parahippocampal place area and the superior temporal cortex, an area that integrates information from the dorsal and ventral streams and is involved in motion processing, might explain why not all motion-processing tasks elicit impaired performance in WS.

Functional brain analysis supports a dorsal-stream deficit in WS, but it also indicates deficits in other areas and atypical connections across brain areas. This demonstrates that given the importance of brain plasticity during development, the WS brain cannot be considered in terms of parts 'intact' and parts 'impaired'. Furthermore, given the emphasis on labelling tasks as 'dorsal' and 'ventral' stream tasks in the behavioural literature, the time is ripe for a cross-syndrome comparison of associated brain activation.

Visuospatial cognition and gene expression

The identification of individuals and families with partial deletions within the Williams syndrome deleted region (the long arm of chromosome 7) has enabled geneticists to isolate candidate genes responsible for specific characteristics in WS (see also Chapter 3). With the exception of the study by Gray et al. (2006), who used a battery of visuospatial tasks, visuospatial-construction performance is typically employed as the behavioural indicator of visuospatial cognitive ability in such individuals.

The first gene implicated in the characteristic visuoconstructive deficit in WS was *LIMK1* (Frangiskakis et al., 1996). However, subsequent discovery of individuals who presented with a partial deletion in the WS region that included *LIMK1* but who did not display visuospatial perceptual or constructive deficits illustrates that deletion of one copy of this gene alone cannot account for visuospatial cognitive deficits in WS (Gray et al., 2006).

More recently, Antonell et al. (2010a, 2010b) referred to the importance of the deleted genes *GTF2I* and *GTF2IRD1* in addition to *LIMK1* (see also Tassabehji, 2003). Furthermore, they report that *MAP1B*, which plays a role in axon guidance during brain development, was overexpressed in lymphoblastoid cell lines from individuals with WS. The authors specifi-cally noted that *GTF2IRD1* was associated with regulating the relationship between all neural layers and the development of the retina in terms of eye size, whereas *LIMK1* deficits were linked to impaired retinal ganglion cells.

Finally, Eckert et al. (2006) predicted an association between *LIMK1* and anomalous development of the pulvinar (part of posterior thalamus) in WS. Antonell et al. (2010a, 2010b) suggested that this combination of deleted genes, all of which are highly expressed in the cortex and the retina, in addition to the overexpression of *MAP1B* could affect the transition of information from photoreceptors in the retina to the optic nerve, thus having an impact on visuospatial ability.

This is potentially an exciting advance in our understanding of genotype–phenotype relationships. However, since these findings arise from transformed lymphocyte cell cultures, it would be important to verify them in human tissue samples. It is also important to note that the suggested neural pathway is responsible for basic low-level visual perception and is only a small contributor to performance on a visuospatial-construction task, the behavioural measure employed. This imbalance between crude measures of behaviour accompanied by precise genetic profiling needs to be addressed; a behavioural methodology in which subtle characteristics of the cognitive profile are assessed (as adopted by Gray et al., 2006) will benefit future understanding of the relationships between genes, brain and behaviour.

Conclusions

Individuals with WS show a complex pattern of visuospatial abilities, which shows atypical functioning from the infant start state (Farran et al., 2007). This has cascading downstream effects on the development of many other domains such as executive function (see Chapter 9) and numeracy (see Chapter 16). Although many of the visuospatial impairments in WS do reflect dorsal-stream vulnerability, the cognitive phenotype of WS involves strengths and weaknesses in behaviours associated with many areas of the brain.

There is merit in using what is known about the emergence and rate of development of cognitive mechanisms in the typical population as a starting point to understand disordered development, regardless of whether the mechanism is associated with dorsal-stream activation. This argument predicts that developmental functions that reach an adult level of ability early in development are less likely to show impairment in a neurodevelopmental disorder, whereas those that emerge later or develop slowly are more vulnerable to atypical development. Figure 12.1 illustrates the level of ability across visuospatial tasks while taking developmental vulnerability into account. Each bar represents the highest age of TD participants who were assessed on that measure. The blue portion of each bar illustrates 'developing' ability, such that development has reached adult-like performance at the top of the blue portion. Therefore, during the red portion of the bar the level of typical ability does not develop further. Black-triangle data points represent WS performance. A comparison across tasks illustrates that knowledge of the pattern of development in the typical population is informative. For example, although adult-like performance is reported for both biological motion and motion coherence, this represents more of a peak in the profile for biological motion because development on this task is ongoing until adulthood in the typical population. By contrast, typical 6-year-olds also show adult-like performance on Reiss et al.'s (2005) motion coherence task, and so it is less surprising that this level was also achieved in WS. Similarly, because susceptibility to visual illusions does not change in typical development from the age of 3 years to adulthood, susceptibility in WS could be claimed to be at the adult level or at the 3-year-old level, both of which purvey different messages of strong and weak performance. This has implications for studies that have employed a matched group design because WS performance might be at or below the age at which adult-level performance on that task is reached in typical development. Knowledge of typical development, therefore, can inform conclusions relating to the level of ability in WS.

Although exploring developmental vulnerability is enticing, the problem remains that this does not necessarily uncover syndrome-specific profiles. Phenotypic characteristics can only be addressed by analysis of error types and completion strategies as indices of neural competence, as well as by exploration of neural activation itself. Such analytic exploration can then be interpreted in the context of a genetic expression and environmental influence. Phenotypic versus generalised characteristics can be further differentiated by cross-syndrome comparison.

Future research should focus on profiling developmental trajectories of a full array of visuospatial abilities. It is notable from Figure 12.1 that studies that have used matched

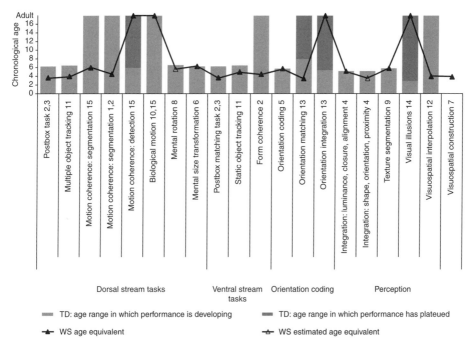

Fig. 12.1 (See also Plate 6) Age equivalents of WS performance across visuospatial cognitive tasks. WS performance is plotted as black triangles. Closed black triangles represent known age equivalents. Where open black triangles are used, WS performance is below the typically developing TD control group, but an exact age equivalent is not known; WS performance is conservatively plotted as 6 months below the mean age of the control group. In order to understand WS performance within the context of typical development, typically developing trajectories are plotted as bars. The extent of each bar represents the highest chronological age for which comparison data were collected. The blue portion of each bar demonstrates the age range within which development was observed for performance on the task. Where present, the red portion of each bar demonstrates a developmental plateau, i.e. performance has reached an adult level. Abbreviations: TD = typically developing; WS = Williams syndrome. Sources: [1] Atkinson et al. 1997; [2] Atkinson et al. (2003, 2006); [3] Dilks et al. (2008); [4] Farran (2005); [5] Farran (2006); [6] Farran & Jarrold (2004); [7] Farran et al. (1999); [8] Farran et al. (2001); [9] Farran & Wilmut (2007); [10] Jordan et al. (2002); [11] O'Hearn et al. (2005); [12] Palomares et al. (2008); [13] Palomares et al. (2009a); [14] Palomares et al. (2009b); [15] Reiss et al. (2005).

group designs do not enable one to determine the sensitivity of a given test to developmental change. Furthermore, accompanying evidence of cortical activation of brain areas and brain networks in TD children will inform our knowledge of precisely how behavioural changes in development map onto cortical changes. It is very notable throughout this chapter that most studies have not explored the actual development of visuospatial function in WS, instead grouping together participants from as young as 8 years with adult participants. However, development is hard to capture in this domain and where development has been explored little or no developmental progression is observed (Atkinson et al., 2006; Farran et al., submitted; Jarrold et al., 2001; Landau & Hoffman, 2005; Nardini et al., 2008; Palomares et al., 2008, 2009a, 2009b). A fruitful approach, therefore, is to observe visuospatial abilities in infants and in the preschool and early school years, as explored by Farran et al., (2007) and Scerif et al. (2004), for comparison with performance in older children and adults with WS. This enables one to determine whether the atypicalities observed in older children and adults are primary deficits or the result of cascading influences of early developmental deficits. Finally, while our understanding of gene–brain–behaviour relations in WS has grown substantially over the past decade, over the next decade it will be exciting to see studies in which behavioural measures are chosen that enable precise mappings to be made.

Editor commentary (Emily K. Farran & Annette Karmiloff-Smith)

Visuospatial cognition is the weakest domain of ability for adults with WS. In this domain, cross-syndrome comparison has advanced the theoretical understanding of WS and autism, meaning that the common hypothesis that both groups display a local processing bias (a bias to process the details of an image over the whole image) can be dissociated when a range of cognitive mechanisms are considered. In typical development, the developmental trajectory approach has demonstrated that different assessments of orientation coding yield different developmental trajectories and different cortical activation patterns. In atypical development, in line with these cortical and behavioural fractionations, relative deficits in complex orientation-coding tasks but not in simple orientation-coding tasks have also been reported in Turner syndrome and autism. The chapter suggested a similar hypothesis for WS. Cross-syndrome comparison across these disorders would, therefore, advance our understanding of the impact of differing genetic influences on the ability to process simple versus complex visual input. Furthermore, and in line with the neuroconstructivist approach, as orientation discrimination is a very early developing ability in typical infants, it is entirely possible that tiny variations in the ability to discriminate orientation in infancy could have a wide-reaching impact on later development of many aspects of cognitive performance.

Poor spatial language in WS and Down syndrome constitutes an interesting cross-syndrome association. Despite different cognitive profiles, both of these atypical groups show poor comprehension of spatial language (e.g. terms such as 'in front of' or 'above'). Although a direct cross-syndrome comparison has not yet been carried out, it seems that similarly impaired spatial language comprehension in the two syndromes stems from a constraint on spatial abilities in WS, but from a constraint on language abilities in Down syndrome, thus supporting the neuroconstructivist view that development proceeds in an integrated manner across domains and that similar behavioural outcomes can emerge from differing developmental trajectories. Clearly, interactions occur across domains and a seemingly specific deficit often turns out to be much more pervasive across domains than first thought.

References

Alivisatos, B., & Petrides, M. (1997). Functional activation of the human brain during mental rotation. *Neuropsychologia*, **35**, 111–18.

Antonell, A., Del Campo, M., Magano, L.F., Kaufmann, L., de la Iglesia, J.M., Gallastegui, F., et al. (2010a). Partial 7q11.23 deletions further implicate GTF2I and GTF2IRD1 as the main genes responsible for the Williams–Beuren syndrome neurocognitive profile. *Journal of Medical Genetics*, **47**, 312–20.

Antonell, A., Vilardell, M., & Perez Jurado, L.A. (2010b). Transcriptome profile in Williams–Beuren syndrome lymphoblast cells reveals gene pathways implicated in glucose intolerance and visuospatial construction deficits. *Human Genetics*, **128**, 27–37.

Atkinson, J., Anker, S., Braddick, O., Nokes, L., Mason, A., & Braddick, F. (2001). Visual and visuo-spatial development in young Williams syndrome children. *Developmental Medicine and Child Neurology*, **43**, 330–37.

Atkinson, J., Braddick, O., Anker, S., Curran, W., Andrew, R., Wattam-Bell, J., et al. (2003). Neurobiological models of visuospatial cognition in children with Williams syndrome: measures of dorsal-stream and frontal function. *Developmental Neuropsychology*, **23**, 139–72.

Atkinson, J., Braddick, O., Rose, F.E., Searcy, Y.M., Wattam-Bell, J., & Bellugi, U. (2006). Dorsal-stream motion processing deficits persist into adulthood in Williams syndrome. *Neuropsychologia*, **44**, 828–33.

Atkinson, J., King, J., Bradick, O., Nokes, L., Anker, S., & Braddick, F. (1997). A specific deficit of dorsal stream function in Williams syndrome. *Neuroreport: Cognitive Neuroscience and Neuropsychology*, **8**, 1919–22.

Bellugi, U., Marks, S., Bihrle, A., & Sabo, H. (1988a). Dissociation between language and cognitive functions in Williams syndrome. In D. Bishop & K. Mogford (Eds), *Language Development in Exceptional Circumstances* (pp. 177–89). Hove: Psychology Press.

Bellugi, U., Sabo, H., & Vaid, J. (1988b). Spatial deficits in children with Williams syndrome. In J. Stiles-Davis, U. Kritchevshy & U. Bellugi (Eds), *Spatial Cognition: Brain Bases and Development* (pp. 273–97). Hillsdale, NJ: Lawrence Erlbaum.

Benton, A.L., Varney, N.R., & Hamsher, K. d. (1978). Visuospatial judgement: a clinical test. *Archives of Neurology*, **35**, 364–67.

Bertone, A., Mottron, L., Jelenic, P., & Faubert, J. (2005). Enhanced and diminished visuo-spatial information processing in Autism depends on stimulus complexity. *Brain*, **128**, 2430–41.

Braddick, O., Atkinson, J., & Wattam-Bell, J. (2003). Normal and anomalous development of visual motion processing: motion coherence and 'dorsal stream vulnerability'. *Neuropsychologia*, **41**, 1769–83.

Bullens, J., Igloi, K., Berthoz, A., Postma, A., & Rondi-Reig, L. (2010). Developmental time course of the acquisition of sequential egocentric and allocentric navigation strategies. *Journal of Experimental Child Psychology*, **107**, 337–50.

Clark, H.H. (1973). Space, time, semantics, and the child. In T.E. Moore (Ed.), *Cognitive Development and the Acquisition of Language* (pp. 27–63). New York, NY: Academic Press.

Curran W, Braddick O J, Atkinson J, Wattam-Bell J, & Andrew, R. (1999). Development of illusory-contour perception in infants, *Perception*, **28**, 527–38.

Deruelle, C., Rondan, C., Mancini, J., & Livet, M.-O. (2006). Do children with Williams syndrome fail to process visual configural information? *Research in Developmental Disabilities*, 27, 243–53.

Dilks, D.D., Hoffman, J.E., & Landau, B. (2008). Vision for perception and vision for action: normal and unusual development. *Developmental Science*, 11, 474–86.

Doeller, C.F., King, J.A., & Burgess, N. (2008). Parallel striatal and hippocampal systems for landmarks and boundaries in spatial memory. *Proceedings of the National Academy of Sciences of the USA*, 105, 5915–20.

Dupont, P., Vogels, R., Vandenberghe, R., Rosier, A., Cornette, L., Bormans, G., et al. (1998). Regions in the brain activated by simultaneous orientation discrimination: a study with positron emission tomography. *European Journal of Neuroscience*, 10, 3689–99.

Eckert, M.A., Galaburda, A.M., Mills, D.L., Bellugi, U., Korenberg, J.R., & Reiss, A.L. (2006). The neurobiology of Williams syndrome: cascading influences of visual system impairment? *Cellular and Molecular Life Sciences*, 63, 1867–75.

Eckert, M.A., Hu, D., Eliez, S., Bellugi, U., Galaburda, A., Korenberg, J., et al. (2005). Evidence for superior parietal impairment in Williams syndrome. *Neurology*, 64, 152–53.

Eden, G.F., VanMeter, J.W., Rumsey, J.M., Maisog, J.M., Woods, R.P., & Zeffiro, T.A. (1996). Abnormal processing of visual motion in dyslexia revealed by functional brain imaging. *Nature*, 382, 19–20.

Elgar, K., & Campbell, R. (2001). Annotation: the cognitive neuroscience of face recognition: implications for developmental disorders. *Journal of Child Psychology and Psychiatry*, 42, 705–717.

Elliot, C.D. (1990). *Differential Ability Scales*. New York, NY: The Psychological Corporation.

Faillenot, I., Sunaert, S., Van Hecke, P., & Orban, G.A. (2001). Orientation discrimination of objects and gratings compared: an fMRI study. *European Journal of Neuroscience*, 13, 585–96.

Farran, E.K. (2005). Perceptual grouping ability in Williams syndrome: evidence for deviant patterns of performance. *Neuropsychologia*, 43, 815–22.

Farran, E.K. (2006). Orientation coding: a specific deficit in Williams syndrome? *Developmental Neuropsychology*, 29, 397–414.

Farran, E.K., Blades, M., Boucher, J., & Tranter, L.J. (2010). How do individuals with Williams syndrome learn a route in a real world environment? *Developmental Science*, 13, 454–68.

Farran, E.K., & Brosnan, M.J. (2011). Perceptual grouping abilities in individuals with autism spectrum disorder; exploring patterns of ability in relation to grouping type and levels of development. *Autism Research*, 4, 283–92.

Farran, E.K., Brown, J.H., Cole, V.L., Houston-Price, C., & Karmiloff-Smith, A. (2007). The development of perceptual grouping in infants with Williams syndrome. *European Journal of Developmental Science*, 1, 253–71.

Farran, E.K., & Cole, V.L. (2008). Perceptual grouping and distance estimates in Williams syndrome: comparing performance across perception, drawing and construction tasks. *Brain and Cognition*, 68, 157–65.

Farran, E.K., Courbois, Y., Van Herwegen, J., & Blades, M. (submitted). How useful are landmarks when learning a route in a virtual environment? Evidence from typical development and Williams syndrome.

Farran, E.K., & Jarrold, C. (2003). Visuospatial cognition in Williams syndrome: reviewing and accounting for the strengths and weaknesses in performance. *Developmental Neuropsychology*, 23, 175–202.

Farran, E.K., & Jarrold, C. (2004). Exploring block construction and mental imagery: evidence of atypical orientation discrimination in Williams syndrome. *Visual Cognition*, 11, 1019–40.

Farran, E.K., & Jarrold, C. (2005). Evidence for unusual spatial location coding in Williams syndrome: an explanation for the local bias in visuo-spatial construction tasks? *Brain and Cognition*, 59, 159–72.

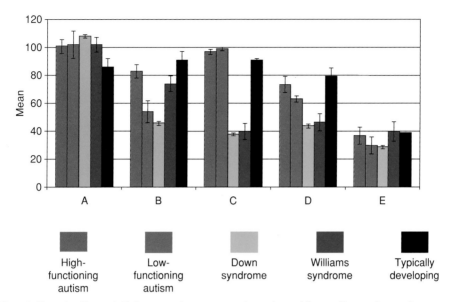

Plate 1 (See also Figure 1.1) Cross-syndrome comparison of cognitive profiles on four tasks. (A) Mean chronological age (in months). (B) Age equivalent (in months) according to the British Picture Vocabulary Scale. (C) Age equivalent (in months) according to the Pattern Construction subtest of the British Abilities Scales II. (D) Age equivalent (in months) according to the Copying subtest of the British Abilities Scales II. (E) Raw test scores on the Benton Facial Recognition Test. Results are shown for children with high-functioning autism (n=16, 5-11 years of age), low-functioning autism (n=17, 5-11 years of age), Down syndrome (n=15, 6-13 years of age), or Williams syndrome (n=15, 5-12 years of age) and for typically developing children (n=25, 3-12 years of age). Note that the typically developing group had a lower mean chronological age than the disorder groups. The error bars show the standard error of the mean. Data from Annaz (2006).

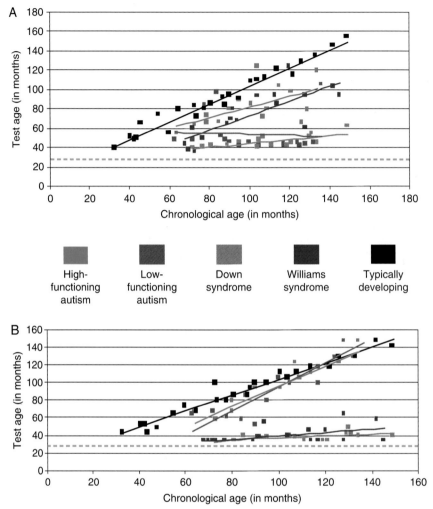

Plate 2 (See also Figure 1.2) Developmental trajectories for the five groups described in Figure 1.1. (A) British Picture Vocabulary Scale. (B) Pattern Construction subtest of the British Abilities Scales II. The dashed line depicts 'floor' performance on the task. Data from Annaz (2006).

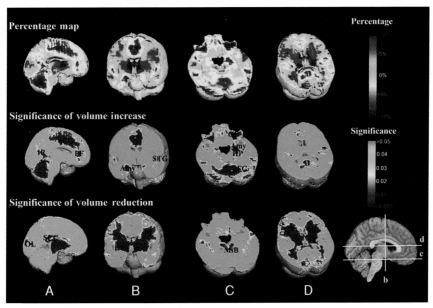

Plate 3 (See also Figure 2.1) Volumetric maps of the brain in Williams syndrome, derived from magnetic resonance imaging. WS and control brain volumes were compared in the ICBM space to adjust for individual differences in total brain volumes. The ratio of the mean JICBM space in WS to the mean JICBM in control subjects was computed voxel-wise to map the three-dimensional profile of brain volume increases (colour-coded as red) or reductions (colour-coded as blue) (first row). Panels (A) to (D) show relative preservation of the volume (which is shown as increase in the volume percentage maps) in prefrontal and orbitofrontal areas, anterior cingulate gyrus, inferior parietal regions at the parieto-occipital junction, superior temporal gyrus, amygdala and part of hippocampus (especially on the right side), fusiform gyrus, and cerebellum. Occipital areas, parietal lobes close to temporo-parietal junction, splenium and posterior body of the corpus callosum, thalamus and the basal ganglia (including globus pallidus, putamen, and caudate nucleus), and midbrain are disproportionally reduced. The Mann–Whitney U test was used to obtain the significance maps for the volume increase (second row) or reduction (third row). Abbreviations: aCG = anterior cingulate gyrus; Amy = amygdala; BG = basal ganglia; FG = fusiform gyrus; HP = hippocampus; IP = inferior parietal region; JICBM = Jacobian determinant in the ICBM space; MiB = midbrain; OF = orbitofrontal area; OL = occipital lobe; PF = prefrontal area; PL = parietal lobe; SCC = splenium of the corpus callosum; STG = superior temporal gyrus; TL = thalamus. Reprinted from *NeuroImage*, **36** (4), Ming-Chang Chiang, Allan L. Reiss, Agatha D. Lee, Ursula Bellugi, Albert M. Galaburda, Julie R. Korenberg, et al, 3D pattern of brain abnormalities in Williams syndrome visualized using tensor-based morphometry, pp. 1096–1109, Copyright (2007), with permission from Elsevier.

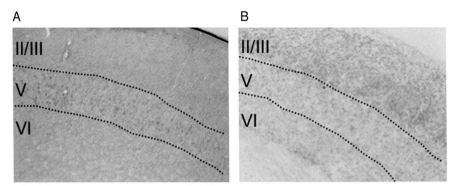

Plate 4 (See also Figure 3.2) Patterns of TFII-IRG1 and TFII-I expression. (A) Coronal sections (50 μm) from the medial prefrontal cortex from *Gtf2ird1*$^{Gt(Xs0608)Wtsl}$ adult mice. (B) Coronal sections (50 μm) from the medial prefrontal cortex from *Gtf2i*$^{Gt(YTA365)Byg}$ adult mice. Expression of the LacZ fusion protein in sections from each mouse line was visualised by X-gal staining. The Roman numerals indicate layers of the cortex.

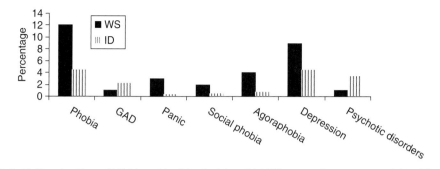

Plate 5 (See also Figure 5.1) Mental health of adults with Williams syndrome versus adults with intellectual disabilities. Abbreviations: GAD = generalised anxiety disorder; ID = intellectual disabilities; WS = Williams syndrome.

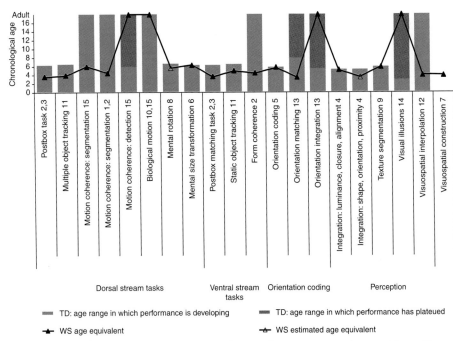

Plate 6 (See also Figure 12.1) Age equivalents of WS performance across visuospatial cognitive tasks. WS performance is plotted as black triangles. Closed black triangles represent known age equivalents. Where open black triangles are used, WS performance is below the typically developing TD control group, but an exact age equivalent is not known; WS performance is conservatively plotted as 6 months below the mean age of the control group. In order to understand WS performance within the context of typical development, typically developing trajectories are plotted as bars. The extent of each bar represents the highest chronological age for which comparison data were collected. The blue portion of each bar demonstrates the age range within which development was observed for performance on the task. Where present, the red portion of each bar demonstrates a developmental plateau, i.e. performance has reached an adult level. Abbreviations: TD = typically developing; WS = Williams syndrome. Sources: [1] Atkinson et al. 1997; [2] Atkinson et al. (2003, 2006); [3] Dilks et al. (2008); [4] Farran (2005); [5] Farran (2006); [6] Farran & Jarrold (2004); [7] Farran et al. (1999); [8] Farran et al. (2001); [9] Farran & Wilmut (2007); [10] Jordan et al. (2002); [11] O'Hearn et al. (2005); [12] Palomares et al. (2008); [13] Palomares et al. (2009a); [14] Palomares et al. (2009b); [15] Reiss et al. (2005).

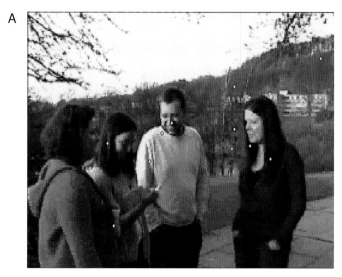

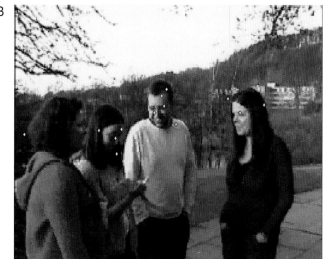

Plate 7 (See also Figure 14.1) Fixation scatters for individuals attending to a frame showing four adults during a social encounter. (A) Individuals on the autistic spectrum (of varying degrees of functioning capacity). (B) Individuals with Williams syndrome. Each small dot represents a fixation. The frame has been taken from a movie. For the movie overall, individuals with Williams syndrome spent significantly longer than typically developing individuals fixating on the face regions, whereas those with autism spent significantly less time than typical attending to the same regions. For full details see Riby & Hancock (2009).

Farran, E.K., Jarrold, C., & Gathercole, S.E. (September 1999). Visuo-spatial cognition in Williams syndrome: an uneven profile of abilities. Presented at the British Psychological Society Developmental Section Annual Conference, Nottingham.

Farran, E.K., Jarrold, C., & Gathercole, S.E. (2001). Block design performance in the Williams syndrome phenotype: a problem with mental imagery? *Journal of Child Psychology and Psychiatry*, **42**, 719–28.

Farran, E.K., Jarrold, C., & Gathercole, S.E. (2003). Divided attention, selective attention and drawing: processing preferences in Williams syndrome are dependent on the task administered, *Neuropsychologia*, **41**, 676–87.

Farran, E.K., & Wilmut, K. (2007). Texture segmentation in Williams syndrome. *Neuropsychologia*, **45**, 1009–1018.

Farroni, T., Valenza, E., & Simion, F. (2000). Configural processing at birth: evidence for perceptual organisation. *Perception*, **29**, 355–72.

Formby, S.C., & Farran, E.K. (September 2010). Williams syndrome and developmental coordination disorder: examining visual search for ventral and dorsal stimuli. Presented at the British Psychological Society Developmental Section Annual Conference, London.

Frangiskakis, J.M., Ewart, A.K., Morris, C.A., Mervis, C.B., Bertrand, J., Robinson, B.F., Klein, B.P., et al. (1996). LIM-kinase1 hemizygosity implicated in impaired visuospatial constructive cognition. *Cell*, **86**, 59–69.

Galaburda, A., Holinger, D.P., Bellugi, U., & Sherman, G.F. (2002). Williams syndrome: neuronal size and neuronal-packing density in primary visual cortex. *Achives of Neurology*, **59**, 1461–67.

Goldenberg, G. (2009). Apraxia and the parietal lobes. *Neuropsychologia*, **47**, 1449–59.

Gray, V., Karmiloff-Smith, A., Funnell, E., & Tassabehji, M. (2006). In-depth analysis of spatial cognition in Williams syndrome: a critical assessment of the role of the LIMK1 gene. *Neuropsychologia*, **44**, 679–85.

Grice, S.J., de Haan, M., Halit, H., Johnson, M.H., Csibra, G., Grant, J., et al. (2003). ERP abnormalities of illusory contour perception in Williams syndrome. *Neuroreport*, **14**, 1773–77.

Hansen, P.C., Stein, J.F., Orde, S.R., Winter, J.L., & Talcott, J.B. (2001). Are dyslexics' visual deficits limited to measures of dorsal stream function? *Neuroreport* **12**, 1527–30.

Hoffman, J.E., Landau, B., & Pagani, B. (2003). Spatial breakdown in spatial construction: evidence from eye fixations in children with Williams syndrome. *Cognitive Psychology*, **46**, 260–301.

Hirai, M., Nakamura, M., Kaneoke, Y., & Kakigi, R. (2009). Intact point-light walker processing in Williams syndrome: a magnetoencephalography study. *Neuroreport*, **20**, 267–72.

Hermer, L., & Spelke, E. (1996). Modularity and development: the case of spatial reorientation. *Cognition*, **61**, 195–232.

Hudson, K., & Farran, E.K. (2011). Drawing the line: graphic strategies for simple and complex shapes in Williams syndrome and typical development. *British Journal of Developmental Psychology*, **29**, 687–705.

Jarrold, C., Baddeley, A.D., Hewes, A.K., & Phillips, C. (2001). A longitudinal assessment of diverging verbal and non-verbal abilities in the Williams syndrome phenotype. *Cortex*, **37**, 423–31.

Jordan, H., Reiss, J., Hoffman, J.E., & Landau, B. (2002). Intact perception of biological motion in the face of profound spatial deficits: Williams syndrome. *Psychological Science*, **13**, 162–67.

Kesler, S.R., Haberecht, M.F., Menon, V., Warsofsky, I.S., Dyer-Friedman, J., Neely, E.K., et al. (2004). Functional neuroanatomy of spatial orientation processing in Turner syndrome. *Cerebral Cortex*, **14**, 174–80.

Koldewyn, K., Whitney, D., & Rivera, S.M. (2010). The psychophysics of visual motion and global form processing in Autism. *Brain*, **133**, 599–610.

Kitada, R., Kito, T., Saito, D.N., Kochiyama, T., Matsumura, M., Sadato, N., et al. (2006). Multisensory activation of the intraparietal area when classifying grating orientation: a functional magnetic resonance imaging study. *The Journal of Neuroscience*, **26**, 7491–7501.

Laing, E., & Jarrold, C. (2007). Comprehension of spatial language in Williams syndrome: evidence for impaired spatial representation of verbal descriptions. *Clinical Linguistics and Phonetics*, **21**, 689–704.

Lakusta, L., Dessalegn, B., & Landau, B. (2010). Impaired geometric reorientation caused by genetic defect. *Proceedings of the National Academy of Sciences of the USA*, **107**, 2813–17.

Landau, B., & Hoffman, J.E. (2005). Parallels between spatial cognition and spatial language: evidence from Williams syndrome. *Journal of Memory and Language*, **53**, 163–85.

Landau, B., & Lakusta, L. (2009). Spatial representation across species: geometry, language, and maps. *Current Opinion in Neurobiology*, **19**, 12–19.

Laws, G. (2002). Working memory in children and adolescents with Down syndrome: evidence from a colour memory experiment. *Journal of Child Psychology and Psychiatry*, **43**, 353–64.

Laws, G., & Lawrence, L. (2001). Spatial representation in the drawings of children with Down's syndrome and its relationship to language and motor development: a preliminary investigation. *British Journal of Developmental Psychology*, **19**, 453–73.

Li, P., & Gleitman, L. (2002). Turning the tables: language and spatial reasoning. *Cognition*, **83**, 265–94.

Levinson, S.C., Kita, S., Haun, D.B., & Rasch, B.H. (2002). Returning the tables: language affects spatial reasoning. *Cognition*, **84**, 155–88.

Lewis, T.L., Kingdon, A., Ellemberg, D., & Maurer, D. (2007). Orientation discrimination in 5-year-olds and adults tested with luminance-modulated and contrast-modulated gratings. *Journal of Vision*, **7**, 1–11.

Lovegrove, W.J., Garzia, R.P., & Nicholson, S.B. (1990). Experimental evidence for a transient system deficit in specific reading disability. *Journal of American Optomology Association*, **61**, 137–46.

McIntosh, R.D., & Schenk, T. (2009). Two visual streams for perception and action: current trends. *Neuropsychologia*, **47**, 1391–96.

Mercuri, E., Atkinson, J., Braddick, O., Rutherford, M., Cowan, F., Counsell, S., et al. (1997). Chiari I malformation in asymptomatic young children with Williams syndrome: clinical and MRI study. *European Journal of Paediatric Neurology*, **1**, 177–81.

Mervis, C.B., & John, A.E. (2008). Vocabulary abilities of children with Williams syndrome: strengths, weaknesses, and relation to visuospatial construction ability. *Journal of Speech, Language, and Hearing Research*, **51**, 967–82.

Mervis, C.B., Morris, C.A., Bertrand, J., & Robinson, B.F. (1999). Williams syndrome: findings from an integrated program of research. In H. Tager-Flusberg (Ed.), *Neurodevelopmental Disorders: Contributions to a New Framework from the Cognitive Neurosciences* (pp. 65–110). Cambridge, MA: MIT Press.

Meyer-Lindenberg, A., Kohn, P., Mervis, C.B., Kippenhan, J.S., Olsen, R.A., Morris, C.A., et al. (2004). Neural basis of genetically determined visuospatial construction deficit in Williams syndrome. *Neuron*, **43**, 623–31.

Meyer-Lindenberg, A., Mervis, C.B., Sarpal, D., Koch, P., Steele, S., Kohn, P., et al. (2005). Functional, structural, and metabolic abnormalities of the hippocampal formation in Williams syndrome. *Journal of Clinical Investigation*, **115**, 1888–95.

Milner, A.D., & Goodale, M.A. (1995). *The Visual Brain in Action*. Oxford: Oxford Psychological Press.

Milner, A.D., & Goodale, M.A. (2008). Two visual systems re-viewed. *Neuropsychologia*, **46**, 774–85.

Mobbs, D., Eckert, M.A., Menon, V., Mills, D., Korenberg, J., Galaburda, A.M., et al. (2007). Reduced parietal and visual cortical activation during global processing in Williams syndrome. *Developmental Medicine and Child Neurology*, **49**, 433–38.

Montfoort, I., Frens, M.A., Hooge, I.T.C., Lagers-van Haselen, G.C., & Van der Geest, J.N. (2007). Visual search deficits in Williams-Beuren syndrome. *Neuropsychologia*, 45, 931–38.

Navon, D. (1977). Forest before trees: the precedence of global features in visual perception. *Cognitive Psychology*, 9, 353–83.

Nardini, M., Atkinson, J., Braddick, O., & Burgess, N. (2008). Developmental trajectories for spatial frames of reference in Williams syndrome. *Developmental Science*, 11, 583–95.

O'Hearn, K., Landau, B., & Hoffman, J.E. (2005). Multiple object tracking in people with Williams syndrome and normally developing children. *Psychological Science*, 16, 905–912.

Palomares, M., Landau, B., & Egeth, H. (2008). Visuospatial interpolation in typically developing children and in people with Williams syndrome. *Vision Research*, 48, 2439–50.

Palomares, M., Landau, B., & Egeth, H. (2009a). Orientation perception in Williams syndrome: discrimination and integration. *Brain and Cognition*, 70, 21–30.

Palomares, M., Ogbonna, C., Landau, B., & Egeth, H. (2009b). Normal susceptibility to visual illusions in abnormal development: evidence from Williams syndrome. *Perception*, 38, 186–99.

Pani, J.R., Mervis, C.B., & Robinson, B.F. (1999). Global spatial organization by individuals with Williams syndrome. *Psychological Science*, 10, 453–58.

Phillips, C., Jarrold, C., Baddeley, A., Grant, J., & Karmiloff-Smith, A. (2004). Comprehension of spatial language terms in Williams syndrome: evidence for an interaction between domains of strength and weakness. *Cortex*, 40, 85–101.

Porter, M.A., & Coltheart, M. (2006). Global and local processing in Williams syndrome, autism, and Down syndrome: perception, attention, and construction. *Developmental Neuropsychology*, 30, 771–89.

Reiss, A.L., Eckert, M.A., Rose, F.E., Karchemskiy, A., Kesler, S., Chang, M., et al. (2004). An experiment of nature: brain anatomy parallels cognition and behavior in Williams syndrome. *Journal of Neuroscience*, 24, 5009–5015.

Reiss, J.E., Hoffman, J.E., & Landau, B. (2005). Motion processing specialization in Williams syndrome. *Vision Research*, 45, 3379–90.

Rondan, C., Santos, A., Mancini, J., Livet, M.O., & Deruelle, C. (2008). Global and local processing in Williams syndrome: drawing versus perceiving. *Child Neuropsychology*, 14, 237–48.

Rossen, R., Klima, E.S., Bellugi, U., Bihrle, A., & Jones, W. (1996). Interaction between language and cognition: evidence from Williams syndrome. In J. Beitchman, N. Cohen, M. Konstantareas & R. Tannock (Eds), *Language, Learning and Behaviour Disorders: Developmental, Behavioural and Clinical Perspectives* (pp. 367–92). New York, NY: Cambridge University Press.

Sarpal, D., Buchsbaum, B.R., Kohn, P.D., Kippenhan, J.S., Mervis, C.B., Morris, C.A., et al. (2008). A genetic model for understanding higher order visual processing: functional interactions of the ventral visual stream in Williams syndrome. *Cerebral Cortex*, 18, 2402–2409.

Scerif, G., Cornish, K., Wilding, J., Driver, J., & Karmiloff-Smith, A. (2004). Visual search in typically developing toddlers and toddlers with fragile X or Williams syndrome. *Developmental Science*, 7, 116–30.

Schmitt, J.E., Eliez, S., Bellugi, U., Galaburda, A., & Reiss, A.L. (2002). Increased gyrification in Williams syndrome: evidence using 3D MRI methods. *Developmental Medicing and Child Neurology*, 44, 292–95.

Shah, A., & Frith, U. (1993). Why do autistic individuals show superior performance on the Block design task? *Journal of Child Psychology and Psychiatry*, 34, 1351–64.

Smith, A.D., Gilchrist, I.D., Hood, B., Tassabehji, M., & Karmiloff-Smith, A. (2009). Inefficient search of large-scale space in Williams syndrome: further insights on the role of LIMK1 deletion in deficits of spatial cognition. *Perception*, 38, 694–701.

Spencer, J., O'Brien, J., Riggs, K., Braddick, O., Atkinson, J., Wattam-Bell, J. (2000). Motion processing in autism: evidence for a dorsal stream deficiency. *Cognitive Neuroscience and Neuropsychology* 11, 2765–67.

Stinton, C., Farran, E.K., & Courbois, Y. (2008). Mental rotation in Williams syndrome: an impaired imagery ability. *Developmental Neuropsychology*, **33**, 565–83.

Tassabehji, M. (2003). Williams-Beuren syndrome: a challenge for genotype–phenotype correlations. *Human Molecular Genetics*, **12**, 229–37.

Taylor, N.M., Jakobson, L.S., Maurer, D., & Lewis, T.L. (2009). Differential vulnerability of global motion, global form, and biological motion processing in full-term and preterm children. *Neuropsychologia*, **47**, 2766–78.

Van der Geest, J.N., & Frens, M.A. (2005). Visual depth processing in Williams-Beuren syndrome. *Experimental Brain Research*, **166**, 200–209.

Van Essen, D.C., Anderson, C.H., & Felleman, D.J. (1992). Information processing in the primate visual system: an integrated systems perspective. *Science*, **255**, 419–23.

Wang, P.P., Doherty, S., Rourke, S.B., & Bellugi, U. (1995). Unique profile of visuo-perceptual skills in a genetic syndrome. *Brain and Cognition*, **29**, 54–65.

Wechsler, D. (1992). *Wechsler Intelligence Scale for Children Third Edition UK*. London: The Psychological Corporation.

Wechsler, D. (2004). *Wechsler Intelligence Scale for Children Fourth Edition UK*. London: The Psychological Corporation.

Williams, C., Happé, F., & Jarrold, C. (2008). Intact inner speech use in autism spectrum disorder: evidence from a short-term memory task. *Journal of Child Psychology and Psychiatry*, **49**, 51–58.

Witkin, H.A., Oltman, P.K., Raskin, E., & Karp, S.A. (1971). *Children's Embedded Figures Test*. Palo Alto, CA: Consulting Psychologists Press.

Yoon, J.M.D., & Johnson, S.C. (2009). Biological motion displays elicit social behavior in 12-month-olds. *Child Development*, **80**, 1069–75.

Chapter 13

Spatial cognition, visuomotor action and attention

Janette Atkinson and Oliver Braddick

Introduction

The brain mechanisms of vision are intimately linked to the systems that use visual information for the control of actions, spatial cognition and executive control, all of which are modulated by the networks that control and maintain visual attention. The emergence of these interconnected functional brain networks is a key issue in both typical and atypical development. In particular, problems of attention and control are implicated in many areas of learning difficulty.

In the first part of this chapter, we outline a neurobiological model of visual mechanisms (and their development) that provides the neural underpinnings of the infant and young child's visual, attentional and spatial abilities. We discuss the links between attention and the child's other cognitive abilities, including planning and executing actions, and how these dynamic developmental interactions between different neural systems may be altered in atypical development from birth through early childhood. A key concept is the broad division of the visual brain into 'ventral' and 'dorsal' cortical streams, with the dorsal-stream processing visual information for the behavioural goals of controlling actions and understanding spatial relationships and the ventral-stream processing information for the recognition of objects and faces (Mishkin et al., 1983; Milner & Goodale, 1995). This distinction is sometimes described as a dorsal 'Where?' or 'How?' system versus a ventral 'What?' or 'Who?' system, although realistically these should be described as a plurality of both dorsal and ventral streams. We discuss the idea of dorsal-stream vulnerability, found across a number of neurodevelopmental disorders, which can be identified through effects on motion perception, but which may be associated with knock-on effects on tasks of visual attention, spatial cognition and visuomotor coordination throughout development.

Dorsal-stream deficits are consistent with the characteristic visuocognitive profile found in Williams syndrome (WS), although dorsal-stream problems are certainly not unique to this disorder. In the second part of this chapter, we will present some evidence on the form these problems take in the visuospatial and visuomotor abilities in children with WS.

Lastly we discuss the overlap between the brain networks controlling action systems and those involved in attention. This means that when we consider visuospatial deficits, these may be associated with deficits of attention. The hypothesis that areas within the dorsal streams heavily overlap with networks for controlling attention and that these functions develop in an interlocking way throughout infancy and late into childhood is discussed more fully in Chapter 6.

Neurobiological model of brain development underpinning visuomotor and visuospatial abilities

Early models of infant visual development started from the idea of two visual systems: a phylogenetically older retinotectal system (subcortical) for orienting to visual stimuli and a newer geniculostriate system (cortical) for recognising objects (Bronson, 1974).

Later models (e.g. Atkinson, 1984, 2000; Atkinson & Braddick, 2003) have refined this two-system model in two major ways that are relevant for understanding neurodevelopmental disorders. First, specific processes have been identified through which developing, selective cortical systems come to modulate and control more automatic subcortical systems. In particular, newborns show orientation of the eyes and head towards salient stimuli, but cannot readily disengage from a centrally viewed stimulus that has captured their fixation when a second object appears in the periphery. The ability to make prompt shifts of fixation away from a fixated central target to a second newly appearing target under conditions of competition (i.e. when both central and peripheral targets are visible together) develops from 3-4 months onwards (Atkinson et al., 1992). It is unilaterally absent in infants who have had one cerebral hemisphere surgically removed (hemispherectomy), with subcortical visual systems intact bilaterally, confirming its cortical basis (Braddick et al., 1992; Morrone et al., 1999). This fixation shift test has been shown to be sensitive to cerebral injury and predictive of neurocognitive outcome in children with perinatal brain damage (Mercuri et al., 1999; Atkinson et al., 2008). As discussed below, it is proposed that fixation shift under competition requires the integration of attentional systems in the parietal lobe and frontal eye fields to modulate the subcortical orienting system, which includes the superior colliculus and the oculomotor nuclei.

A second major development has come from behavioural and electrophysiological (visual evoked potentials/visual event-related potentials [VERP]) studies in typically developing infants that have made it possible to identify the development of specific selective specialised systems in the visual cortex. Visual cortical neurons respond selectively to changes in various stimulus attributes, such as the change in a stimulus in slant or orientation, and this selectivity has been found to emerge progressively in the period between 1-5 months (Atkinson, 2000; Atkinson & Braddick, 2003) with responses emerging first to discriminate changes in contour orientation, followed by discrimination of changes in the direction of motion and, later still, changes in depth, signalled by changes in binocular disparity. These selective properties are all found in the primary visual cortex (V1), but they reflect input from different classes of neurons in the pathway leading from the retina to V1; in particular, directional responses are associated with input to the cortex from the magnocellular pathway and processing within the cortex by the dorsal stream (Livingstone & Hubel, 1988). By contrast, the channel for orientation selectivity, which becomes functional relatively early in an infant's life, can be regarded as the first stage of the pattern of processing required for shape and object recognition, which is largely a function of the ventral stream. This latter pathway arises from parvocellular layers within the lateral geniculate nucleus (Atkinson, 1992).

Orientation and direction selectivity are properties found in the neurons of the primary visual cortex, area V1. Information from these neurons is integrated and elaborated in extrastriate visual areas such as V4 (in the ventral stream) and V5/MT (in the dorsal stream). We have assessed these integrative processes with measures of global coherence using both VERP and behavioural methods (eye fixations in preferential looking). This involves measuring the sensitivity to global structures, such as line segments arranged in concentric circles to form a static circular shape (for the assessment of global form or shape processed in the ventral stream) or dots moving on concentric paths in a circle to form a rotating circular shape (for the assessment of global coherent motion processed in the dorsal stream). Both types of global processing can be demonstrated in typically developing infants by around 5-6 months of age, although in general global coherence for motion is relatively more mature and starts to function earlier than global coherence for static forms (Braddick & Atkinson, 2007; Wattam-Bell et al., 2010). Of course, within the dorsal coherent motion stimulus there is also information concerning form and some have considered this a 'shape from motion' discrimination task that may involve some integration of information from both dorsal and ventral streams.

Figure 13.1 shows our summary of the major elements of visual brain development in the first year of life and their relation to some major behavioural milestones (Atkinson, 2000; Atkinson & Braddick, 2003). These milestones—orienting head and eyes, visually directed reaching and grasping, and locomotion—are functions of specific visuomotor modules within the dorsal stream that extract the visual information needed to guide these actions and translate them into the form required for motor planning and control (Rizzolatti et al., 1997). In some cases, the components of these modules have been identified in neurophysiological and neuropsychological studies (in adult patients or in nonhuman primates) as specific areas in the dorsal-stream network in parietal and frontal lobes, as shown in Figure 13.2 (Atkinson & Braddick, 2000; based on the extensive reviews of Milner and Goodale, 1995, and Jeannerod, 1997).

An important point within both Figures 13.1 and 13.2 is the relationship between these dorsal-stream systems and attention. Many aspects of attention can be regarded as selection for action (Allport, 1989; Rizzolatti, 1983; Berthoz, 1996). Actions such as reaching, grasping and locomotion require attentional modulation to select and initiate the appropriate behaviour, to direct it towards a selected goal object and to inhibit actions that are inappropriate for the current goal. It is therefore not surprising that many brain structures that have been implicated as part of attention networks are within the dorsal streams or closely interconnected with these 'spatial action' networks.

The sequence of development in early infancy indicates that the initial development of the dorsal-stream pathway may be slower than that of the parvocellular/ventral pathway, which specialises in the processing of form (orientation or slant) and colour discrimination (Atkinson & Braddick, 1990). However, the maturation of higher-level aspects of the dorsal

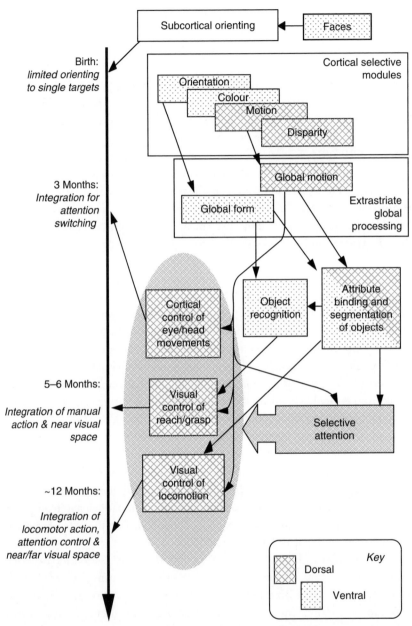

Fig. 13.1 Model of visuospatial development in the first year of life, with behavioural milestones and brain processes in dorsal and ventral streams that become functional at different stages of development. Developed from Atkinson (2000) and Atkinson & Braddick (2003). With kind permission from Springer Science+Business Media: *Motion Vision*, Gaze control: A developmental perspective, 2000, pp. 219–225. Atkinson, J., & Braddick, O.

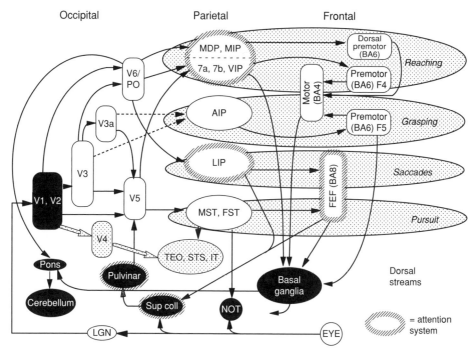

Fig. 13.2 Brain areas involved in visuomotor modules and their connections, for four aspects of the development of visually controlled behaviour. Areas involved in spatial attention networks are highlighted by hatched borders. Abbreviations: AIP = anterior intraparietal; FEF = frontal eye fields; FST = fundal superior temporal; IT = inferotemporal; LGN = lateral geniculate nucleus; LIP = lateral intraparietal; MDP = medial dorsal parietal; MIP =medial intraparietal; MST = medial superior temporal; NOT = nucleus of the optic tract; PO = parieto-occipital; STS = superior temporal sulcus; sup coll = superior colliculus; TEO = a posterior region of the inferotemporal cortex; VIP = ventral intraparietal. Based on data reviewed by Jeannerod (1988), Milner and Goodale (1995) and Rizzolatti et al. (1997). With kind permission from Springer Science+Business Media: *Motion Vision*, Gaze control: A developmental perspective, 2000, pp. 219–225. Atkinson, J., & Braddick, O.

stream, which serves the global integration of motion information, proceeds rapidly and at age 5 months it is more developmentally advanced than the equivalent response to the global structure of static forms (Braddick & Atkinson, 2007; Wattam-Bell et al., 2010).

Later, in middle childhood, thresholds for global form and motion structure can be measured and compared in two behavioural tests. In one test, the threshold for detecting static form or pattern coherence is estimated. In the other, the threshold for detecting global motion coherence is estimated. Results from these tests indicate that global form processing (ventral) reaches adult levels earlier (between ages of 4 and 10 years) than does global motion processing (dorsal).

The developmental trajectories for ventral- and dorsal-stream function, therefore, have a complex and changing relationship (Braddick et al., 2003). It is not yet known which stages of this developmental relationship are responsible for the differential vulnerability of dorsal-stream function in neurodevelopmental disorders (discussed in the next section) and, of course, in different disorders different areas within this developing dynamic network may be abnormally functioning or delayed in development.

Dorsal-stream vulnerability: form and motion coherence in Williams syndrome and other disorders

The tasks mentioned previously that have been used to compare dorsal and ventral-stream function are designed to be as comparable as possible in general cognitive demands apart from the specifics of the stimuli used. For global motion, the child has to spot a distinctive coherently moving region in a display of moving dots. The region can be defined as an oscillating strip moving contrary to the surrounding strips (the 'road in the snowstorm' task, Atkinson et al., 1997) or as a set of dots moving in arcs around a common centre (Atkinson & Braddick, 2005). In either case, the coherently moving dots are mixed with a variable percentage of randomly moving 'noise' dots, and a threshold coherence (e.g. identifying the region where 20% of the dots share the coherent motion) can be measured. The form coherence task ('finding the ball in the grass') is similar, except that the coherent elements are static short arcs with the same concentric structure and the noise elements are static, randomly oriented arcs. Each task can be presented as a computer game that children with a mental age as young as 4 years can perform successfully. Neuroimaging and VERP experiments with similar stimuli in adults indicate that they are processed by independent brain networks, although these do not seem to be neatly divided between classic areas within dorsal and ventral streams (i.e. temporal lobe areas for ventral stream and parietal lobe areas for dorsal stream) (Braddick et al., 2000; Wattam-Bell et al., 2010).

As part of their uneven profile of neuropsychological development, children with WS show severe impairments across many areas of spatial construction and cognition (see for example Bellugi et al., 1988, 1999; Klein & Mervis, 1999; Pezzini et al., 1999; Chapter 12). By contrast, they are relatively unimpaired on visual recognition and, in particular, perform well on face recognition tests (e.g. Bellugi et al., 1999; Chapter 14). Children with WS also reach motor milestones later than typically developing children. They are often delayed in learning to walk, in the development of fine motor skills and on a standardised test of motor function (Movement ABC; Henderson & Sugden, 1992). Children with WS under 13 years of age showed an average delay of at least 2 years below their chronological age (Atkinson et al., 1996). Their problems include uncertainty when negotiating stairs or uneven surfaces (Atkinson et al., 1996; Cowie, 2007; Cowie et al., in press), awkward gait (in some children; Kaplan et al., 1989; Pober, 2010) and difficulty with the use of everyday tools (Dilts et al., 1990). Although WS children have a high incidence of basic visual disorders (e.g. strabismus, refractive errors), their visuospatial performance does not seem to be well correlated with these visual disorders (Atkinson et al., 2001) but is a central feature of the neural developmental pathway of this syndrome.

The described profile is consistent with what would be expected from a developmental deficit of dorsal-stream functions with relatively intact ventral-stream processes. This hypothesis was tested with the global form and motion coherence thresholds described earlier, which confirmed that children with WS showed much poorer performance on motion than on static form coherence tests, compared with typically developing children who were matched not on chronological age but on verbal mental age (Atkinson et al., 1997). Although the extent of this deficit is found to be quite variable in children with WS (Atkinson et al., 2003), it persists into adulthood in WS and so cannot be characterised as a simple delay in development (Atkinson et al., 2006).

Another indicator designed to compare dorsal and ventral-stream function is the postbox task developed by Milner & Goodale (1995) from the work of Perenin & Vighetto (1988). Milner and Goodale's patient, with specific brain damage in an area considered to be part of the ventral stream, performed at chance when asked to indicate the orientation of a slot by turning a card to be aligned with it. However, she performed accurately and fluently when asked simply to post the card through the slot. Thus, visual orientation information was available for the control of action (dorsal) but inaccessible for an explicit perceptual matching judgement (ventral). Children with WS have been found to show the opposite pattern (Atkinson et al., 1997): in posting the card, they frequently approached the slot at a wrong angle, with trial and error attempts to insert it. In some cases, older WS children made an extremely slow approach, apparently matching the orientation by a much more cautious and deliberate action than the fluent, unreflective action by typically developing children. The differential deficit between the two postbox tasks in WS has been confirmed by Dilks et al. (2008). This is the pattern that would be expected if the dorsal-stream translation of visuospatial information into action was impaired. It was also notable that the participants with WS often made very awkward wrist rotations in the course of finding the right angle for posting. We will return to the issue of motor planning for 'end-state comfort' in a later section of this chapter.

The idea that there are anomalies of the dorsal pathway in WS that affect spatial cognition has been supported by neuroimaging studies. Meyer-Lindenberg et al. (2004) made functional magnetic resonance imaging measurements on a small group of relatively high-functioning adults with WS while they performed tasks requiring either shape matching, or mental rotation of the same shapes to decide if they fitted together. A dorsal-stream area in the parietal lobe showed differential activation, compared with controls, in the latter task but not the former. Meyer-Lindenberg et al. (2004) also found a structural difference in grey-matter density in a region that would connect extrastriate visual areas to the parietal area showing this functional deficit. (It should be noted, however, that a wide variety of structural differences has been reported between WS and control brains and, of course, that functional brain differences are not limited to spatial cognition, with major effects in areas involved in processing social stimuli; see for example Meyer-Lindenberg et al., 2005a).

Since the original WS study on form and motion coherence thresholds, this comparison between form and motion coherence has been used to study a wide variety of neurodevelopmental disorders, using identical or similar stimuli and tasks. The relative deficit in global motion processing has been found to be far from unique to WS. A similar pattern has been reported in autism (Spencer et al., 2000; Milne et al., 2005), in hemiplegia (Gunn et al., 2002), in subsets of dyslexia (Cornelissen et al., 1995; Hansen et al., 2001;

Ridder et al., 2001) and in fragile X syndrome (Kogan et al., 2004). Other indicators of dorsal-stream function, such as the postbox task, have been less extensively explored. However, a study of a wide variety of neurocognitive functions in a group of children aged 5-7 years who were born prematurely (Atkinson & Braddick, 2007) demonstrated that, in addition to having more difficulty with motion coherence tests than with form coherence tests, the children showed the greatest deficits in spatial, visuomotor and attentional tasks—the areas of function that we have argued involve largely dorsal-stream networks rather than ventral-stream networks. However, we would not want to claim that many of these tasks are totally controlled by either dorsal-stream networks or ventral-stream networks; most involve some processing within classically ventral-stream areas and the problem may be integration between information extracted from each stream to achieve a common goal.

Thus, dorsal-stream function seems to be particularly vulnerable to the effects of neurodevelopmental disorders, whether genetic (WS, fragile X syndrome, probably autism) or acquired (hemiplegia, related to prematurity) in origin. We have speculated on the reasons for this vulnerability (Braddick et al., 2003), which may be associated with the high demands for precision on neural timing of motion processing and visuomotor transformation. The severe problems of spatial cognition seen in WS do not, however, occur so generally across neurodevelopmental disorders, although fragile X syndrome shows some similarities (Cornish et al., 1998). Thus, the profile of WS must presumably involve some developmental interactions between this general dorsal-stream vulnerability and other neural effects of the WS genotype, which determine how the impaired dorsal-stream information is used downstream in tasks with spatial-cognitive, motor and attentional demands. We will now outline some findings in these areas, although attentional deficits associated with WS are discussed in detail in Chapter 6.

Motor control and planning in spatial tasks

Motor skills are often poor in WS and these difficulties are quite evident in everyday life (see also Chapter 9). In particular, difficulty in stepping down stairs or at a change of level such as a kerb is often commented on by families as an area of extreme difficulty, even in adults with WS. These types of everyday tasks are often associated with anxiety.

The control of action requires, first, the selection and maintenance of a goal. This is closely related to the discussions of spatial attention in Chapters 6 and 18, and given that there will generally be alternative goal objects available, it is also closely related to the deficit in the inhibitory control processes discussed earlier in this chapter and in Chapter 6. Second, it requires the acquisition of visuospatial information relevant to the goal of the action and its translation into a motor programme. This is the classic function of dorsal-stream networks as illustrated in Figure 13.2. Third, given that most goals require more than one action element (e.g. reaching towards an object and forming an appropriate grasp), they generally require planning a sequence of actions, some of which may not be immediately directed to the goal. Neuroimaging and neural recording evidence (Cavina-Pratesi et al., 2006; Tanji et al., 2007) indicate that this kind of planning involves activity in the premotor and prefrontal areas of the brain.

An example of the second requirement, sensory–motor translation, is in the control of the limbs during step descent. Typical individuals anticipate the depth of the step by swinging the lower leg and foot inwards with a timing that is related to the anticipated moment of contact with the step below (Cowie et al., 2008). This use of visual information is apparent, albeit not fully mature, in typically developing children as young as 3 years (Cowie et al., 2010). Many older children with WS show poorly organised translation of visual cues into motor actions in this stepping-down task, although there is large variability across individuals. In general, the overall stepping speed of children with WS is low and, in particular, some major kinematic measures do not show the relation to visually determined step height that is found in typically developing 3-year-olds (Cowie et al., in press). An analogous deficit of visuomotor control is seen in WS control in reaching for an object, where inadequate use of information concerning the estimation of depth and distance has been reported (Elliott et al., 2006).

These motor control problems indicate neural deficits in occipitoparietal and parieto-frontal systems. However, a wide range of other brain structures are involved in motor control, for example the cerebellum. Morphological differences in the cerebellum and parietal lobe have been found in a study of two very young children with WS (Mercuri et al., 1997), indicating that these cerebellar abnormalities are present very early in development. Such abnormalities (notably enlargement of the cerebellar tonsils) have also been identified in adults with WS in a number of other studies (Jernigan & Bellugi, 1990; Wang et al., 1992; Galaburda et al., 1994). However, the relationship between cerebellar morphology and the cognitive and visuomotor characteristics of WS is not yet understood.

An example of the third aspect of control of motor action, motor planning, is exemplified by a task based on the work of Rosenbaum et al. (1992) and has been investigated in a developmental context by Smyth & Mason (1997). It is best explained by imagining the example of picking up a wine glass with a stem: if you intend to place the glass onto a table, you will grasp the stem with your thumb at the top, but if you intend to place the glass base-up on a shelf, you will grasp it with your thumb down, so that your wrist is at a comfortable angle at the end of the action. This planning for end-state comfort is tested by asking the child to grasp a handle in order to rotate an attached pointer from various starting positions to a specified location on a clock face, indicated by a light or a particular coloured mouse picture. Adults select a thumb-up or thumb-down grasp so as to achieve a comfortable rotation of the wrist at the target location (Rosenbaum et al., 1992). Young children (6 years or younger) tend to adopt a stereotypical 'thumb-towards' strategy, with the thumb pointing in the direction of the pointer regardless of the end-state position this will lead to. Between 6 and 8 years, they progress to the adult-like pattern (Smyth & Mason, 1997). It is proposed that the thumb-towards strategy results from the action being linked to the immediate visual properties of the object: the pointer is the focus of the intended action and determines the grasp. The end-state comfort strategy requires this link to be over-ridden by the longer-term goal.

The awkward wrist postures of children with WS during the postbox task, mentioned earlier, indicated to Newman (2001) that it would be interesting to study their performance on this pointer-rotation task. At no age (investigated chronological age: 5-14 years; the mental age was assessed through vocabulary scores) did children with WS show either the thumb-towards pattern seen in typically developing very young children or the adult end-state comfort pattern, although there was a weak trend towards increasing end-state-comfort responses with increasing mental age in the WS group. Behaviour on this task was very variable both across individuals and across the group as a whole, but a significantly larger proportion (compared with typically developing children of any age) showed a stereotyped response pattern in which the handle was grasped with the thumb up, regardless of either the starting position or the target position of the pointer. Thus, children with WS at all ages are relatively weak either in the translation of the visual properties of the object into a grasp pattern (the thumb-towards pattern of typically developing children aged 4-5 years) or in the more sophisticated translation of visually specified locations into anticipated motor states (the end-state comfort pattern of typical 8-year-olds and adults). The first of these deficits is consistent with other evidence, discussed earlier in this chapter, for poor immediate visuomotor translation by the dorsal stream; the second implies problems in the more frontal preparation of goal-directed actions. However, Newman (2001) looked for, and failed to find, a significant correlation between end-state comfort pattern in his participants with WS and their performance on a set of frontal-lobe tasks, perhaps because the results were confounded by variability in the earlier parietal visuomotor translation.

Remembering and transforming spatial information

We have discussed aspects of behaviour that require the transformation of visuospatial information that is immediately present in the field of view. Another aspect of spatial processing, also required for effective direction of spatial actions, is the registration in memory of information about locations and its transformation for the purposes of later performance. The spatial layout of our environment is acquired in egocentric coordinates, a frame of reference related to the viewpoint from our current body position. However, we may subsequently need to refer to this location from a different viewpoint because we may move through the environment, and so have to transform the information into an allocentric frame of reference related to spatial features of the external world. Alternative reference frames may also be possible; for example, the location of objects on a movable tray could be specified relative to the array of objects on the tray or relative to features of the fixed environment, that is, the room in which the display tray is placed.

Typically developing young children show a steady progression in the use of these multiple frames and of translation between them (Nardini et al., 2006). Tested in finding a toy that they see hidden under one of multiple cups on a display tray, 3-year-olds can succeed either from their original viewpoint (egocentric frame) or from a different viewpoint to which they have walked (allocentric, based on room landmarks or on updating by registering the path taken through space). However, if the tray is rotated within the room, they are much worse at finding the remembered location relative to the array of objects on the tray; the ability to use this frame of reference does not emerge until around 5 years of age in typical development.

In similar testing with WS individuals, there was a marked overall delay, with children with WS aged 5-11 years showing higher error rates than typical 3-year-olds, even in purely egocentric localisation (Nardini et al., 2008). Even adults with WS were generally poor at using the local array as a frame of reference and showed a pattern of error rates across the conditions that was similar to that seen in typical 4-year-olds. Adolescents (12-15 years) with WS showed similar patterns to even younger typically developing children. Furthermore, the nature of errors by participants with WS showed greater disorganisation than for even the youngest typically developing children: the latter, when faced with the rotated array, tend to make errors of inappropriately using an egocentric or room-based frame of reference, whereas the participants with WS showed spatially random behaviour without any pattern that could be ascribed to using an earlier-emerging frame of reference. Individuals with WS have also been found to show deficits in searching for objects in a room-sized space (Smith et al., 2009) and in way-finding and route learning (Atkinson et al., 2001; Farran et al., 2010).

Can these deficits in remembering and processing spatial locations be ascribed to the dorsal stream and the parietofrontal system discussed in earlier sections? A different brain structure, the hippocampus, has a critical role in human navigation and landmark use (Burgess et al., 2002) and this structure shows much reduced responses to visual stimuli in individuals with WS (Meyer-Lindenberg et al., 2005b). Spatial memory tasks of course require appropriate encoding of the stimulus information, and it is plausible that the particular difficulty shown by individuals with WS in referencing a location to local landmarks might be because the spatial relations between objects are poorly represented in dorsal-stream processing, which provides an input to the hippocampus. However, Meyer-Lindenberg et al. (2005b) did consider this argument and provided evidence that face stimuli, which are primarily processed in the ventral cortical stream, also activated the hippocampus much more weakly in individuals with WS than in controls.

One question that arises in all of these studies of spatial tasks is whether any improvement can be seen following extensive practice or alternative training strategies. Although there are no formal tests of practice effects for many of these tests, one strategy that has been tried informally with some of the families with children with WS has been to accompany visuomotor tasks with verbal instructions, phrases or rhythms. One success story for a child who was always having difficulty with dressing (i.e. putting his clothes on in the correct order) was to use a song to cue the order of the sequence with clothes labels for each piece of clothing.

Conclusions

The neurocognitive anomalies of WS are quite pervasive and include many areas dealt with in this volume, for example social cognition, behaviour and affect (see Chapter 15), which are outside the scope of this chapter. The areas we have considered form a diverse but connected set of problems. Atypical development of dorsal-stream function, including a profoundly disordered ability to generally process spatial information, seem to underlie many of the difficulties faced by individuals with WS. Problems with functions such as memory, motor control and executive function may not be exclusively visuospatial but are certainly strongly coloured by this disorder in spatial and motion processing.

In attempting to understand the links between the components of cognitive and behavioural anomaly in WS, it is important to keep in mind that this is a neurodevelopmental disorder. The genetic abnormality of WS is well explored. However, we know little about how the expression of these genes, starting in prenatal brain development but perhaps continuing through the lifespan, leads to a cascade of neural events whose developmental consequences appear over the course of infancy, childhood and beyond. Only thorough cross-sectional and longitudinal developmental study, starting in infancy, will resolve which brain and behavioural effects occur initially. We will then have to unravel the chain of dependency by which interaction of these effects with each other, and with the child's physical and social environment, leads to the wide-ranging and unique WS profile.

The evidence we have discussed indicates that anomalous development of the dorsal stream plays a key part in this sequence, but it remains to be shown how far these anomalies are primary and which other parts of the WS pattern are knock-on effects of a disordered dorsal cortical stream. The research considered in this chapter has emphasised a common theme of dorsal-stream deficits in WS. However, this is not the endpoint. We have pointed out the overlap between dorsal-stream brain networks (which must be part of the underpinnings for visuomotor spatial tasks) and brain networks for controlling both bottom-up and top-down control of attention. So, ideas in this chapter are heavily connected to those in Chapter 6, where development of attention and its neural underpinnings are discussed more fully.

One area which remains wide open for future research is the study of the immense variety of possibilities for strategies of treatment, individualised for each child with WS. We hope that future researchers will carry this further.

Editor commentary (Emily K. Farran & Annette Karmiloff-Smith)

One specific measure of attention in infancy—fixation shift—is predictive of neurocognitive outcome in children with another neurodevelopmental disorder: perinatal brain damage. This illustrates the role of attentional mechanisms in cognitive development and supports the neuroconstructivist view that early impairments in the infant start state can have cascading impacts on later development. This chapter considered the effects of attention on the visual brain, with a particular focus on the distinction between the dorsal visual stream and the ventral visual stream. The chapter explored the development of the two visual streams in the first year of life and discussed how visual milestones relate to visuomotor milestones of the dorsal visual stream, highlighting that many visuomotor actions (e.g. reaching, grasping and locomotion) require attentional modulation. During middle childhood, dorsal-stream functions reach adult levels of ability later than ventral-stream functions.

Although dorsal-stream vulnerability does not seem to be unique to WS, the chapter noted that the spatial difficulties observed in this group are indeed syndrome-specific. The authors proposed that general dorsal-stream vulnerability interacts with syndrome-specific genetic expression patterns and with neural and behavioural development in WS to produce the phenotypic outcome. Examples were given, first of impaired motor control and planning in WS (e.g. reaching and grasping, staircase descent), which the chapter associated with impaired interaction between the dorsal visual stream and the parietofrontal cortex, and potentially the cerebellum, and second, of impaired spatial memory and spatial transformation (e.g. navigating around an environment, using landmarks to find objects and places), which are associated with impaired interaction between the dorsal visual stream and the hippocampus, involved in episodic memory and navigation. As we observed in Chapter 2 these areas show both structural and functional impairments in WS. These examples highlight the fact that the brain is a very interactive system and illustrate why it is important to focus on networks of activation.

This provides a useful framework in which to consider other neurodevelopmental disorders purported to display a dorsal-stream deficit (e.g. dyslexia, fragile X syndrome, autism). Cross-syndrome comparison may help to elucidate the modulating effects of overlapping networks and reveal how these differ across syndromes. For example, both cerebellar dysfunction and a dorsal-stream deficit are reported in WS and fragile X syndrome. Multilevel comparison across these two disorders would be particularly fruitful to determine the behavioural outcome associated with syndrome-specific characteristics of these overlapping networks.

References

Allport, A. (1989). Visual attention. In M.I. Posner (Ed.), *Foundations of Cognitive Science* (pp. 631–82). Cambridge, MA: MIT Press.

Atkinson, J. (1984). Human visual development over the first six months of life. A review and a hypothesis. *Human Neurobiology*, **3**, 61–74.

Atkinson, J. (1992). Early visual development: differential functioning of parvocellular and magnocellular pathways. *Eye*, **6**, 129–35.

Atkinson, J. (2000). *The Developing Visual Brain*. Oxford: Oxford University Press.

Atkinson, J., Anker, S., Braddick, O., Nokes, L., Mason, A., & Braddick, F. (2001). Visual and visuo-spatial development in young Williams syndrome children. *Developmental Medicine & Child Neurology*, **43**, 330–37.

Atkinson, J. & Braddick, O.J. (1990). The developmental course of cortical processing streams in the human infant. In C. Blakemore (Ed.) *Vision: Coding and Efficiency* (pp. 247–53). Cambridge: Cambridge University Press.

Atkinson, J., & Braddick, O. (2000). Gaze control: a developmental perspective. In J.M. Zanker & J. Zeil (Eds.), *Motion Vision* (pp. 219–25). Berlin: Springer Verlag.

Atkinson, J., & Braddick, O. (2003). Neurobiological models of normal and abnormal visual development. In M. De Haan & M.H. Johnson (Eds.) *The Cognitive Neuroscience of Development* (pp. 43–71). Hove: Psychology Press.

Atkinson, J., & Braddick, O. (2005). Dorsal stream vulnerability and autistic disorders: the importance of comparative studies of form and motion coherence in typically developing children and children with developmental disorders. *Cahiers de psychologie cognitive/Current Psychology of Cognition*, **23**, 49–58.

Atkinson, J., & Braddick, O. (2007). Visual and visuocognitive development in children born very prematurely. *Progress in Brain Research*, **164**, 123–49.

Atkinson, J., Braddick, O., Anker, S., Curran, W., & Andrew, R. (2003). Neurobiological models of visuospatial cognition in children with Williams syndrome: measures of dorsal-stream and frontal function. *Developmental Neuropsychology*, 23, 141–74.

Atkinson, J., Braddick, O., Anker, S., Ehrlich, D., Macpherson, F., Rae, S., et al. (1996). *Development of Sensory, Perceptual, and Cognitive Vision and Visual Attention in Young Williams Syndrome Children.* Presented at the Seventh International Professional Conference on Williams Syndrome, King of Prussia, PA.

Atkinson, J., Braddick, O., Anker, S., Nardini, M., Birtles, D., Rutherford, M., et al. (2008). Cortical vision, MRI and developmental outcome in preterm infants. *Archives of Disease in Childhood: Fetal Neonatal Edition*, 93, F292–97.

Atkinson, J., Braddick, O., Rose, F.E., Searcy, Y.M., Wattam-Bell, J., & Bellugi, U. (2006). Dorsal-stream motion processing deficits persist into adulthood in Williams syndrome. *Neuropsychologia*, 44, 828–33.

Atkinson, J., Hood, B. Wattam-Bell, J. & Braddick, O.J. (1992). Changes in infants' ability to switch visual attention in the first three months of life. *Perception*, 21, 643–53.

Atkinson, J., King, J., Braddick, O., Nokes, L., Anker, S. & Braddick, F. (1997). A specific deficit of dorsal visual stream function in Williams syndrome. *NeuroReport*, 8, 1919–22.

Bellugi, U., Lichtenberger, L., Mills, D., Galaburda, A. & Korenberg, J.R. (1999). Bridging cognition, the brain, and molecular genetics: evidence from Williams syndrome. *Trends in Neurosciences*, 22, 197–207.

Bellugi, U., Sabo, H. & Vaid, J. (1988). Spatial deficits in children with Williams syndrome. In J. Stiles-Davis, M. Kritchevsky & U. Bellugi (Eds.) *Spatial Cognition: Brain Bases and Development* (pp. 273–97). Hillsdale, NJ: Lawrence Erlbaum.

Berthoz, A. (1996). Neural basis of decision in perception and the control of movement. In A.R. Damasio, H. Damasio, & Y. Christen (Eds.) *Neurobiology of Decision Making* (pp. 83–100). Berlin: Springer.

Braddick, O., & Atkinson, J. (2007). Development of brain mechanisms for visual global processing and object segmentation. *Progress in Brain Research*, 164, 151–68.

Braddick, O., Atkinson, J., Hood, B., Harkness, W., Jackson, G., & Vargha-Khadem, F. (1992). Possible blindsight in babies lacking one cerebral hemisphere. *Nature*, 360, 461–63.

Braddick, O., Atkinson, J., & Wattam-Bell, J. (2003). Normal and anomalous development of visual motion processing: motion coherence and 'dorsal stream vulnerability'. *Neuropsychologia*, 41, 1769–84.

Braddick, O.J., O'Brien, J.M.D., Wattam-Bell, J., Atkinson, J. & Turner, R. (2000). Form and motion coherence activate independent, but not dorsal/ventral segregated, networks in the human brain. *Current Biology*, 10, 731–34.

Bronson, G.W. (1974). The postnatal growth of visual capacity. *Child Development*, 45, 873–90.

Burgess, N., Maguire, E.A., & O'Keefe, J. (2002). The human hippocampus and spatial and episodic memory. *Neuron*, 35, 625–41.

Cavina-Pratesi, C., Valyear, K.F., Culham, J.C., Köhler, S., Obhi, S.S., Marzi, C.A., et al. (2006). Dissociating arbitrary stimulus-response mapping from movement planning during preparatory period: evidence from event-related functional magnetic resonance imaging. *Journal of Neuroscience*, 26, 2704–13.

Cornelissen, P., Richardson, A., Mason, A., Fowler, S., & Stein, J.F. (1995). Contrast sensitivity and coherent motion detection measured at photopic luminance levels in dyslexics and controls. *Vision Research*, 35, 1483–94.

Cornish, K.M., Munir, F., & Cross, G. (1998). The nature of the spatial deficit in young females with Fragile-X syndrome: a neuropsychological and molecular perspective. *Neuropsychologia*, 36, 1239–46.

Cowie, D. (2007). *Development of Visually Guided Locomotion.* DPhil Thesis, University of Oxford.

Cowie, D., Atkinson, J., & Braddick, O. (2010). Development of visual control in stepping down. *Experimental Brain Research*, 202, 181–88.

Cowie, D., Braddick, O., & Atkinson, J. (2008). Visual control of action in step descent. *Experimental Brain Research*, 186, 343–48.

Cowie, D., Braddick, O., & Atkinson, J. (in press). Visually guided locomotion in children with Williams syndrome. *Developmental Science.*

Dilks, D.D., Hoffman, J.E., & Landau, B. (2008).Vision for perception and vision for action: normal and unusual development. *Developmental Science*, 11, 474–86.

Dilts, C.V., Morris, C.A., & Leonard, C.O (1990). Hypothesis for development of a behavioral phenotype in Williams syndrome. *American Journal of Medical Genetics, Supplement*, 6, 126–31.

Elliott, D., Welsh, T.N., Lyons, J., Hansen, S., & Wu, M. (2006). The visual regulation of goal-directed reaching movements in adults with Williams syndrome, Down syndrome, and other developmental delays. *Motor Control*, 10, 34–54.

Farran, E.K., Blades, M., Boucher, J. & Tranter, L.J. (2010). How do individuals with Williams syndrome learn a route in a real-world environment? *Developmental Science*, 13, 454–68.

Galaburda, A.M., Wang, P.P., Bellugi, U., & Rossen, M. (1994). Cytoarchitectonic anomalies in a genetically based disorder. *NeuroReport*, 5, 753–57.

Gunn A, Cory E, Atkinson J, Braddick O, Wattam-Bell J, Guzzetta A, et al. (2002). Dorsal and ventral stream sensitivity in normal development and hemiplegia. *NeuroReport.* 13, 843–47.

Hansen, P.C., Stein, J.F., Orde, S.R., Winter, J.L., & Talcott, J.B.(2001). Are dyslexics' visual deficits limited to measures of dorsal stream function? *Neuroreport*, 12, 1527–30.

Henderson, S.E., & Sugden, D.A. (1992). *The Movement ABC Manual*. The Psychological Corporation, London.

Jeannerod, M. (1988). *The Neural and Behavioural Organization of Goal Directed Movements*. Oxford: Oxford University Press.

Jeannerod, M. (1997). *The Cognitive Neuroscience of Action*. Oxford: Blackwell.

Jernigan, T., & Bellugi, U. (1990). Anomalous brain morphology on magnetic resonance images in Williams syndrome and Down syndrome. *Archives of Neurology*, 47, 529–33.

Kaplan, P., Kirschner, M., Watters, G. & Costa, M.T. (1989). Contractures in patients with Williams syndrome. *Pediatrics*, 84, 895–99.

Klein, B.P., & Mervis, C.B. (1999). Contrasting patterns of cognitive abilities of 9 and 10-year- olds with Williams syndrome or Down syndrome. *Developmental Neuropsychology*, 16, 177–96.

Kogan, C.S., Boutet, I., Cornish, K., Zangenehpour, S., Mullen, K.T., Holden, J.J.A., et al. (2004). Differential impact of the FMR1 gene on visual processing in fragile X syndrome. *Brain*, 127, 591–601.

Livingstone, M. & Hubel, D.H. (1988). Segregation of form, color, movement and depth: anatomy, physiology and perception. *Science*, 240, 740–49.

Mercuri, E., Atkinson, J., Braddick, O., Rutherford, M., Cowan, F., & Counsell, S. (1997). Chiari I malformation and white matter changes in asymptomatic young children with Williams syndrome: clinical and MRI study. *European Journal of Paediatric Neurology*, 1, 177–81.

Mercuri, E., Haataja, L., Guzzetta, A., Anker, S., Cowan, F., Rutherford, M., et al. (1999). Visual function in term infants with hypoxic-ischaemic insults: correlation with neurodevelopment at 2 years of age. *Archives of Diseases in Childhood*, 80, F99–F104.

Meyer-Lindenberg, A., Hariri, A.R., Munoz, K.E., Mervis, C.B., Mattay, V.S., Morris, C.A., et al. (2005a). Neural correlates of genetically abnormal social cognition in Williams syndrome. *Nature Neuroscience*, 8, 991–93.

Meyer-Lindenberg, A., Kohn, P., Mervis, C.B., Kippenhan, J.S., Olsen, R.K., Morris, C.A., et al. (2004). Neural basis of genetically determined visuospatial construction deficit in Williams syndrome. *Neuron*, 43, 623–31.

Meyer-Lindenberg, A., Mervis, C.B., Sarpal, D., Koch, P., Steele, S., Kohn, P., et al. (2005b). Functional, structural, and metabolic abnormalities of the hippocampal formation in Williams syndrome. *Journal of Clinical Investigation*, 115, 1888–95.

Milne, E., Swettenham, J., & Campbell, R. (2005). Motion perception and autistic spectrum disorder: a review. *Cahiers de Psycologie Cognitive/Current Psychology of Cognition*, 23, 3–36.

Milner, A.D. & Goodale, M.A. (1995). *The Visual Brain in Action*. Oxford: Oxford University Press.

Mishkin, M., Ungerleider, L., & Macko, K.A. (1983). Object vision and spatial vision: two cortical pathways. *Trends in Neuroscience*, 6, 414–17.

Morrone, M.C., Atkinson, J., Cioni, G., Braddick, O.J., & Fiorentini, A. (1999). Developmental changes in optokinetic mechanisms in the absence of unilateral cortical control. *NeuroReport* 10, 1–7.

Nardini, M., Atkinson, J., Braddick, O., & Burgess, N. (2008). Developmental trajectories for spatial frames of reference in Williams syndrome. *Developmental Science*, 11, 583–95.

Nardini, M., Burgess, N., Breckenridge, K., & Atkinson, J. (2006). Differential developmental trajectories for egocentric, environmental and intrinsic frames of reference in spatial memory. *Cognition*, 101, 153–72.

Newman, C. (2001). *The Planning and Control of Action in Normal Infants and Children with Williams Syndrome*. PhD Thesis, University of London.

Perenin, M.T., & Vighetto, A. (1988). Optic ataxia: a specific disruption in visuomotor mechanisms.I. Different aspects of the deficit in reaching for objects. *Brain* 111, 643–74.

Pezzini, G., Vicari, S., Volterra, V., Milani, L., & Ossella, M.T. (1999). Children with Williams syndrome: is there a single neuropsychological profile? *Developmental Neuropsychology*, 15, 141–55.

Pober, B.R. (2010). Williams-Beuren syndrome. *New England Journal of Medicine*, 362, 239–52.

Ridder, W.H.I., Borsting, E., & Banton, T. (2001). All developmental dyslexic subtypes display an elevated motion coherence threshold. *Optometry and Vision Science*, 78, 510–17.

Rizzolatti, G. (1983). Mechanisms of selective attention in mammals. In J.P. Ewert, R.R. Capranica, & D.J. Ingle (Eds.) *Advances in Vertebrate Neuroethology* (pp. 261–97). Amsterdam: Elsevier.

Rizzolatti, G., Fogassi, L., & Gallese, V. (1997). Parietal cortex: from sight to action. *Current Opinion in Neurobiology*, 7, 562–67.

Rosenbaum, D.A., Vaughan, J., Barnes, HJ, Marchak, F., & Slotta JD. (1992). Timecourse of movement planning: selection of handgrips for object manipulation. *Journal of Experimental Psychology: Learning, Memory and Cognition*, 18, 1058–73.

Smith, A.D., Gilchrist, I.D., Hood, B., Tassabehji, M., & Karmiloff-Smith, A. (2009). Inefficient search of large-scale space in Williams syndrome: further insights on the role of LIMK1 deletion in deficits of spatial cognition. *Perception*, 38, 694–70.

Smyth, M.M., & Mason, U.M. (1997). Planning and execution of action in children with and without developmental co-ordination disorder. *Journal of Child Psychology and Psychiatry*, 38, 1023–27.

Spencer, J., O'Brien, J., Riggs, K., Braddick, O., Atkinson, J., & Wattam-Bell, J., (2000). Motion processing in autism: evidence for a dorsal stream deficiency, *NeuroReport*, 11, 2765–67.

Tanji, J., Shima, K., & Mushiake, H. (2007). Concept-based behavioral planning and the lateral prefrontal cortex. *Trends in Cognitive Sciences*, 12, 528–34.

Wang, P.P., Hesselink, J.R., Jernigan, T.L., Doherty, S., & Bellugi, U. (1992). Specific neurobehavioral profile of Williams syndrome is associated with neocerebellar hemispheric preservation. *Neurology*, 42, 1999–2002.

Wattam-Bell, J., Birtles, D., Nyström, P., von Hofsten, C., Rosander, K., Anker, S., et al. (2010). Reorganization of global form and motion processing during human visual development. *Current Biology*, 20, 411–15.

Part 4c

Social Domain

Chapter 14

Face processing and social interaction

Deborah M. Riby

Introduction

The human face is unique in that it is extraordinarily rich in socially important cues from which a multitude of information can be extracted (Kanwisher & Moscovitch, 2000). As 'typical' adults, not only can we distinguish friends from strangers when viewing them at various angles and lighting conditions, but we can also make social evaluations such as deciphering feelings, assessing trustworthiness and deciding whether to approach or avoid a person from their face. Adults have a dedicated, specialised neural network for processing this type of information that is based on the involvement of multiple, bilateral brain regions (Haxby et al., 2000).

For individuals with Williams syndrome (WS), it is highly likely that face perception does not occur in a typical manner, that the neural underpinnings of these skills do not function in a typical way and that the development of face skills follows atypical trajectories. In this chapter, we explore two important concepts related to face perception in WS: first, that some face-processing skills may seem to be a relative strength/weakness; and second, that some face-processing skills are likely to develop along an atypical trajectory. The chapter moves through three sections, from considering structural encoding to the interpretation of communicative face cues and finally to considering attention to faces throughout development. Along the way, the existing data will be used to probe the two concepts that have just been outlined. The quantity and quality of existing data will vary across the three sections in terms of how well they can begin to answer the key concepts of development and face skills.

Face recognition and structural encoding atypicalities

During the 1990s, initial exploration of the cognitive profile associated with WS indicated an 'island of sparing' with relation to face perception. That evidence predominantly focused on face recognition skills of adults with the disorder. Bellugi and colleagues (1999) reported 'near normal' performance levels for individuals with WS using the Benton Test of Face Recognition (Benton et al., 1978). Although there was great variability between participants, 10 out of 16 performed within the range expected for typically developing (TD) individuals of the same age. The Benton task is a standardised assessment involving the simultaneous matching of face exemplars across viewpoints and/or lighting conditions. Individuals with WS typically perform better on this task than might be expected compared with their other visuospatial skills (Bellugi et al., 1999). Critically, however, ceiling effects (especially for TD controls) make it difficult to evaluate claims of age-appropriate performance and it has also been suggested that the Benton task can be completed using non-face information (Duchaine & Weidenfeld, 2003).

Although this research provided an ideal starting point for further investigation of face perception in WS, many questions remained. In this section, we probe how subsequent research delved deeper to question whether these near-normal scores result from typical or atypical developmental processes and whether typical or atypical neural substrates are involved.

The previously mentioned evidence suggesting intact face recognition skills did not reveal exactly how individuals with WS process faces. Structural encoding refers to the way in which a face is coded perceptually and the set of descriptions produced for each face (see Bruce & Young, 1986). Although task performance may seem to be within a typical range in WS, this does not mean the face has been encoded in a typical manner. For example, we might encode the individual features of a person's face or alternatively use the spatial relationship between features. Typical adults process faces based on their configuration rather than their individual features (Young et al., 1987), and for TD children configural processing develops with age and expertise (Carey, 1981). Younger children rely more on featural processing (Mondloch et al., 2003). Importantly, between the ages of about 6 and 10 years, TD individuals begin to use configural information in a systematic way (Mondloch et al., 2002).

So what do we mean by these terms? Configural information refers to the spatial relationship between features (Bruce, 1988). Specifically, first-order relationships define a face as a face (e.g. the eyes are above the nose, which is in turn above the mouth; see Diamond & Carey, 1986). Second-order relationships define the spatial relations of the face (e.g. the distance between the eyes). However, some researchers judge the specific distance between features to be of little importance and believe that we process a face as a holistic image (e.g. Tanaka & Farah, 1993). This is considered an extreme alternative to featural processing and the holistic view considers that a 'template' is used for recognition. Having considered these possible encoding styles, how does this fit with face perception in WS?

Taking a matched-groups approach, research has involved a large mix of age groups to explore group differences of structural encoding in WS compared with typical development. Deruelle and colleagues (1999; experiment 2) explored the use of configural and featural strategies as participants with WS (n=12, age range: 7-23 years) and two groups of TD participants of comparable chronological and mental age detected whether two simultaneously presented faces or houses were the same or different. Half the trials were upright, whereas the other half were inverted. The rationale for including inverted faces was that inversion disrupts the use of configural processing but not of featural processing (Leder & Bruce, 2000). The face inversion effect refers to a performance reduction when faces are inverted compared with when they are upright (Yin, 1969). Deruelle and colleagues (1999) found that both groups of TD participants were more accurate for upright than for inverted trials. However, the group with WS was less affected by inversion (exact figures for accuracy per condition were not provided). The study was taken as evidence that individuals with

WS did not rely on configural information. However, it should be noted that although some studies reported a reduced inversion effect in WS (e.g. Deruelle et al., 1999), other studies have reported a more typical effect of inversion (e.g. Rose et al., 2006; Riby et al., 2009a). Feeding into the concept of typical/atypical face-processing skills in WS, there is certainly evidence at a group level that faces may not be processed using typical mechanisms.

Another way to explore the encoding of face information involves the detection of subtle face manipulations. Deruelle et al. (1999; experiment 3) used schematic (drawn) faces to discriminate between featural and configural transformations. A configural transformation was a trial involving a change in the spacing of face features, whereas featural transformations involved a change of a single feature. Participants with WS made more configural errors than TD participants of comparable mental or chronological age. Critically, however, error rates were very low and the images did not represent real human faces. It could be proposed that the relative contribution of featural and configural information to face recognition differs between schematic images and real human faces, both in typical development and, critically, in WS.

Here, we are able to begin to probe the second concept of interest in this chapter, namely the development of face-processing skills. Face recognition skill is to date the only aspect of face perception in WS that has benefited from the consideration of a developmental trajectory approach. Karmiloff-Smith et al. (2004; experiment 3) explored this issue using schematic and geometric stimuli to examine the importance of developmental changes of processing strategy in WS (n=12, mean age: 27 years, age range: 15-52 years) and typical development. It could be proposed that in WS, structural encoding strategies change with age in an atypical manner. Developmental trajectories were built for a task exploring the use of featural and configural face information according to chronological age. Participants had to make 'same' or 'different' judgements for faces where half had been manipulated with featural or configural modifications. The group with WS showed developmental delay in the ability to process face configurations, which remained when controlling for their face recognition ability according to the Benton task. The authors concluded that face processing in WS showed evidence not only of developmental delay but also of an atypically reduced reliance upon configural processing throughout development. Therefore, the development of configural processing strategies is seen to follow an atypical developmental trajectory in WS compared with typical development.

To explore these effects using human faces and to investigate in more detail the developmental trajectory of face skills in WS, Karmiloff-Smith et al. (2004; experiment 1) used real faces and implemented face modifications (feature versus configuration). Participants with WS detected subtle manipulations as detailed previously and indicated whether two faces were exactly the same or slightly different. When detecting a spacing change that had been made to an upright face (i.e. a configural change), the participants with WS performed significantly less accurately than TD controls. This group difference did not emerge for the trials involving a feature change. Taking into consideration the evidence from schematic and human faces, Karmiloff-Smith et al. (2004) concluded that configural processing in WS remains qualitatively different with age. Therefore, individuals with WS rely on their use of featural processing strategies.

The final component of structural encoding to consider is the use of holistic processing. In this account, the face is recognised as a whole image and template matching may be used as a rapid route to recognition (see Tanaka & Farah, 1993). Holistic processing in WS was first assessed by Tager-Flusberg and colleagues (2003) in a group of adolescents and adults with WS and a TD group matched for chronological age. The researchers used a part–whole paradigm in which the participants learnt a set of target faces and associated names and then identified features from one of the target faces that were presented either in isolation (e.g. 'Which is Bill's nose?') or in the context of a whole face (e.g. 'Which person is Bill?'). The participants with WS performed less accurately than TD participants of comparable chronological age. Importantly, though, the same results pattern was evident across groups. The authors noted that a whole-face advantage for upright but not inverted images was indicative of holistic face processing in both WS and typical development.

Annaz et al. (2009) followed up this finding and applied a developmental perspective to explore how WS shapes the development of holistic face perception. The participants with WS (n=15; age range 5-12 years) showed the same pattern as TD individuals in the same study in that they recognised facial features in isolation better than facial features in the context of a whole face, and they performed better for upright than for inverted trials. However, developmental trajectory analyses suggested that young people with WS showed a slow rate of development for holistic face perception skills, especially when compared with TD individuals and participants who were high-functioning on the autistic spectrum. In this case, the application of a developmental trajectory approach has unearthed a possible developmental delay of holistic processing, even though overall task performance later in development may seem relatively typical.

The studies reported here emphasise the importance of exploring the nature of development and changes of face skill with age in WS. The development of configural processing proficiency (which TD children tend to master between the ages of 6 and 8 years) is qualitatively different in WS and remains so throughout development and into adulthood. Similarly, holistic processing shows a slower rate of development in WS, although group performance may seem somewhat typical for older participants. These studies emphasise that comparable performance at a developmental end state does not necessarily result from the same process of development, and this is the case for the development of structural encoding strategies used for face recognition in WS.

These face recognition tasks reveal nothing about the neural mechanisms underpinning performance. It is highly likely that atypicalities of these mechanisms exist in WS and also play a role in shaping the nature of face recognition (e.g. Mobbs et al., 2004). Mills et al. (2000) revealed that despite similar scores on a face recognition task between adults with WS and adults who had developed typically, those with WS showed different event-related potentials (ERPs). In WS, the ERP was characterised by an abnormally large spike in the N200 (discrimination/categorisation) component and an abnormally small N100 (pre-attentive) component. These differences in ERP components are indicative of increased attention to faces. In recent work (as discussed in Chapter 2), Golarai et al. (2010) reported enhanced responsiveness to faces in the fusiform gyrus of adults with WS compared with adults who had developed typically (but see also Meyer-Lindenberg et al.,

2006; Mobbs et al., 2004; Sarpal et al., 2008, who report no such difference). Golarai and colleagues (2010) also reported a significantly enlarged fusiform face area volume in WS compared with typical development that is associated with equivalent performance across groups on the Benton recognition task. The question of exactly how these atypicalities contribute to shaping face recognition and encoding strategies in WS remains for further investigation.

Communicative face skills

As noted by Knapp (1978), the 'face is rich in communicative potential'. As well as identifying people we know from those we do not know, we must decipher communicative cues from faces. Understanding communicative signals such as expressions of emotion or eye gaze is critical for successful interpersonal communication. These signals serve a number of functions: regulating turn taking, expressing intimacy, directing attention and exercising social control (Kleinke, 1986). In this section, we focus on communicative face skills by exploring the processing of expressions of emotion. It is important to note that although the studies conducted in this area are able to probe concepts of strengths/weaknesses of face skills associated with WS, to date they are not able to provide insight into the developmental trajectory of such skills. Indeed, communicative face skills have yet to be included in a developmental trajectory approach of face perception in WS. Furthermore, it is also highly likely that great individual variability exists and that this variability plays a central role in variations of social competence within WS.

In terms of a personality profile, individuals with WS are often described as sensitive, caring and empathetic (e.g. Klein-Tasman & Mervis, 2003; Gosch & Pankau, 1997). It could therefore be hypothesised that individuals with WS are especially good at deciphering socioemotive cues from other people and at responding to those cues in a sensitive manner. Some researchers have proposed that WS is characterised by relative strength when deciphering socioperceptual cues (see Karmiloff-Smith et al., 1995; Tager-Flusberg et al., 1998; Riby & Back, 2010). When interpreting complex emotions (e.g. flirtatious, worried, disinterested) from the faces of actors, individuals with WS perform well, especially if they have the whole face available for interpretation and the face presents the target emotion dynamically (Riby & Back, 2010). However, when using a static black-and-white strip-of-the-eye region (see stimuli from Baron-Cohen et al., 2001) that does not mirror the type of face cue available during everyday situations, individuals with WS have rather more difficulty (Plesa Skwerer et al., 2006).

How about basic expressions of emotion? Great variability of findings exists in this area. The published work has focused on the processing of basic facial expressions such as happy, sad and angry. In studies of emotion recognition, researchers have repeatedly found performance at a level characteristic of individuals with other forms of intellectual difficulty (Gagliardi et al., 2003; Plesa Skwerer et al., 2006). When discriminating basic expressions (e.g. happy, sad) from schematic faces, individuals with WS (aged 9-23 years) performed near ceiling, at a level comparable with TD children matched for mental age (Karmiloff-Smith et al., 1995). Slightly more complex tasks, such as sorting basic expressions

(Tager-Flusberg & Sullivan, 2000) and recognising basic expressions from moving faces (Gagliardi et al., 2003), proved more challenging. Indeed, across a range of emotion perception tasks (e.g. labelling, matching, identification), individuals with WS (aged 6-15 years) performed worse than TD individuals of comparable verbal ability (Lacroix et al., 2009). Therefore, across the range of methods and differences in stimuli and group characteristics (e.g. age-matched comparison group) used to assess expression perception in WS, there is little evidence to suggest that this is a particular strength, although when directly compared, performance is stronger than that among individuals with autism (e.g. Riby et al., 2008) or Down syndrome (e.g. Porter et al., 2007).

Although the interpretation of basic expressions of emotion is important to social behaviour (e.g. monitoring our own behaviour towards another person), as discussed in Chapter 15, these cues alone are rarely pivotal to social interactions. However, it has been suggested that problems rating faces appropriately for approachability are entwined with problems correctly inferring basic expressions (Porter et al., 2007). So, when individuals with WS have problems making emotion judgements from faces, this may lead to an inappropriate evaluation of approachability (see Jones et al., 2000). Indeed, research has suggested that individuals with WS fail to give attentional priority to angry faces (Santos et al., 2010; Dodd & Porter, 2010) but show increased attentional bias towards happy faces (Dodd & Porter, 2010). These attentional biases may link emotion perception to other aspects of WS (for discussion see Santos et al., 2010) and may contribute to shaping the nature of social behaviours associated with the disorder.

One benefit of recent research has been insight into the neural underpinnings linked to emotional understanding. For example, the amygdala, a structure in the medial temporal lobes, is considered to be an important neural substrate of emotional processing (e.g. Adolphs et al., 1994). Several studies have reported structural and/or functional alterations of the amygdala in WS (e.g. Mobbs et al., 2004; Reiss et al., 2004; Meyer-Lindenberg et al., 2005; Tager-Flusberg et al., 2006; Sarpal et al., 2008; Haas et al., 2009) (see also Chapters 2 and 15). For example, functional magnetic resonance imaging studies have demonstrated a reduced amygdala response to fearful facial expressions compared with TD controls (Haas et al., 2009; Meyer-Lindenberg et al., 2005). Although much of the work addressing the role of the amygdala has focused on the neural substrate for atypicalities of approachability (e.g. Martens et al., 2009; Jawaid et al., 2010; Haas et al., 2010), it is also highly relevant to the mechanisms that shape basic emotion perception. In view of the link between amygdala functioning and fear/threat perception, further work is required to follow up the suggestions that individuals with WS have problems interpreting negative emotions (see Plesa Skwerer et al., 2006), that they do not give attentional priority to some negative expressions (see Santos et al., 2010) and that this may be linked to a tendency to approach people indiscriminately (e.g. Bellugi et al., 1999; Jones et al., 2000; Martens et al., 2009).

Looking at faces and social interactions

So far, this chapter has considered structural encoding of faces for recognition purposes and communicative face signals in terms of emotion perception. In both these sections, we have noted atypicalities that relate more widely to sociocognitive processing. In terms of face recognition, we have evidence of atypical use of configural processing that links to the deviant and delayed development of this skill. In terms of communicative face skills (particularly emotion), we have evidence that, at a group level, there are problems inferring emotional states. However, to date research has not applied a developmental trajectory approach to investigate the development of these communicative face skills. In the current section, we consider attention to faces as a possible insight into what may have shaped peculiarities of face perception in this population (throughout development).

Individuals with WS show an extreme interest in looking at people and their faces, and this interest is present in infancy (Mervis et al., 2003) and persists into adolescence and adulthood (Riby & Hancock, 2008, 2009). Research with toddlers who have WS revealed that during encounters with their geneticist, nearly all (23 out of 25) showed atypically prolonged gaze towards the geneticist's face (Mervis et al., 2003). This behaviour contrasted with that of TD infants of the same chronological age. Indeed, young infants with WS preferred to look at people rather than objects (Laing et al., 2002). Similarly, adolescents and adults with the disorder tended to fixate on faces in social scenes and movies for significantly longer than TD individuals, as evident through tracking eye movements (Riby & Hancock, 2008, 2009). This prolonged facial attention was especially apparent towards the eye region. For example, when attending to faces within a social scene, individuals with WS spent over half their time (58% of their face gaze) attending to the eye region and this was significantly longer than in TD individuals of the same age (36%; Riby & Hancock, 2008). Interestingly, in the same study, participants with autism only allocated 17% of their face gaze towards the eyes, indicating differences between neurodevelopmental disorders. Figure 14.1 shows fixation locations for individuals with WS and autism who attended to one specific frame of a movie containing an interaction between four adults. Whereas individuals with WS predominantly attended to the faces of the actors in this frame, those with autism showed more scattering of fixations and very few individuals attended to the face regions. Atypical development has a divergent impact upon attention to faces in WS and autism.

Atypically prolonged attention to faces from a young age in WS may have implications and may in fact link to atypicalities of perceptual ability or social functioning. Recent studies may provide clues to the way in which atypically prolonged attention to the eye region has negative implications for processing information from other face regions, and may help to explain why increased attention to the eye region does not equate to enhanced processing ability when using the eyes for sociocognitive cues.

To make the first of these points, we turn to research by Riby and Back exploring the interpretation of complex emotions from dynamic faces. When adolescents and adults with WS had access to a whole moving face, they performed at a level appropriate for their chronological age (Riby & Back, 2010). However, the researchers manipulated the face stimuli to explore the source of mental state information; parts of the face (eyes or mouth) remained neutrally frozen, whereas other regions were expressive (e.g. worried). Participants with WS showed an atypically large performance decrement when the eye region was neutrally

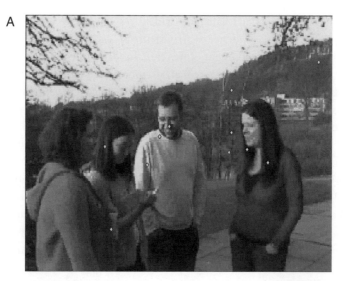

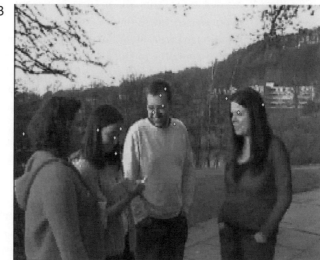

Fig. 14.1 (See also Plate 7) Fixation scatters for individuals attending to a frame showing four adults during a social encounter. (A) Individuals on the autistic spectrum (of varying degrees of functioning capacity). (B) Individuals with Williams syndrome. Each small dot represents a fixation. The frame has been taken from a movie. For the movie overall, individuals with Williams syndrome spent significantly longer than typically developing individuals fixating on the face regions, whereas those with autism spent significantly less time than typical attending to the same regions. For full details see Riby & Hancock (2009).

expressive and they had to rely upon the mouth region. It could be proposed that a propensity towards increased attention to the eyes throughout development has led to increased reliance upon eye region cues. A similar pattern was seen for identity matching. A study requiring participants to match two faces by identity showed that covering the eye region with sunglasses slowed reaction times for adolescents and adults with WS significantly more than for TD participants (Riby, 2010). This pattern was not evident when the mouth region was covered with a scarf (Riby, 2010) and therefore does not relate to a general slowing when any face region is covered. Increased attention to the eyes throughout development may have led individuals with WS to first direct their attention to that region (even if it is not informative) before needing to shift attention to process information elsewhere.

So, does increased attention to faces and the eye region lead to expertise in processing cues from these regions in WS? Riby et al. (2009b) combined eye tracking and performance on a gaze-cueing task to explore this issue. Although individuals with WS spent significantly longer than TD individuals attending to faces and the eyes of actors in social scenes, they were less able to interpret gaze cues from those faces and name the item being attended to by the actor. This pattern of performance may relate to deficits of joint attention in WS (Laing et al., 2002). The participants with WS looked at faces for longer, but could not transform that into greater proficiency on a gaze-cueing task. It could be proposed that in WS, too much (in terms of facial attention) can be as dysfunctional as too little in autism (see Minshew, 2010; see also Chapter 15).

In summary, increased attention to faces during development may shape the nature of some face perception atypicalities and does not increase expertise. This increased attention to faces may also have shaped the neural mechanisms involved in a range of skills outlined in this chapter (or vice versa). For example, an atypical attentional motivation towards faces from a very early age may influence the nature of cortical specialisation or neural mechanisms such as the increased activation towards faces seen by adults with the disorder (e.g. Haas et al., 2010) or the atypicalities associated with making social judgements (e.g. amygdala atypicalities; Martens et al., 2009; see also Jawaid et al., 2010). Many questions remain to be answered in this domain, but researchers now have the methods (e.g. tracking eye movements, neuropsychological insights) available to them to make such advances to our current knowledge.

Conclusions

At the beginning of this chapter, we suggested face perception was considered a possible 'island of sparing' in relation to WS cognition. Throughout this chapter, it has been made clear that face-processing skills are far from typical. We have considered evidence from tasks exploring strengths and difficulties of face skills, research applying developmental trajectory approaches and informative cross-syndrome comparisons. The latter of these methodologies is, to date, restricted to the exploration of face recognition and structural encoding approaches. The wider application of these methods would be particularly beneficial for understanding the relation between communicative face skills and wider issues of the WS social and cognitive phenotypes. Finally, with advances in our understanding of the neural mechanisms involved in face perception and social functioning associated with WS, much work remains to explore the nature of face perception in this population.

Editor commentary (Emily K. Farran & Annette Karmiloff-Smith)

Initial exploration led many researchers to suggest that face processing is 'spared' in WS. This chapter demonstrated the neuroconstructivist view that this is unlikely to be the case.

Although tests of face recognition in WS often yield scores in the normal range, individuals with WS encode faces in an atypical manner, characterised by a reduced reliance on configural processing and a stronger reliance on featural processing relative to typical development. The chapter highlighted the need for research to determine the direction of the interactions between atypical functioning of the amygdala in WS and the profile of emotional expression processing abilities in WS, as well as between atypical neurophysiological activation and increased attention to faces in WS. Cascading developmental impacts of any of these factors might, for example, lead to the tendency observed in WS to approach people indiscriminately (a problem also reported in Down syndrome that presumably arises as a result of qualitatively different developmental interactions).

The chapter concluded by discussing the possibility that increased attention to faces from infancy through to adulthood might shape the profile of face-processing skills described earlier in the chapter. It also demonstrated that although individuals with WS attend predominantly to the eye region of a face, this is not beneficial to social interaction. Consistent with the argument put forward in Chapter 15, individuals with WS have difficulty interpreting gaze cues referentially even in adolescence and adulthood. A comparison with autism illustrates the neurocontructivist stance that different mechanisms can lead to a similar behavioural outcome: whereas decreased attention to faces in autism can be detrimental to social interaction, increased attention to faces in WS can have a similar effect.

References

Adolphs, R., Tranel, D., Damasio, H., & Damasio, A. (1994). Impaired recognition of emotion in facial expressions following bilateral damage to the human amygdala. *Nature*, **372**, 669–72.

Annaz, D., Karmiloff-Smith, A., Johnson, M.H., & Thomas, M.S.C. (2009). A cross-syndrome study of the development of holistic face recognition in children with autism, Down syndrome, and Williams syndrome. *Journal of Experimental Child Psychology*, **102**, 456–86.

Baron-Cohen, S., Wheelwright, S., & Hill, J. (2001). The 'reading the mind in the eyes' test revised version: a study with normal adults, and adults with Asperger syndrome or high functioning autism. *Journal of Child Psychology and Psychiatry*, **42**, 241–51.

Bellugi, U., Lichtenberger, E., Mills, D., Galaburda, A., & Korenberg, J.R. (1999). Bridging cognition, brain, and molecular genetics: evidence from Williams syndrome. *Trends in Neuroscience*, **5**, 197–208.

Benton, A., VanAllen, M., Hamsher, K., & Levin, H. (1978). *Test of Facial Recognition Manual*. Iowa City, IA: Benton Laboratory of Neuropsychology.

Bruce, V. (1988). *Recognising Faces*. Hillsdale, NJ, England: Lawrence Erlbaum.

Bruce, V., & Young, A. (1986). Understanding face recognition. *British Journal of Psychology*, **77**, 305–27.

Carey, S. (1981). The development of face perception. In G. Davies, H. Ellis, & J. Shepherd (Eds), *Perceiving and Remembering Faces* (pp. 9–38). London: Academic Press.

Deruelle, C., Mancini, J., Livet, M., Cassé-Perrot, C., & de Schonen, S. (1999). Configural and local processing of faces in children with Williams syndrome. *Brain and Cognition*, **41**, 276–98.

Diamond, R., & Carey, S. (1986). Why faces are and are not special: an effect of expertise, *Journal of Experimental Psychology: General*, **2**, 107–117.

Dodd, H.F., & Porter, M.A. (2010). I see happy people: attention towards happy but not angry facial expressions in Williams syndrome. *Cognitive Neuropsychiatry*, **15**, 549–67.

Duchaine, B.C., & Weidenfeld, A. (2003). An evaluation of two commonly used tests of unfamiliar face recognition. *Neuropsychologia*, **41**, 713–20.

Gagliardi, C., Frigerio, E., Burt, D.M., Cazzaniga, I., Perrett, D.I., & Borgatti, R. (2003). Facial expression recognition in Williams syndrome, *Neuropsychologia*, **41**, 733–38.

Golarai, G., Hong, S., Haas, B.W., Galaburda, A.M., Mills, D.L., Bellugi, U., et al. (2010). The fusiform face area is enlarged in Williams syndrome. *The Journal of Neuroscience*, **30**, 6700–6712.

Gosch, A., & Pankau, R. (1997). Personality characteristics and behavior problems in individuals of different ages with Williams syndrome. *Developmental Medicine and Child Neurology*, **39**, 527–33.

Haas, B.W., Hoeft, F., Searcy, Y.M., Mills, D., Bellugi, U., & Reiss, A. (2010). Individual differences in social behaviour predict amygdala response to fearful facial expressions in Williams syndrome. *Neuropsychologia*, **48**, 1283–88.

Haas, B.W., Mills, D., Yam, A., Hoeft, F., Bellugi, U., & Reiss, A. (2009). Genetic influences on sociability: heightened amygdala reactivity and event-related responses to positive social stimuli in Williams syndrome. *Journal of Neuroscience*, **29**, 1132–39.

Haxby, J.V., Hoffman, E.A., & Gobbini, M.I. (2000). The distributed human neural system for face perception. *Trends in Cognitive Sciences*, **4**, 223–33.

Jawaid, A., Riby, D.M., Egridere, S., Schmolck, H., Kass, J.S., & Schulz, P.E. (2010). Approachability in Williams syndrome. *Neuropsychologia*, **48**, 1521–23.

Jones, W., Bellugi, U., Lai, Z., Chiles, M., Reilly, J., Lincoln, A., et al. (2000). Hypersociability in Williams syndrome. *Journal of Cognitive Neuroscience*, **12**, 30–46.

Kanwisher, N. & Moscovitch, M. (2000). The cognitive neuroscience of face processing: an introduction. *Cognitive Neuropsychology*, **17**, 1–11.

Karmiloff-Smith, A., Klima, E., Bellugi, U., Grant, J., & Baron-Cohen, S. (1995). Is there a social module? Language, face processing, and theory of mind in individuals with Williams syndrome. *Journal of Cognitive Neuroscience*, **7**, 196–208.

Karmiloff-Smith, A., Thomas, M., Annaz, D., Humphreys, K., Ewing, S., Brace, N., et al. (2004). Exploring the Williams syndrome face processing debate: The importance of building developmental trajectories. *Journal of Child Psychology and Psychiatry*, **45**, 1258–74.

Kleinke, C.L. (1986). Gaze and eye contact: a research review. *Psychological Bulletin*, **100**, 78–100.

Klein-Tasman, B.P., & Mervis, C.B. (2003). Distinctive personality characteristics of children with Williams syndrome. *Developmental Neuropsychology*, **23**, 271–92.

Knapp, M.L. (1978). *Nonverbal Communication in Human Interaction*, 2nd edn. Holt, Rinehart and Winston, USA.

Lacroix, A., Guidetti, M., Rogéb, B., & Reilly, J. (2009). Recognition of emotional and nonemotional facial expressions: a comparison between Williams syndrome and autism. *Research in Developmental Disabilities*, **30**, 976–85.

Laing, E., Butterworth, G., Ansari, D., Gsodl, M., Longhi, E., Panagiotaki, G., et al. (2002). Atypical development of language and social communication in toddlers with Williams syndrome. *Developmental Science*, **5**, 233–46.

Leder, H., & Bruce, V. (2000). Inverting line drawings of faces. *Swiss Journal of Psychology*, **59**, 159–69.

Martens, M.A., Wilson, S.J., Dudgeon, P., & Reutens, D.C. (2009). Approachability and the amygdala: insights from Williams syndrome. *Neuropsychologia*, **47**, 2446–53.

Mervis, C.B., Morris, C.A., Klein-Tasman, B.P., Bertrand, J., Kwitny, S., Appelbaum, L.G., et al. (2003). Attentional characteristics of infants and toddlers with Williams syndrome during triadic interactions. *Developmental Neuropsychology*, **23**, 243–68.

Meyer-Lindenberg, A., Hariri, A.R., Munoz, K.E., Mervis, C.B., Mattay, V.S., Morris, C.A., et al. (2005). Neural correlates of genetically abnormal social cognition in Williams syndrome. *Nature Neuroscience*, **8**, 991–93.

Meyer-Lindenberg, A., Mervis, C.B., & Berman, K.F. (2006). Neural mechanisms in Williams syndrome: a unique window to genetic influences on cognition and behavior. *Nature Reviews Neuroscience*, **7**, 380–93.

Mills, D.L., Alvarez, T.D., St. George, M., Appelbaum, L.G., Bellugi, U., & Neville, H. (2000). Electrophysiological studies of face processing in Williams syndrome. *Journal of Cognitive Neuroscience*, **12**, 47–64.

Minshew, N.J. (2010). Neuroimaging of developmental disorders: commentary. In M. Shenton & B. Turestsky (Eds), *Understanding Neuropsychiatric Disorders: Insights from Neuroimaging* (pp. 555–58). Cambridge: Cambridge University Press.

Mobbs, D., Garrett, A., Menon, V., Rose, F., Bellugi, U., & Reiss, L. (2004). Anomalous brain activation during face and gaze processing in Williams syndrome. *Neurology*, **62**, 2070–76.

Mondloch, C.J., Le Grand, R. & Maurer, D. (2002). Configural face processing develops more slowly than featural face processing. *Perception*, **31**, 553–66.

Mondloch, C.J., Geldart, S., Maurer, D., & Le Grand, R. (2003). Developmental changes in face processing skills. *Journal of Experimental Child Psychology*, **86**, 67–84.

Plesa Skwerer, D., Verbalis, A., Schofield, C., Faja, S., & Tager-Flusberg, H. (2006). Social-perceptual abilities in adolescents and adults with Williams syndrome. *Cognitive Neuropsychology*, **23**, 338–49.

Porter, M.A., Coltheart, M., & Langdon, R. (2007). The neuropsychological basis of hypersociability in Williams and Down syndrome. *Neuropsychologia*, **45**, 2839–49.

Reiss, A.L., Eckert, M.A., Rose, F.E., Karchemskiy, A., Kesler, S., Chang, M., et al. (2004). An experiment of nature: brain anatomy parallels cognition and behaviour in Williams syndrome. *Journal of Neuroscience*, **24**, 5009–5015.

Riby, D.M. (2010). Show me your eyes: evidence from Williams syndrome. *Visual Cognition*, **18**, 801–815.

Riby, D.M., & Back, E. (2010). Can individuals with Williams syndrome interpret mental states from moving faces? *Neuropsychologia*, **48**, 1914–22.

Riby, D.M., Doherty-Sneddon, G., & Bruce, V. (2008). Exploring face perception in disorders of development: evidence from Williams syndrome and autism. *Journal of Neuropsychology*, **2**, 47–64.

Riby, D.M., Doherty-Sneddon, G., & Bruce, V. (2009a). The eyes or the mouth? Feature salience and unfamiliar face processing in Williams syndrome and autism. *Quarterly Journal of Experimental Psychology*, **62**, 189–203.

Riby, D.M., & Hancock, P.J.B. (2008). Viewing it differently: social scene perception in Williams syndrome and Autism. *Neuropsychologia*, **46**, 2855–60.

Riby, D.M., & Hancock, P.J.B. (2009). Looking at movies and cartoons: eye-tracking evidence from Williams syndrome and autism. *Journal of Intellectual Disability Research*, **53**, 169–81.

Riby, D.M., Hancock, P.J.B., & Jones, N. (July 2009b). Tracking eye movements proves informative for studying gaze detection in Williams syndrome and Autism. Presented at a meeting of the Experimental Psychology Society, York.

Rose, F.E., Lincoln, A.J., Lai, Z., Ene, M., Searcy, Y.M., & Bellugi, U. (2006). Orientation and affective expression effects on face recognition in Williams syndrome and autism. *Journal of Autism and Developmental Disorders*, **37**, 513–22.

Sarpal, D., Buchsbaum, B.R., Kohn, P.D., Kippenhan, J.S., Mervis, C.B., Morris, C.A., et al. (2008). A genetic model for understanding higher order visual processing: functional interactions of the ventral visual stream in Williams syndrome. *Cerebral Cortex*, **18**, 2402–2409.

Santos, A., Silva, C., Rosset, D., & Deruelle, C. (2010). Just another face in the crowd: evidence for decreased detection of angry faces in children with Williams syndrome. *Neuropsychologia*, **48**, 1071–78.

Tager-Flusberg, H., Boshart, J., & Baron-Cohen, S. (1998). Reading the windows to the soul: evidence of domain-specific sparing in Williams syndrome. *Journal of Cognitive Neuroscience*, **10**, 631–39.

Tager-Flusberg, H., Plesa-Skwerer, D., Faja, S. & Joseph, R.M. (2003). People with Williams syndrome process faces holistically. *Cognition*, **89**, 11–24.

Tager-Flusberg, H., Plesa Skwerer, D., & Joseph, R.M. (2006). Model syndromes for investigating social cognitive and affective neuroscience: a comparison of autism and Williams syndrome. *Social, Cognitive and Affective Neuroscience*, **1**, 175–82.

Tager-Flusberg, H., & Sullivan, K. (2000). A componential view of theory of mind: evidence from Williams syndrome. *Cognition*, **76**, 59–89.

Tanaka, J.W., & Farah, M.J. (1993). Parts and wholes in face recognition. *Quarterly Journal of Experimental Psychology*, **46**, 225–45.

Yin, R.K. (1969). Looking at upside down faces. *Journal of Experimental Psychology*, **81**, 141–45.

Young, A.W., Hellawell, D., & Hay, D.C. (1987). Configural information in face perception. *Perception*, **16**, 747–59.

Chapter 15

Mental state understanding and social interaction

Ruth Campos and María Sotillo

Introduction

Cognitive psychology establishes a fundamental dissociation between social and nonsocial processing. From cognitive neuropsychology, the strongest point supporting this dichotomy is the existence of two neurodevelopmental disorders that exemplify a double dissociation between the two domains. The clinical groups of autism spectrum disorder (ASD) and Williams syndrome (WS) offer a privileged setting to analyse the specificity of the development of social comprehension. The two groups have been described as clinical opposites regarding social interaction: ASD is characterised by serious deficits in this domain, whereas social interaction seems to be a strength of individuals with WS.

The study of social comprehension competences in individuals with WS and in those with ASD enables us to consider the possibility of the existence of a specific cognitive mechanism for social interaction that could be altered selectively and that could also function within the context of severe deficits in other areas of cognition. Although their phenotypes have been reported as an example of a double dissociation between the social and nonsocial domains (Baron-Cohen, 1998; Baron-Cohen, 1999; Reilly et al., 1990; Tager-Flusberg & Sullivan, 2000), other descriptions also indicate some commonalities in their behavioural patterns at different developmental time points (Gillberg & Rasmussen, 1994; Klein-Tasman et al., 2007; Lincoln et al., 2007). Both the dissociations and the associations between the two syndromes can shed light on the development of social comprehension abilities.

The neuroconstructivist perspective proposes the need to go beyond the behavioural level to understand psychological functioning. Inferences on cognitive processes cannot be made directly from behaviours because even if individuals with neurodevelopmental disorders obtain a level of performance similar to one obtained by typically developing (TD) individuals, it does not necessarily mean that the processes leading to attainment are, in fact, the same. Relationships between behaviour and genetics or neurobiological bases are also mediated by a dynamic environment and the individual's own behaviour (Karmiloff-Smith, 1998). In this chapter, therefore, we consider the development of social interaction and comprehension of various mental states in WS in relation to the different levels of description of psychological functioning (i.e. cognitive, environmental, neurological and genetic), and we suggest some implications with respect to clinical intervention.

Development of social interaction and mental state comprehension in Williams syndrome

Social interaction in Williams syndrome: the more the better?

People with WS are interested in interacting with others (Mervis et al., 1999; Mervis et al., 2003), and this hypersociability distinguishes them from other clinical groups and from TD individuals (Jones et al., 2000). However, this sociability seems to be more compulsive than selected (Frigerio et al., 2006) and tends to imply a social mismatch caused by an increased tendency of approachability toward strangers.

In experimental situations, individuals with WS judge unknown people as more approachable than do TD individuals (Bellugi et al., 1999; Jones et al., 2000; Martens et al., 2008; Porter et al., 2007; Frigerio et al., 2006). However, this approachable and overly friendly behaviour rarely leads to the attainment of fulfilling interpersonal relationships necessary for adequate quality of life. In an extensive study of 70 adults with WS, 96% of them reported having difficulty making friends, and 73% were described as being socially isolated and having no friends of their own (Howlin et al., 1998; see also Chapter 5).

People with WS are generally reported as empathic and attentive to others' feelings (Tomc et al., 1990; Tager-Flusberg & Sullivan, 2000; Klein-Tasman & Mervis, 2003) and in experimental settings they also show greater concern for others (Tager-Flusberg & Sullivan, 2000). However, they sometimes seem to miss relevant cues regarding the mechanisms of interactions. Their hypersensitivity to emotions and their insistence in asking others about their feelings towards them is a sign of their difficulty in decoding contextual information from close antecedents or from other people's behaviours.

To understand what others do or say, we have to attribute beliefs, intentions, desires and emotions to their actions; it is necessary to realise that others—and we ourselves—can have different mental states with respect to the same content; namely, it is necessary to have developed a theory of mind (ToM).

A different way to construct a theory of mind

Developing a ToM involves developing the abilities to attribute epistemic and emotional mental states and to use them when communicating with others. In this section, we will summarise research on emotion understanding, belief attribution and communicative competences of individuals with WS. Whenever it is possible, we will offer information from behavioural, cognitive, brain and genetic levels of explanation of psychological functioning.

The feeling mind

Mental state attribution implies the comprehension of emotions. Furthermore, from an ontogenetic perspective, it is not possible to understand this development without taking into account the subjective nature of contact with others as an origin and motive for mental state attribution (Hobson, 2002; Trevarthen & Aitken, 2001).

The performance of individuals with WS in tasks that assess emotional processing is similar to that of individuals of the same developmental level (both compared with younger TD children and with groups with intellectual disability). These tasks draw on different emotion classification abilities (Tager-Flusberg & Sullivan, 2000; Campos, 2009). Tasks such as facial and vocal emotion identification (Gagliardi et al., 2003; Plesa-Skwerer et al., 2006a) and mental state attribution from the facial area of the eyes are evaluated (Plesa-Skwerer et al., 2006b; Tager-Flusberg et al., 1998). In a recent study with dynamic facial stimuli, the WS group (age range: 8 years 6 months to 23 years 6 months) was as able as same-age peers to infer mental states, but their performance was particularly affected when the eye region was uninformative (Riby & Back, 2010). In the same procedure, adolescents with ASD (age range: 10 years 8 months to 14 years 9 months) were also able to recognise mental states based on the information conveyed by the eyes (Back et al., 2007; see also Chapter 14).

When the two groups are directly compared, the results are inconsistent. In a number of studies, individuals with WS perform better than the group with ASD on tasks that assess the detection of mental states from gaze and the identification of emotional facial expressions, both as children (6 years 0 months to 15 years 10 months) (Riby et al., 2008) and from early adolescence to adulthood (10 years 0 months to 44 years 3 months) (Rose et al., 2007). However, the opposite pattern has also been reported for children with WS (6 years 1 month to 15 years 3 months) and children with ASD (4 years 9 months to 8 years 0 months) (Lacroix et al., 2009).

Apart from assessing gaze interpretation and identification of emotional expression, to understand emotions it is necessary to relate them to their causes. Children with WS (4 years 11 months to 15 years 6 months) are as able as TD children with the same mental age to attribute basic emotions according to the eliciting events. However, individuals with WS have more difficulty when attributing complex emotions such as surprise, shame, pride and guilt (Campos, 2009). They also have difficulty inferring the emotion based on a character's desire when this desire is distinct from their own (Campos, 2009).

From this set of data, it seems that individuals with WS experience difficulties in the attribution of some emotions, and their performance is not better than the performances exhibited by groups with other neurodevelopmental disorders. However, some peculiarities have been found in WS that could be related to their characteristic pattern of social relations. It has been suggested that the hypersociability associated with individuals with WS could be related to their difficulty in attributing certain emotions (Porter et al., 2007). Individuals with WS have greater difficulty attributing negative than positive emotions (Santos et al., 2010), perhaps because they rely more on superficial cues that are normally observed as positive at the expense of more subtle social cues. For example, an individual with WS may interpret a mischievous-looking smirk for a happy smile (Jones et al., 2000). In addition, individuals with WS, from childhood to adulthood, use features other than the eyes and mouth to decide the approachability of strangers, and they tend to comment more on peripheral cues (Martens et al., 2009; Porter et al., 2007).

From a neurobiological perspective, this hypersociability and the atypical emotion attribution have been related to both structural (Galaburda & Bellugi, 2000; Martens et al., 2009) and functional (Haas, et al., 2010; Jawaid et al., 2008) characteristics of the amygdala. A higher reactivity of the amygdala to positive social stimuli (i.e. emotional expressions of happiness) and an attenuated response to negative social stimuli (i.e. emotional expressions of fear) have been recorded in adults with WS relative to TD adults (Haas et al., 2009). Adults with WS show decreased amygdala activation in response to threatening faces but increased activation in response to potentially dangerous scenes, relative to matched typical controls. Moreover, in WS, in contrast to TD, the processing of these threatening stimuli does not activate the orbitofrontal cortex (Meyer-Lindenberg et al., 2005). In relation to the lower specificity of processing potentially dangerous social stimuli in WS, this group showed increased amygdala reactivity relative to TD controls when processing nonsocial stimuli (Muñoz et al., 2010). It is possible that atypical responses in the way that WS individuals judge unfamiliar faces are directly related to the likelihood of WS individuals approaching those unfamiliar people.

Facial stimuli processing, as discussed in detail in Chapter 14, has been referred to as an atypical autonomic response in WS for two different stimuli, which are both relevant for social interaction. Both dynamic stimuli of facial expressions (Plesa Skwerer et al., 2009) and stimuli of face-to-face interactions (Doherty-Sneddon et al., 2009) produce an automatic hypoarousal in adolescents and adults with WS relative to the TD group, whereas children with ASD show a hyperactivation to similar stimuli (Hirstein et al., 2001). These data can be related to the evidence presented in Chapter 14 on the processing of social stimuli in WS and ASD individuals, which, in general, suggests atypical patterns in both groups when compared with typical development with longer fixation times to faces for WS individuals and shorter fixation times for individuals with ASD.

From a genetic level of explanation, it has been suggested that only individuals with the typical deletion 7q11.23 have this unusual gaze profile as a phenotypic characteristic (Mervis et al., 2003). From the study of a patient with an atypical deletion, it was concluded that the gene *GTF2I* could influence social behaviour in WS individuals, including the profile of intense gaze and strong attention to strangers (Dai et al., 2009). *GTF2I* could be related to the regulation of oxytocin, a neurohormone linked to social functioning that, in ASD, facilitates the processing of emotional stimuli (Hollander et al., 2007; Andari et al., 2010). Further evidence towards an understanding of the relationship between genes deleted in WS and social behaviour comes from patients with a duplication of the WS critical region. These individuals show a severe language delay, difficulties in social interactions and restrictive interests—a pattern similar to the one exhibited by individuals with ASD (Somerville, et al., 2005; Berg et al., 2007).

However, from a developmental perspective, the existence of a gene, or a set of genes, responsible for the behaviour of gazing intensely or, in a more general way, for the personality profile in WS individuals does not seem likely. Indeed, deletion of *GTF2I* has also been implicated in the visual problems experienced in WS (see Chapter 12). Behavioural features are a manifestation of a developmental process including relations between the genetic profile and all other levels (cortical and subcortical brain networks, cognitive processing and environmental influences).

The thinking mind

The hallmark of representational ToM is false belief attribution. There is little research on first- and second-order belief comprehension in individuals with WS, and the existing studies show discrepant results. Some studies conclude an acceptable performance on belief attribution tasks (Karmiloff-Smith et al., 1995). Other studies show similar functioning to that obtained by children of the same mental age with other neurodevelopmental disorders (Tager-Flusberg et al., 1997). Still another set of data indicates a deficit relative to general cognitive ability in individuals with WS (Sullivan & Tager-Flusberg, 1999; Tager-Flusberg & Sullivan, 2000; Sotillo et al., 2007; Campos, 2009).

The variable developmental level of the sample seems essential in the explanation of the conflicting results. In the study concluding good ToM competences, the sample consisted mainly of adults with WS, and tasks employed were generally solved by TD children between 4 and 5 years of age (Karmiloff-Smith et al., 1995). However, in other studies (Tager-Flusberg & Sullivan, 2000), samples included children with WS showing developmental ages much lower than that necessary to solve false beliefs (below 4 years of age). This suggests two important reflections from a developmental perspective: first, the need to reconsider arguments with respect to mentalising functions independent of other cognitive functions, and their 'preservation' from the general cognitive deficit observed in WS; and second, the conflicting results confirm the importance of studying the development of these abilities. Two ways of studying this development include examining competences prior to the comprehension of belief such as desire or knowledge and considering different approaches to test belief attribution.

In a study involving the variables 'level of representational redescription' (the children were asked explicitly or implicitly about a person's mental state) and 'availability of clues' (the children were provided with mental state information related to the person they were asked about), it was found that children and adolescents with WS (chronological age range: 4 years 11 months to 15 years 6 months) are more capable of attributing beliefs when they are not required to give an explicit explanation on the mental state (i.e. 'What does she think?') than when they are asked about the emotion linked to a character's belief (i.e. 'How does she feel?'). On the other hand, in questions on belief, WS children benefited from having a clue about the character's emotion based on their belief (i.e. 'Before opening the package, she is happy. What does she think is inside?') (Campos, 2009).

People with WS are empathetic and quite able to read the mental states from a person's face and to attribute basic expressions of emotions to emotional contexts; however, they experience greater difficulty understanding complex mental states such as having to attribute beliefs or thoughts. This relatively dissociated pattern in mentalising competences of WS individuals led researchers to propose a componential model of ToM (Tager-Flusberg & Sullivan, 2000; this was partially questioned afterwards by the same authors [Plesa-Skwerer et al., 2006b]). This model describes the existence of two components of ToM abilities: a cognitive component that performs complex cognitive inferences on the content of mental states, and a perceptive component that makes quick judgements on mental states based on facial expression or body language. The dissociation between the two behavioural components is supported by different neurobiological substrates, distinct ontogenesis, different degrees of impairment in diverse populations (WS and ASD), and the dependence of both on different cognitive skills.

The communicative mind

The development of ToM abilities is closely related to the acquisition of language. Given that linguistic development in WS presents some peculiarities (see Chapters 10 and 11), their difficulties in epistemic mental state attribution could be related to the verbal demands of the tasks. However, the same difficulties have been replicated in nonverbal tasks (Porter et al., 2008; Santos & Deruelle, 2009). Furthermore, performance levels of individuals with WS are higher in verbal than in nonverbal ToM tasks (Santos & Deruelle, 2009).

Because of the failure to find a relationship between the performance of people with WS in belief attribution tasks and some general linguistic measurements, it has been suggested that general language measures are perhaps not gathering the most relevant aspects of semantic and syntactic development for mind-reading competences (Tager-Flusberg & Sullivan, 2000).

From the lexical point of view, it has been considered that mental state comprehension is a prerequisite to using linguistic forms for expressing these concepts (Tager-Flusberg, 1993). In their narrations and spontaneous discourse, individuals with WS use terms that reflect higher cognitive states to a lesser extent than TD individuals do (Reilly et al., 1990; Jones et al., 2000; Losh et al., 2000).

However, representations of mental states are not only coded through the semantics of mental verbs, but also through the syntax allowed by those verbs. Sentences containing mental verbs can include a direct-object completive clause in such a way that the information in the subordinate clause cannot be judged independent of the mental verb on which it depends. It has been proposed that children are not able to develop a representational ability to understand propositional attitudes necessary for the comprehension of false belief until they can use linguistic forms of completive subordination (de Villiers & de Villiers, 2000; de Villiers & Pyers, 2002). This development occurs from 3 years 6 months to 4 years 6 months approximately. Children with WS (4 years 11 months to 15 years 6 months) have difficulty understanding these linguistic completive structures even when they do not imply a verb of belief but rather a verb of desire ('want'), of communication ('say') or of a nonmental representation ('paint') (Campos et al., 2009).

In narrative or free conversation situations, children with WS usually refer to characters' emotional states and make use of lexical evaluative devices and vocal prosody (Reilly et al., 1990; Jones et al., 2000). However, they have difficulty understanding and expressing emotions through prosody (Martínez-Castilla et al., 2010; see Chapter 11 for further discussion of prosody), and they do not consider the interlocutor's knowledge state in their narratives (Losh et al., 2000; Reilly et al., 2004) or in referential communication tasks (John et al., 2009).

Individuals with WS also demonstrate a poor comprehension of nonliteral statements such as idiomatic expressions (Lacroix et al., 2010), metaphors (Thomas et al., 2010) or jokes (Sullivan et al., 2003). The inability to differentiate the intention in jokes or in deceptions will necessarily hinder their social exchanges.

Social setting: learning to interact with others

Together with neurobiological structures and, in this case, genetic profiles, the environment of a person with a neurodevelopmental disorder is also atypical. The neuroconstructivist perspective emphasises the critical role of the environment, which is modified by the active processing of the child. Besides the constraints imposed by the physical properties of the environment, social aspects of the environment also affect, and are affected by, the individual's behaviour.

Hodapp (2004) differentiates between direct and indirect effects of a genetic disorder linked to intellectual disability. The indirect effects can be divided into those arising from having a neurodevelopmental disorder and those linked to the specific aetiology of each diagnosis. Regarding the general effects of exhibiting a neurodevelopmental disorder, it could be that once carers know the child is developing atypically, the input they offer is different. It is possible, for instance, that people with developmental disabilities have fewer opportunities to obtain information from situations that involve mentalistic reasoning. In addition, they may have fewer opportunities to interact with peers, and these relationships are usually more mediated by others than relationships in the typical population. The behaviour of other people in these relationships could also be different; people might tend to play jokes or use ironic or sarcastic statements to a lesser extent with individuals with neurodevelopmental disorders or use a discourse involving lower-level mental concepts and more descriptions in terms of behaviour.

In addition to conversation within daily situations, various contexts offer valuable information for the development of human mind reading: literature, cinema, theatre and so on are settings to practise our comprehension of mental states. It is likely that difficulties for people with WS in extracting relevant information and in giving coherence to events in narrative contexts could make it difficult for them to benefit from these settings. Facilitating the understanding of these narrative sequences, for example highlighting the relevant events, could be a useful strategy to help individuals with WS to make an explicit reflection on characters' mental states. Similar strategies could be used to help them understand situations involving misunderstandings, jokes, irony or deception. As significant curricula adaptations are made for people with intellectual disabilities so as to favour the learning of academic contents (i.e. in the classroom), it is also necessary to make adaptations to facilitate the acquisition of certain competences in nonformal contexts of interaction (i. e. on the playground).

The indirect effects of a neurodevelopmental disorder on relationships with others can be linked to specific features of the aetiology. When mother–child interactions during a visuospatial-construction task were compared in dyads in which children had different developmental conditions, mothers with children with WS helped and reinforced their children more than mothers of children with Prader–Willi syndrome (Hodapp, 2004). There was a relationship between their behaviour and the diagnosis of their child regardless of the child's competence; attribution of ability to the child was at least as important as the child's actual competence. Furthermore, mothers of children with WS were more intrusive and more goal-oriented. It would be interesting to study whether this goal-oriented behaviour also occurs in other situations, because a reflection on the process rather than on the goal could be more effective when trying to promote mentalistic reasoning.

Behavioural outcomes of genetic disorders, even those specific to some aetiologies, will change during development and therefore their effects on social environment will also change.

Children with WS are sociable and uninhibited, which could facilitate relationships with adults. This same lack of inhibition in older individuals could make strangers feel suspicious. Therefore, even if initially their personality profile triggers approachability behaviours, later in development it can lead to greater isolation.

In addition, going back to the first level of psychological functioning, behavioural variations among individuals with the same diagnosis will mean that not all individuals demonstrate the expected pattern. In this sense, from the description of the general psychological profile of people with WS, they are described as sociable and affectionate, and although this is often the case, it is possible that some people with WS do not fit this pattern or do not do so throughout their entire development. Rather than concluding a weakness or deficit in the use of interaction tools, their families could give an interpretation of purpose to their behaviours. Furthermore, generalisation of the description of this profile of social func-tioning may, as a consequence, lead one to determine that it is not necessary to intervene in these competences. Thus, it is necessary to analyse the functioning and necessities of people with WS at different time points in their development and in different settings.

Social cognition in Williams syndrome: a developmental view

From a neuroconstructivist perspective, it is essential to adopt a sixth level of analysis—in addition to the other five levels of explanation of psychological functioning (i. e. behavioural, cognitive, environmental, neurological and genetic)—that interacts with the others: development itself. It is necessary to acknowledge social comprehension competences from the earliest points of development but also to adopt this developmental perspective throughout the individual's life.

The marked social interest of people with WS appears very early in development: at the age of 18 months, children with WS show less intense negative responses when the attached adult leaves them with a stranger than observed in typical children (Jones et al., 2000). They are also more interested in establishing contact with strangers and show patterns of longer and more intense gazing at others' faces than do same-age children without WS (Jones et al., 2000). Other data indicate, however, that the affiliation behaviour of children with WS cannot be explained only by their attention to faces, because they were more willing than TD children to engage with a stranger in a play situation even when the stranger's face could not be seen (Dodd et al., 2010).

Their behaviours suggest positive consequences: toddlers with WS show more behaviours of empathy and comfort (Mervis et al., 2003). However, sustained attention to faces, to the near exclusion of objects or actions, can also result in fewer possibilities to learn about the world. This early atypical gaze pattern has important implications for the development of first communicative behaviours. Children with WS are better at dyadic than at triadic interactions and exhibit atypical development of joint attention (Laing et al., 2002; Mervis et al., 1999; Chapter 10).

Social behaviours, tested through diagnostic tests for ASD, suggest shared symptoms between WS and ASD clinical groups especially in terms of joint attention, pointing, gestures, showing, and integrating eye contact with other communicative behaviours, as well as shared difficulties with functional and symbolic play and repetitive behaviours. However, children with WS (2-5 years old) made more efforts to engage others than did children with ASD (Klein-Tasman et al., 2007; Lincoln, et al., 2007). In spite of the idea that the two groups exhibit opposite patterns, it is noteworthy that more than half of the children with WS met the criteria for autism on some of the measures of the diagnostic scales (Klein-Tasman et al., 2007).

ASD scales have been applied to preschool children with WS, but it is possible that other features of the ASD psychological profile could emerge at distinct developmental time points. Together with other shared features between the two diagnostic groups, this observation could point to the hypothesis of a continuum between neurodevelopmental disorders (Karmiloff-Smith, 1998) and would be evidence against the view of polar opposites for WS and autism.

As previously explained, the neuroconstructivist perspective states the need to study the development of processes from infancy while also adopting a developmental view throughout ontogenesis. From this ontogenetic logic, it is important to understand when and how certain competences are acquired. Thus, it is essential to attend to the mechanisms of change in development. A developmental approach must, apart from making a proposal on the ontogenesis of the functional architecture of the mind, take a stance on the development of knowledge acquisition. The neuroconstructivist perspective is fundamentally a model on the genesis of the functional organisation of the mind, but it also accepts the principles of Karmiloff-Smith's model on knowledge acquisition. Karmiloff-Smith (1992) defined development on the basis of two parallel processes: a progressive modularisation and a gradual representational redescription. ToM is acquired implicitly, but its development demands the progressive explicitation of its representations. In TD children, implicit functioning of mentalising competences develops earlier than explicit functioning (Clements & Perner, 1994; Clements et al., 2000; Garnham & Perner, 2001; Perner & Clements, 2000).

Children with WS perform better on implicit questions with respect to the attribution of beliefs and desires and experience greater difficulties with explicit questions than TD children of the same level of development (Campos, 2009). The distinction between implicit and explicit functioning distinguishes between the developmental trajectories in WS and ASD. Whereas children with WS benefit from an implicit approach to the mental state, individuals with ASD perform better in explicit ToM tasks than in implicit ones (Ruffman et al., 2001; Senju et al., 2009). These differences in mental processing demand distinct ways of supporting the development of mental state attribution in both groups.

Conclusions and implications for intervention

The description of social comprehension competences in WS does not uphold the argument for preserved social functioning independent of other cognitive processes. On the contrary, the development of social cognition in WS is atypical from the outset and throughout the individual's life. Their attribution of emotions is not better than expected by their general level of development, and they have difficulty understanding epistemic mental states and using pragmatic cues in communication.

Developmental trajectories in WS differ from those associated with typical development or with other neurodevelopmental disorders. Social interaction competence in individuals with WS is in many aspects different from that of individuals with ASD, but the two disorders should not be regarded as polar opposites in terms of functioning (Brock et al., 2008; Tager-Flusberg et al., 2006). In this sense, it is important to consider the possibility of comorbidity between the syndromes when diagnosing, to ensure that the child will gain adequate access to specific services for both WS and ASD if required (Klein-Tasman et al., 2007).

Apart from aspects establishing dissociation, associations among symptoms of the two conditions are illustrative and suggest the importance of understanding the notion of an intra- and intersyndrome continuum. The concept of a spectrum disorder could be extended to WS because both ASD and WS imply significant variability in phenotypic manifestations and thus enable the establishment of different behavioural patterns within the same diagnosis. Within WS, various cognitive profiles have been identified, one of which is characterised by a specific deficit in emotion perception and false belief attribution (Porter & Coltheart, 2005; Porter et al., 2008). In ASD, the 'active but odd' subtype of social functioning (Wing & Gould, 1979; Beglinger & Smith, 2001) involves a peculiar social relationship tendency to actively search for social relationships despite the difficulties individuals with ASD have with social conventions, communication and eye contact, features also shared by people with WS.

It is necessary to go into further depth with respect to intergroup analyses by means of direct comparisons with the same procedures and an adequate selection of samples to have groups that are as homogeneous as possible. Cases of double diagnoses (WS and ASD) offer a very appealing opportunity to study intergroup associations and dissociations. These cases would also be ideal for rigorous intragroup analyses that focus on the individual variabilities within the group so as to establish and identify differential patterns of social functioning within a diagnosis of WS. In both types of analyses, different levels of psychological functioning and the relationships among them should be considered.

From a developmental perspective, it is crucial to collect data from longitudinal studies that offer detailed information of changes in the behaviour of the same participants over time. It is also necessary to use fine-grained assessment measures, to differentiate among processes on the basis of behaviours that can be similar and to perform an analysis of the mechanisms of change in acquisition of social comprehension competences. In this analysis, the way of inquiring about the mental states can offer relevant information: differentiation between explicit and implicit approaches can distinguish between typical development and development consistent with WS or ASD (Ruffman et al., 2001; Senju et al., 2009; Campos, 2009).

To further explore mental state understanding, it would be interesting to assess the comprehension of mental states in WS by means of even more implicit indicators than by asking questions about emotion, such as by investigating gaze direction, performance of motor action, emotional reaction or empathic response. As mentioned earlier, when children with WS are provided with a clue about a person's emotion, their performance on false belief attribution improves. The influence of various types of clues could be studied in different situations, or one could even develop a research programme with an evaluation–intervention–evaluation design. It could also be interesting to analyse the competences in WS with respect to real situations that require an understanding of mental states. Everyday situations involving misunderstandings, jokes and the management of information in natural contexts would offer valuable information that would complement the findings garnered from the laboratory studies.

The neuroconstructivist perspective considers two fundamental aims in the study of neurodevelopmental disorders: 'to use disorders to help our understanding of the normal processes of development' and 'to identify appropriate methods of remediation' (Mareschal et al., 2007). However, work on psychological functioning in WS (as in other neurodevelopmental disorders) sometimes refers only to the importance of identifying the implications from the results for intervention, and almost none develop these implications beyond explaining the need to carry out future studies along those lines.

Intervention in neurodevelopmental disorders suggests in-depth analysis of the genesis of the cognitive processes implied. Intervention always has to be set in the microgenesis (the online development of psychological functions) because only from here are processes going to be modified. People with WS do not start by having problems in social abilities; rather, developmental studies indicate that the processes behind apparently good interaction behaviours are somehow different and that these processes imply future difficulties in establishing relationships. Therefore, it seems necessary to provide these individuals with the requisite tools to improve their interactions with others from the outset. As the diagnosis is often made early on, it is essential to intervene in these and other areas as soon as possible, even before behavioural deficits are evident.

Clinical intervention is frequently based solely on behavioural measures without considering the possibility that a similar behaviour may rely on different processes. In some cases, discovering these underlying processes should be the main objective of remediation because the generalisation and adaptability of behaviour may only be guaranteed if we use them as the basis for intervention. In our opinion, neuroconstructivism's radical rejection of the isolated segmentation of Marr's levels of analysis (Mareschal et al., 2007) could be extended to the need to consider more than just the behavioural level in the design, implementation and assessment of intervention programmes. Only from a perspective of assuming that the interrelation of biological factors and experience has an influence throughout development is it going to be possible to tackle treatment beyond behavioural symptoms.

In general, maturational models will see the influence in just one sense. The neuroconstructivist perspective's opposition to the modular approaches of development can be argued not only from its theoretical consequences but also from its effect on clinical decisions. From the implicit theories of maturation, data reporting an extremely sociable profile in WS might conclude, as a consequence, the questionable futility of the application of programmes aimed at improving social competences in this group. However, data from research are far removed from this picture of intact social functioning and indicate that people with WS demonstrate serious lapses in their relationships with others, which interferes negatively on their quality of life both by its influence on the acquisition of other cognitive skills and by the anxiety implied by awareness of these difficulties.

From the essential assumption that research results must lead to intervention, it is critical that diverse developmental trajectories should result in different methods of remediation. Intervention in neurodevelopmental disorders usually requires the teaching of some functions that are normally acquired implicitly (i.e. language or ToM) through explicit instruction. Results from programmes on social comprehension abilities are of varying success. Often, participants are able to learn how to solve tasks involving emotional processing and false belief attribution, but they cannot generalise this learning to other contexts or other mental states (Hadwin et al., 1997; Howlin et al., 1999). Individuals with ASD must follow this slow, 'cold' and strained route. However, if the data point to better implicit functioning in WS, perhaps a strategy based on using the implicit identification with the other as a shortcut to one's beliefs could be more effective in this group.

These considerations can be extended to testing. ToM tasks normally suggest explicit questions that may not reflect tacit knowledge that the child could be using. In this sense, it is important to consider the relationship between performance in mind-reading tasks and social interaction competence. It seems that the explicit route, so successful for individuals with high-functioning ASD in solving false belief tasks, does not enable these individuals to develop a social functioning that individuals with WS can attain implicitly. For intervention with individuals with WS, it is possible that—together with activities that make mental functioning explicit—it is efficient to intervene using their phenotypic strengths of intersubjectivity and empathy and to exploit their genuine interest in establishing social relationships so as to provide them with social strategies. To use empathy and put ourselves in others' shoes is another way of understanding others' mental worlds and also our own.

We assert that it is essential to extend the accumulated knowledge of the functioning profile of WS and the theoretical assumptions of the neuroconstructivist framework for intervention with the aim of improving the quality of life for people with WS. However, it should be a two-way street. Research of the most appropriate clinical strategies for developmental conditions should have theoretical implications that promote a more in-depth study of the developmental processes and the mechanisms that channel ontogeny.

Editor commentary (Emily K. Farran & Annette Karmiloff-Smith)

A prominent characteristic of individuals with WS is their hypersociability or overfriendliness. This chapter probed deeper into the social domain to explore mental state understanding and social interaction. We learnt that individuals with WS often miss contextual cues in social interactions and that, relatedly, hypersociability can lead to isolation. When basic emotions are considered, individuals with WS are able to attribute expressions of emotions to emotional contexts. However, the chapter suggested that individuals with WS rely on more superficial cues at the expense of subtle cues. Taking a multidisciplinary examination of atypical social behaviour, the chapter pointed to atypical structure and functional activation of the amygdala in WS, and to the *GTF2I* gene. Importantly, the chapter discussed these interactions between brain, genes and behaviour within the context of development and environmental influences. Taking a neuroconstructivist approach, as in Chapter 14, the chapter considered that a strong interest in faces at the expense of objects in infancy might lead to the later atypical development of triadic interactions and, in turn, to the pragmatic deficits discussed in Chapter 11. Cross-domain influences of the verbal domain were also discussed. Impairments in the linguistic domain in WS, such as difficulty understanding prosody, can thus have a negative impact on mental state understanding within the social domain. A theme throughout the chapter is the interesting cross-syndrome comparison between WS and autism. On first look, these two disorders seem to present with opposite profiles of social interaction. Yet, in fact, they show both some overlapping and some opposing social abilities. This is yet another striking demonstration that developmental disorders cannot be described in terms of 'parts intact' and 'parts impaired' and that development can proceed along multiple alternative trajectories.

References

Andari, E., Duhamel, J., Zalla, T., Herbrecht, E., Leboyer, M., & Sirigu, A. (2010). Promoting social behavior with oxytocin in high-functioning autism spectrum disorders. *Proceedings of the National Academy of Sciences of the USA*, **107**, 4389–94.

Back, E., Ropar, D., & Mitchell, P. (2007). Do the eyes have it? Inferring mental states from animated faces in autism. *Child Development*, **78**, 397–411.

Baron-Cohen, S. (1998). Does the study of autism justify minimalist innate modularity? *Learning and Individual Differences*, **10**, 179–91.

Baron-Cohen, S. (1999). The extreme male-brain theory of autism. In H. Tager-Flusberg (Ed.), *Neurodevelopmental Disorders* (pp. 401–429). Cambridge, MA: MIT Press.

Beglinger, L., & Smith, T. (2001). A review of subtyping in autism and proposed dimensional classification model. *Journal of Autism and Developmental Disorders*, **31**, 411–22.

Bellugi, U., Lichtenberger, L., Mills, D., Galaburda, A., & Korenberg, J.R. (1999). Bridging cognition, the brain and molecular genetics: evidence from Williams syndrome. *Trends in Neurosciences*, **22**, 197–207.

Berg, J.S., Brunetti-Pierri, N., Peters, S.U., Kang, S.H., Fong, C.T., Salamone, J., et al. (2007). Speech delay and autism spectrum behaviors are frequently associated with duplication of the 7q11.23 Williams-Beuren syndrome region. *Journal of Medical Genetics*, **9**, 427–41.

Brock, J. Einav, S., & Riby, D. (2008). The other end of the spectrum? Social cognition in Williams syndrome. In T. Striano & V. Reid (Eds), *Social Cognition: Development, Neuroscience and Autism* (pp. 281–300). Oxford: Blackwell.

Campos, R. (2009). *Construyendo mentes: desarrollo de la comprensión de estados mentales en niños con síndrome de Williams y en desarrollo típico.* Doctoral thesis, Universidad Autónoma de Madrid.

Campos, R., Sotillo, M., & Martínez-Castilla, P. (November 2009). Development of sentential complementation in children with Williams syndrome. Presented at the II Congreso Internacional de Lingüística Clínica, Madrid.

Clements, W.A., & Perner, J. (1994). Implicit understanding of belief. *Cognitive Development*, **9**, 377–95.

Clements, W.A., Rustin, C.L., & McCallum, S. (2000). Promoting the transition from implicit to explicit understanding: a training study of false belief. *Developmental Science*, **3**, 81–92.

Dai, L., Mills, D., Bellugi, U., & Korenberg, J.R. (2009). Is it Williams syndrome? GTF2IRD1 implicated in visual-spatial construction and GTF2I in sociability revealed by high resolution arrays. *American Journal of Medical Genetics*, **149**, 302–314.

Dodd, H.F., Porter, M.A., Peters, G.L., & Rapee, R.M. (2010). Social approach in pre-school children with Williams syndrome: the role of the face. *Journal of Intellectual Disability Research*, **54**, 194–203.

Doherty-Sneddon, G., Riby, D.M., Calderwood, L., & Ainsworth, L. (2009). Stuck on you: face-to-face arousal and gaze aversion in Williams syndrome. *Cognitive Neuropsychiatry*, **14**, 510–23.

Frigerio, E., Burt, D.M., Gagliardi, C., Cioffi, G., Martelli, S., Perrett, D.I., et al. (2006). Is everybody always my friend? Perception of approachability in Williams syndrome. *Neuropsychologia*, **44**, 254–59.

Gagliardi, C., Frigerio, E., Burt, D.M., Cazzaniga, I., Perrett, D.I., & Borgatti, R. (2003). Facial expression recognition in Williams syndrome. *Neuropsychologia*, **41**, 733–38.

Galaburda, A.M., Bellugi, U. (2000). Multi-level analysis of cortical neuroanatomy in Williams syndrome. *Journal of Cognitive Neuroscience*, **12 Supplement 1**, 74–88.

Garnham, W.A., & Perner, J. (2001). Actions really do speak louder than words - but only implicitly: young children's understanding of false belief in action. *British Journal of Developmental Psychology*, **19**, 413–32.

Gillberg, C., & Rasmussen, P. (1994). Four case histories and a literature review of Williams syndrome and autistic behavior. *Journal of Autism and Developmental Disorders*, **24**, 381–93.

Haas, B.W., Hoeft, F., Searcy, Y.M., Mills, D., Bellugi, U., & Reiss, A. (2010). Individual differences in social behavior predict amygdala response to fearful facial expressions in Williams syndrome. *Neuropsychologia*, **48**, 1283–88.

Haas, B.W., Mills, D., Yam, A., Hoeft, F., Bellugi, U., & Reiss, A.L. (2009). Genetic influences on sociability: heightened amygdala reactivity and event-related responses to positive social stimuli in Williams syndrome. *Journal of Neuroscience*, **29**, 1132–39.

Hadwin, J., Baron-Cohen, S., Howlin, P. & Hill, K. (1997). Podemos enseñar a comprender emociones, creencias o ficciones a los niños autistas. In A. Riviere & J. Martos (Eds), *El Tratamiento Del Autismo* (pp. 586–623). Madrid: Asociación de Padres de Niños Autistas - Inserso.

Hirstein, W., Iversen, P., & Ramachandran, V.S. (2001). Autonomic responses of autistic children to people and objects. *Proceedings of Biological Sciences*, **268**, 1883–88.

Hobson, P. (2002). *The Cradle of Thought. Exploring the Origins of Thinking*. London: Macmillan.

Hodapp, R.M. (2004). Studying interactions, reactions, and perceptions: can genetic disorders serve as behavioral proxies? *Journal of Autism and Developmental Disorders*, **34**, 29–34.

Hollander, E., Bartz, J., Chaplin, W., Phillips, A., Sumner, J., Soorya, L., et al. (2007). Oxytocin increases retention of social cognition in autism. *Biological Psychiatry*, **61**, 498–503.

Howlin, P., Baron-Cohen, S., & Hadwin, J. (1999). *Teaching Children with Autism to Mind-Read: A Practical Guide*. New York, NY: John Wiley and Sons.

Howlin, P., Davies, M., & Udwin, O. (1998). Cognitive functioning in adults with Williams syndrome. *Journal of Child Psychology and Psychiatry*, **39**, 183–89.

Jawaid, A., Schmolck, H., & Schulz, P.E. (2008). Hypersociability in Williams syndrome: a role for the amygdala? *Cognitive Neuropsychiatry*, **13**, 338–42.

John, A.E., Rowe, M.L., & Mervis, C.B. (2009). Referential communication skills of children with Williams syndrome: understanding when messages are not adequate. *American Journal on Intellectual and Developmental Disabilities*, **114**, 85–99.

Jones, W., Bellugi, U., Lai, Z., Chiles, M., Reilly, J., Lincoln, A., & et al. (2000). Hypersociability in Williams syndrome. *Journal of Cognitive Neuroscience*, **12 Supplement 1**, 30–46.

Karmiloff-Smith, A. (1992). *Beyond Modularity: A Developmental Perspective on Cognitive Science*. Cambridge, MA: MIT Press.

Karmiloff-Smith, A. (1998). Developmental itself is the key to understanding developmental disorders. *Trends in Cognitive Sciences*, **2**, 389–98.

Karmiloff-Smith, A., Klima, E., Bellugi, U., Grant, J., & Baron-Cohen, S. (1995). Is there a social module? Language, face processing and theory of mind in individuals with Williams syndrome. *Journal of Cognitive Neuroscience*, **7**, 196–208.

Klein-Tasman, B.P., & Mervis, C.B. (2003). Distinctive personality characteristics of 8-, 9-, and 10-year-olds with Williams syndrome. *Developmental Neuropsychology*, **23**, 269–90.

Klein-Tasman, B.P., Mervis, C.B., Lord, C.E., & Phillips, K.D. (2007). Socio-communicative deficits in young children with Williams syndrome: performance on the Autism Diagnostic Observation Schedule. *Child Neuropsychology*, **13**, 444–67.

Lacroix, A., Aguert, M., Dardier, V., Stojanovik, V., & Laval, V. (2010). Idiom comprehension in French-speaking children and adolescents with Williams syndrome. *Research in Developmental Disabilities*, **31**, 608–616.

Lacroix, A., Guidetti, M., Rogé, B., & Reilly, J. (2009). Recognition of emotional and nonemotional facial expressions: a comparison between Williams syndrome and autism. *Research in Developmental Disabilities*, **30**, 976–85.

Laing, E., Butterworth, G., Ansari, D., Gsödl, M., Longhi, E., Panagiotaki, G., et al. (2002). Atypical development of language and social communication in toddlers with Williams syndrome. *Developmental Science*, **5**, 233–46.

Lincoln, A.J., Searcy, Y.M., Jones, W., & Lord, C. (2007). Social interaction behaviors discriminate young children with autism and Williams syndrome. *Journal of the American Academy of Child and Adolescent Psychiatry*, **46**, 323–31.

Losh, M., Bellugi, U., Reilly, J., & Anderson, D. (2000). Narrative as a social engagement tool: The excessive use of evaluation in narratives from children with Williams syndrome. *Narrative Inquiry*, **10**, 265.

Mareschal, D., Johnson, M.H., Sirois, S., Spratling, M., Thomas, M., & Westermann, G. (2007). *Neuroconstructivism, Vol. I: How the Brain Constructs Cognition*. Oxford: Oxford University Press.

Martens, M.A., Wilson, S.J., Dudgeon, P., & Reutens, D.C. (2009). Approachability and the amygdala: insights from Williams syndrome. *Neuropsychologia*, **47**, 2446–53.

Martens, M.A., Wilson, S.J., & Reutens, D.C. (2008). Williams syndrome: a critical review of the cognitive, behavioral, and neuroanatomical phenotype. *Journal of Child Psychology and Psychiatry*, **49**, 576–608.

Martínez-Castilla, P., Sotillo, M., & Campos, R. (2010). Prosodic abilities of Spanish-speaking adolescents and adults with Williams syndrome. *Language and Cognitive Processes*. DOI: 10.1080/01690965.2010.504058 [advance online publication].

Mervis, C., Morris, C., Bertrand, J., & Robinson, F.R. (1999). Williams syndrome: findings from an integrated program of research. In H. Tager-Flusberg (Ed.), *Neurodevelopmental Disorders: Contribution to a New Framework from the Cognitive Neurosciences* (pp. 65–110). Cambridge, MA: MIT Press.

Mervis, C., Morris, C., Klein-Tasman, B., Bertrand, J., Kwinty, S., Appelbaum, L., et al. (2003). Attentional characteristics of infants and toddlers with Williams syndrome during triadic interactions. *Developmental Neuropsychology*, **23**, 243–68.

Meyer-Lindenberg, A., Hariri, A.R., Munoz, K.E., Mervis, C.B., Mattay, V.S., Morris, C.A., et al. (2005). Neural correlates of genetically abnormal social cognition in Williams syndrome. *Nature Neuroscience*, **8**, 991–93.

Muñoz, K.E., Meyer-Lindenberg, A., Hariri, A.R., Mervis, C.B., Mattay, V.S., Morris, C.A., et al. (2010). Abnormalities in neural processing of emotional stimuli in Williams syndrome vary according to social vs. non-social content. *NeuroImage*, **50**, 340–6.

Perner, J., & Clements, W.A. (2000). From an implicit to an explicit "theory of mind". In Y. Rossetti & A. Revonsuo (Eds), *Beyond Dissociation: Interaction between Dissociated Implicit and Explicit Processing* (pp. 273–93). Amsterdam: John Benjamins.

Plesa Skwerer, D., Borum, L., Verbalis, A., Schofield, C., Crawford, N., Ciciolla, L., et al. (2009). Autonomic responses to dynamic displays of facial expressions in adolescents and adults with Williams syndrome. *Social Cognitive and Affective Neuroscience*, **4**, 93–100.

Plesa-Skwerer, D., Faja, S., Schofield, C., Verbalis, A., & Tager-Flusberg, H. (2006a). Perceiving facial and vocal expressions of emotion in individuals with Williams syndrome. *American Journal on Mental Retardation*, **111**, 15–26.

Plesa Skwerer, D., Verbalis, A., Schofield, C., Faja, S., & Tager-Flusberg, H. (2006b). Social-perceptual abilities in adolescents and adults with Williams syndrome. *Cognitive Neuropsychology*, **23**, 338–49.

Porter, M.A., & Coltheart, M. (2005). Cognitive heterogeneity in Williams syndrome. *Developmental Neuropsychology*, **27**, 275–306.

Porter, M.A., Coltheart, M., & Langdon, R. (2007). The neuropsychological basis of hypersociability in Williams and Down syndrome. *Neuropsychologia*, **45**, 2839–49.

Porter, M.A., Coltheart, M., & Langdon, R. (2008). Theory of mind in Williams syndrome assessed using a nonverbal task. *Journal of Autism and Developmental Disorders*, **38**, 806–814.

Reilly, J., Klima, E., & Bellugi, E. (1990). Once more with feeling: affect and language in atypical populations. *Development and Psychopathology*, **2**, 367–91.

Reilly, J., Losh, M., Bellugi, U., & Wulfeck, B. (2004). 'Frog, where are you?' Narratives in children with specific language impairment, early focal brain injury, and Williams syndrome. *Brain and Language*, **88**, 229–47.

Riby, D.M., & Back, E. (2010). Can individuals with Williams syndrome infer mental states from moving faces? *Neuropsychologia*, **48**, 1914–22.

Riby, D.M., Doherty-Sneddon, G., & Bruce, V. (2008). Exploring face perception in disorders of development: evidence from Williams syndrome and autism. *Journal of Neuropsychology*, **2**, 47–64.

Rose, F.E., Lincoln, A.J., Lai, Z., Ene, M., Searcy, Y.M., & Bellugi, U. (2007). Orientation and affective expression effects on face recognition in Williams syndrome and autism. *Journal of Autism and Developmental Disorders*, **37**, 513–22.

Ruffman, T., Garnham, W., & Rideout, P. (2001). Social understanding in autism: eye gaze as a measure of core insights. *The Journal of Child Psychology and Psychiatry and Allied Disciplines*, **42**, 1083–94.

Santos, A., & Deruelle, C. (2009). Verbal peaks and visual valleys in theory of mind ability in Williams syndrome. *Journal of Autism and Developmental Disorders*, **39**, 651–59.

Santos, A., Silva, C., Rosset, D., & Deruelle, C. (2010). Just another face in the crowd: evidence for decreased detection of angry faces in children with Williams syndrome. *Neuropsychologia*, **48**, 1071–78.

Senju, A., Southgate, V., White, S., & Frith, U. (2009). Mindblind eyes: an absence of spontaneous theory of mind in Asperger syndrome. *Science*, **325**, 883–85.

Somerville, M.J., Mervis, C.B., Young, E.J., Seo, E.-J., del Campo, M., Bamforth, S., et al. (2005). Severe expressive language delay related to duplication of the Williams-Beuren locus. *New England Journal of Medicine*, **353**, 1694–1701.

Sotillo, M., García Nogales, M.A., & Campos, R. (2007). Teoría de la mente y lenguaje: el caso del síndrome de Williams. *Infancia y Aprendizaje*, **30**, 459–74.

Sullivan, K., & Tager-Flusberg, H. (1999). Second-order belief attribution in Williams syndrome: intact or impaired? *American Journal on Mental Retardation*, **104**, 523–32.

Sullivan, K., Winner, E., & Tager-Flusberg, H. (2003). Can adolescents with William syndrome tell the difference between lies and jokes? *Developmental Neuropsychology*, **23**, 85–103.

Tager-Flusberg, H. (1993). What language reveals about the understanding of minds in children with autism. In Baron-Cohen, S., Tager–Flusberg, H., & Cohen, D.J. (Eds), *Understanding Other Minds: Perspectives from Autism.* (pp. 138–57). New York, NY: Oxford Medical Publications.

Tager-Flusberg, H., Boshart, J., & Baron-Cohen, S. (1998). Reading the windows to the soul: evidence of domain-specific sparing in Williams syndrome. *Journal of Cognitive Neuroscience*, **10**, 631–39.

Tager-Flusberg, H., Plesa Skwerer, D., & Joseph, R.M. (2006). Model syndromes for investigating social cognitive and affective neuroscience: a comparison of autism and Williams syndrome. *Social, Cognitive and Affective Neuroscience*, **1**, 175–82.

Tager-Flusberg, H., & Sullivan, K. (2000). A componential view of theory of mind: evidence from Williams syndrome. *Cognition*, **76**, 59–89.

Tager-Flusberg, H., Sullivan, K., & Boshart, J. (1997). Executive functions and performance on false belief tasks. *Developmental Neuropsychology*, **13**, 487–93.

Thomas, M.S.C., Van Duuren, M., Purser, H.R.M., Mareschal, D., Ansari, D., & Karmiloff-Smith, A. (2010). The development of metaphorical language comprehension in typical development and in Williams syndrome. *Journal of Experimental Child Psychology*, **106**, 99–114.

Tomc, S.A., Williamson, N.K., & Pauli, R.M. (1990). Temperament in Williams syndrome. *American Journal Medical Genetics*, **6**, 345–52.

Trevarthen, C., & Aitken, J.A. (2001). Infant intersubjectivity: research, theory and clinical applications. *Journal of Child Psychology and Psychiatry*, **42**, 3–48.

de Villiers, J.G., & de Villiers, P.A. (2000). Linguistic determinism and the understanding of false beliefs. In P. Mitchell & K. Riggs (Eds), *Children's Reasoning about the Mind* (pp. 191–228). Hove: Psychology Press.

de Villiers, J.G., & Pyers, J.E. (2002). Complements to cognition: a longitudinal study of the relationship between complex syntax and false belief understanding. *Cognitive Development*, **17**, 1037–60.

Wing, L., & Gould, J. (1979). Severe impairments of social interaction and associated abnormalities in children: epidemiology and classification. *Journal of Autism and Developmental Disorders*, **9**, 11–29.

Part 4d

Numeracy and Literacy

Chapter 16

Numeracy

Joanne S. Camp, Emily K. Farran and
Annette Karmiloff-Smith

Introduction

Number-relevant information bombards our everyday lives. It is necessary for telling the time, for dealing with money, for changing TV channels, for shopping, for taking local transport and so forth. Interestingly, many other species have number skills, and human children show sensitivity to numerically relevant displays very early in infancy and continue to develop number processing skills and knowledge about number facts throughout childhood. Yet, despite dyscalculia being more prevalent than dyslexia, particularly in children with neurodevelopmental disorders, studies of atypical number development are far less plentiful than those of atypical reading. In this chapter, we examine the neural and cognitive underpinnings of typical and atypical numeracy, in particular numerical cognition in infants, children and adults with Williams syndrome (WS), but also referring to other neurodevelopmental disorders, with particular emphasis on the distinction between numerical sensitivities vis-à-vis small numbers and approximate magnitude computations with large numbers.

The neural bases of typical and atypical numeracy in older children and adults

It is currently considered by many (e.g. Dehaene et al., 2003; Dehaene et al., 2004) that numerical cognition can be described in terms of two purportedly independent systems: an approximate number or magnitude system, which involves estimation of quantities, size or volume and is not related to language, and an exact system, which comprises the use of number facts and learnt rules and is related to language. Dehaene and collaborators (2003) discuss evidence from adult patients with acquired lesions and from neurophysiological and neuroimaging studies to support this distinction. The authors suggest that three areas in the parietal lobe become activated for different aspects of number. The best characterised system is the horizontal segment of the intraparietal sulcus (IPS). This area is activated for tasks that involve the approximate system, that is, estimation and magnitude comparisons. The posterior superior parietal lobule (PSPL) also shows activation during tasks that involve the approximate system, but is less specific to numerical tasks than the IPS. While activation has been shown in the PSPL for magnitude comparison, approximation and counting, this region is also activated for hand reaching, eye orienting, mental rotation and spatial working memory (Corbetta et al., 2000). Dehaene and collaborators (2003) suggest that this area, in light of its role in attention orienting, is activated for tasks than involve the mental number line, that is, the representation of numbers along an axis based on their numerical proximity (Moyer & Landauer, 1967). Finally, the left angular gyrus is activated when number tasks involve verbal processing. For example, activation has been shown for number tasks that call on rote memory of arithmetic facts, such as some forms of mental arithmetic and multiplication, and it is more activated for small additions (sums below 10) than for large ones (Stanescu-Cosson et al., 2000) owing to the ability to call on arithmetic facts for small sums.

Data from both normal and brain-damaged adults have yielded functional distinctions in neural circuitry that have been important for our understanding of number processing in the brain. However, recent exploration of the development of number processing has pointed to the likelihood of qualitatively different neural activation in children relative to adults. Rivera et al. (2005) analysed which regions were activated during a mental arithmetic task in comparison with a control task and assessed whether activation in each of these regions is correlated with chronological age. They report increased activation in left temporoparietal regions with development from 8 to 19 years during mental arithmetic tasks. This resonates with the neuroconstructivist view of gradual specialisation of these regions over developmental time. This was accompanied by evidence of a larger network of neural activation in younger children, involving the dorsolateral and ventrolateral prefrontal cortex and the anterior cingulate cortex. Rivera and colleagues (2005) suggest that this network acts to support the developmental specialisation of parietal areas and points to a stronger involvement of working memory and attention in mental arithmetic problems in young children relative to older children and adults. A particularly interesting finding from the Rivera et al. study is that, with age, there is decreasing activation of the left hippocampus, suggesting that this area, which plays a time-sensitive role in memory formation, is involved early in arithmetic fact encoding but not in the subsequently highly automatised retrieval of facts.

Activation of the inferior frontal cortex has also been demonstrated during magnitude comparison tasks in children (7-year-olds) but not in adults, accompanied by a gradual developmental specialisation of the IPS (Ansari et al., 2005; Ansari & Dhital, 2006; Cantlon et al., 2009; Holloway & Ansari, 2010). Correlated activation between these areas in children, which is not present in adults, supports the assertion of a qualitatively different network of activation in childhood, which scaffolds the development of progressive specialisation over time.

These studies of typical development highlight the importance of taking into account the dynamic nature of behaviour–brain interactions and the gradual specialisation and localisation of function when studying neurodevelopmental disorders (see also Ansari, 2010; Ansari & Karmiloff-Smith, 2002; Karmiloff-Smith, 1998). For example, it is entirely possible that early deficits in working memory and attention in atypical groups could alter developmental trajectories related to number and thus limit later development of neural networks typically associated with number.

In light of the progressive neural changes that have been outlined, the fact that our understanding of the WS brain is based almost exclusively on adult data (see Chapter 2) means that comparisons between regions of impairment in the WS brain and areas known to activate number in typical adults have obvious limitations. This is because subtle differences in infancy can have cascading effects on later development, and we cannot assume that progressive specialisation of neural areas even takes place or follows the same trajectory in neurodevelopmental syndromes compared with the typical case (Karmiloff-Smith, 1998, 2009). However, it is important to recall that many studies have revealed structurally atypical parietal regions in WS, including reduced connectivity to the IPS (Meyer-Lindenberg et al., 2004), and that many of the non-numerical functions also attributed to the PSPL, such as mental rotation (Farran et al., 2001) and attention orienting (Brown et al., 2003), are known to show behavioural impairments in WS (see Chapters 6, 12 and 18). However, while we have structural information about numerically relevant brain regions in WS, there is a distinct paucity of studies that explore functional activation during number processing, even in adults with WS. Establishing brain–behaviour relations has proven fruitful in other disorders that yield numerical deficits. For example, Isaacs et al. (2001) report that in adolescence, children born with very low birth weight can be divided into two distinct groups: those who have no numerical deficits versus those who do have numerical deficits and at the same time show reduced grey matter in an area in the left parietal lobe.

The cognitive bases of numeracy in typical development in infancy

Numerically relevant processing has been explored as early as infancy, initially in typical development, with the aim of determining the developmental origins of the approximate- and exact-number systems. Using the preferential looking or listening techniques, studies have explored infants' ability to discriminate between different numerosities of dots, objects, sounds and events. This has revealed a distinction between the processing involved in discriminating small-number displays compared with large, approximate numerosities. It turns out that even typically developing newborns can distinguish between small-number displays (one, two or three objects). Whether the infant's representation of the display is truly numerical or has more to do with the representation of each object individually, as posited by the 'object file' theory, continues to be a matter of debate (Carey, 2001; Simon, 1997; Uller et al., 1999). According to the object file theory, infants who are confronted with a small-number display represent each object as an individual object file, with a memory limitation of up to three object files. Discrimination is thought to be based on comparing each individual object file in memory with each of the objects on display. Some have argued that the development of the ability to create object files is an important precursor to the development of the exact-number system later in development (Le Corre & Carey, 2007; Feigenson et al., 2004). However, as we shall see later in this chapter, studies on atypical development indicate that it is the approximate magnitude system that is the more important basis for subsequent number development (Karmiloff-Smith, 2011; Karmiloff-Smith et al., submitted).

Large numerosities pose different cognitive demands on infants. From 6 months, they can discriminate between numerosities such as 8 and 16, even when factors such as display size and area are controlled for (Xu & Spelke, 2000), indicating that they are indeed focusing on quantity. However, it turns out to be the ratios between sets rather than the absolute number in each set that constrains performance. For example, Xu et al. (2005) demonstrated the ability of 6-month-old infants to discriminate between 8 and 16 and between 16 and 32, a ratio of 1:2, but the same infants were not capable of discriminating between 8 and 12 or 24 and 32, a ratio of 2:3. Infants require a few more months of development to be able to discriminate the more difficult 2:3 ratio, which they succeed at by 9-10 months (Xu & Arriaga, 2007). Such infant abilities underlie the early development of the approximate magnitude system (Feigenson et al., 2004).

These interesting developmental progressions in typical development between sensitivity to small-number differences and to large, approximate numerosities are of course crucial to examine in atypical development. Indeed, if the different abilities call on different neural processes, we may find some dissociations in children with neurodevelopmental disorders as well as neuroconstructivist clues as to which of the abilities has the most impact on later developing number.

The cognitive bases of numeracy in infants with Williams syndrome

To date, there are fewer than 20 published studies on numerical abilities in WS, and exceedingly few of these are on infancy; yet, it is very apparent that numerical cognition represents a weak area of ability in the WS phenotype. So, what do we know about the small-number and approximate-number systems in atypical infant development? Clearly, an impairment in the early foundations of number may have cascading effects on the later development of numerical cognition. Similarly, as highlighted by the neural evidence outlined earlier in this chapter, the development of number must also be considered in terms of other interacting systems (see Chapter 18). For example, numerical cognition draws upon visuospatial ability, verbal ability, executive function, attention and working memory. Thus, a deficit in any one of these areas could clearly have a developmental impact on later numerical competence. Let us now examine research that has explored the development of early number in WS, adding, where relevant, methodological and theoretical comparisons with other neurodevelopmental disorders in which numerical cognition is also impaired.

The very first study to examine sensitivity to numerical displays in infants with WS was carried out by Paterson and colleagues (Paterson et al., 1999). The authors report results from a small-number discrimination task (2 versus 3), comparing infants with WS, infants with Down syndrome (DS), a typical group matched on chronological age (CA) and another matched on mental age (MA). The children were familiarised over several trials to pairs of cards, each displaying two objects differing in type, colour, size and location. In the test phase, one of the cards still displayed two (new) objects, whereas the other displayed three (new) objects. The idea was to ascertain whether after a certain number of repetitive two-object trials, children would realise that despite all the changes in type of object, its colour, size, location and so on, the common factor in the displays was two-ness. If this was the case, then infants should look longer when presented with a card with three objects. If, by contrast, they looked equally long at the cards displaying two or three objects, they were not sensitive to changes in these small numbers. In other words, novelty preference for three objects, despite the changing features of the displays, would indicate that the infant was sensitive to the numerical aspects of the displays and not merely to the interesting features of the objects. Three of the groups (WS, MA-matched controls and CA-matched controls) all looked at the novel number for significantly longer than the familiar number, indicating that they were sensitive to changes in small numbers and able to discriminate between 2 and 3. This contrasted with the group of infants with DS, who showed no novelty preference. Recall that the infants with WS and DS were matched on general intelligence and performed at an equivalent level on a vocabulary task, indicating that the group disparity was specific to small-number displays and not merely related to a greater domain-general impairment in DS.

In a follow-up study, the same lab (Van Herwegen et al., 2008) replicated the small-exact-number findings in infants with WS but this time also investigated large-approximate-number discrimination. In this study, dot displays were used instead of photos of real objects in order to keep as close as possible to equivalent studies on typical development. As with the Paterson et al. (1999) results, the small-number task (2 versus 3) posed no problem for the infants with WS. However, when tested on large, approximate displays (8 versus 16 dots), they failed to show evidence of discrimination. This dissociation tends to support the argument (Dehaene et al., 2003) that two distinct number processing systems operate in humans and that they do so already in infancy. So, in infants with WS the so-called object file system (a focus on individual objects) operates proficiently, whereas the large approximate system (a focus on quantities) does not.

A more recent study (Karmiloff-Smith et al., submitted) seems to point to the opposite pattern in infants with DS. Replicating the Paterson et al. (1999) finding that infants with DS fail to discriminate small exact numbers in a new set of infants, the new study revealed that these same infants were successful at discriminating large, approximate numbers when the ratio was 1:2 (8 versus 16 dots). Moreover, preliminary analyses of eye tracker data indicate that the scanning patterns of the two syndromes differ. Whereas infants with DS tended to scan the whole array (of, say, 8 dots), those with WS kept their eyes fixated on very few of the dots in the display. This potential double dissociation between the syndromes lends further support to the existence of two separate systems for exact and approximate representations, and provides important potential pointers to the infant start state of the development of small-number and approximate numerosity in WS and DS and to how that might relate to subsequent outcomes, to which we now turn.

The cognitive bases of numeracy in older children and adults with Williams syndrome

Early studies of WS identified particular problems with number within the cognitive profile of WS. Indeed, they report that scores on the Arithmetic subtests of the Wechsler Intelligence Scale for Children (e.g. WISC-R; Wechsler, 1976) and the Wechsler Adult Intelligence Scale (e.g. WAIS-R UK; Wechsler, 1986) were consistently among the lowest subtest scores on the overall tests both for children (Udwin et al., 1987) and for adults (Howlin et al., 1998). More recently, number ability has been explored analytically and the evidence highlights a distinct profile of strengths and weaknesses across numerical tasks (e.g. Ansari et al., 2003; Paterson et al., 2006). As we turn our attention to older children and adults with WS, it becomes appropriate to consider numerical cognition in terms of language-dependent and language-independent systems. This is particularly important in that some syndromes present with relatively stronger language than nonverbal cognition, whereas others present with the opposite pattern.

If the WS cognitive profile of weak visuospatial skills and relatively stronger verbal skills were reflected in their performance on mathematical tasks, one might expect that children and adults with WS would show stronger performance on verbally mediated number tasks than on number tasks that draw on visuospatial processes. The opposite profile in DS, of weaker verbal and relatively stronger nonverbal abilities, would predict the opposite pattern. We will now review studies that have investigated these predictions. In doing so, it is important to bear in mind that development is unlikely to be simply delayed and yet proceed along a typical developmental trajectory, because it is impacted not only by early impairments in the number system itself, but also by atypical interactions with other systems such as attention and working memory.

One of the early studies of numeracy in atypical older children and adults with WS and DS (Paterson et al., 2006) explored number using a battery of tasks designed to tap verbal number competency (exact-number system) and the symbolic distance effect (approximate magnitude judgements). In the magnitude judgement task, older children and adults were presented rapidly with two displays of dots that either had a small difference between them (e.g. 5 versus 6, known as a 'close split') or a large difference between them (e.g. 5 versus 9; a 'far split'). Participants were asked to judge as rapidly as possible which display had the larger number of dots. In typical development, a distance effect emerges whereby displays with a close split elicit longer response times than those with a far split (Moyer & Landauer, 1973). Evidence of this pattern of results indicates a reliance on a mental number line, where numbers very close together are less easy to discriminate than numbers far apart on the line. Paterson and colleagues report that a robust symbolic distance effect emerged for the participants with DS (mean age: 24 years, range: 11-35 years), compared with a much weaker symbolic distance effect for those with WS (mean age: 21 years, range: 10-32 years). The relative difficulty with magnitude comparisons in the WS group compared with the DS group is reminiscent of the findings observed in infancy for large-number discrimination discussed earlier. Thus, it seems that a deficit in large-number discrimination in infancy has cascading effects on the later development of magnitude representation in childhood and adulthood in WS.

The number battery used by Paterson et al. (2006) assessed both general number knowledge and knowledge of arithmetic operations. In the number knowledge section, participants were asked to: count forward and backwards; say which number came before or after a given spoken number; read aloud Arabic numerals; put cards of Arabic numerals or dot patterns into serial order; and match cards with dot displays to Arabic numerals. The arithmetic knowledge section involved asking participants to respond to visually presented addition, subtraction and multiplication questions. The findings across the two groups were interesting. The WS group was able to count forward to 20 and read single digits without making errors, but overall they turned out to perform significantly more poorly than the DS group, as well as the MA- and CA-matched typically developing (TD) control groups. In particular, the WS group was hampered by poor memory for number facts (e.g. when counting from 25 to 35 and in the 'What comes next?' or 'What comes before?' tasks). Interestingly, the weakest performances in the WS group were in the dot seriation task and addition and subtraction. If poor knowledge of number fact retrieval in WS forced them to try to calculate addition and subtraction in real time, then poor performance on all three of these tasks may well be linked to the impaired approximate-number system in WS, with its roots in early infancy.

The error patterns in the more verbal tasks are also interesting to consider. These were characterised in WS by errors of syntax, in which class boundaries were not adhered to and the approximate size of the number was not preserved. For example, participants with WS tended to read 250 as 2500. This again seems to reflect a lack of appreciation of magnitude. Interestingly, similar errors were not observed in the DS group. Although ceiling performance in the DS group precludes a detailed characterisation of their profile of performance, it nonetheless indicates that in this battery of tasks, individuals with DS have superior number abilities relative to individuals with WS. Although approximate-number discrimination seems weak at all ages in WS, support for a relative strength in exact-number representations in WS seems to be task-dependent, reflecting the complex nature of interacting cognitive systems that are drawn upon to complete even a seemingly simple task. Tasks that call on number facts require good rote memory, whereas verbal representation of numbers requires understanding of the semantics and syntax of the number system, both of which are problematic for individuals with WS.

Other research groups have also studied verbal and nonverbal number competencies in WS. Similarly to Paterson and colleagues (2006), Krajcsi and collaborators (2009) measured both exact- and approximate-number discrimination. Participants comprised a WS group (mean age: 17 years 8 months, range: 12-23 years) and three TD groups aged 8, 9 and 10 years, respectively. The symbolic distance effect was measured in a magnitude comparison task, in which participants were asked to judge which of two numerals between 1 and 8 was larger. Exact-number competency was assessed using addition and multiplication tasks, in which participants judged whether visually presented calculations, for example $8 + 2 = 10$, were correct or incorrect. Despite some methodological difficulties (fixed order of task presentation, analysis only of response time and not accuracy), at first blush the results seem to lend some support to the predicted disparity between a stronger language-mediated exact-number system and a weaker nonverbal approximate-number system in WS. All groups of participants showed a symbolic distance effect on the magnitude comparison task, which indicates that the task tapped into approximate-number representation in both the WS and the three TD groups. However, the WS group responded more slowly on this task than the three TD groups. By contrast, performance was in line with the 8- and 9-year-olds in the addition task, and in line with all three TD groups for multiplication judgements. Thus, poorer performance on the magnitude task in WS can be taken as evidence of an impaired (nonverbal) magnitude system but better verbal retrieval ability. However, this is based on response time only. As mentioned, analysis of accuracy was not included, but from examining the published proportions of errors in the WS group it does not seem that there was any within-group difference for accuracy across tasks (the mean error rates were: 15% for magnitude comparison, 14% for addition and 19% for multiplication). It might also be argued that addition can be carried out using a mental number line (see discussion in Dehaene et al., 2003), although the authors do report similar patterns of responses across groups, which provides some indication that the TD and WS groups drew on similar mechanisms to complete the tasks.

Taking a more standardised approach to mathematical cognition, O'Hearn and Landau (2007) administered the Test of Early Mathematical Ability Second Edition (TEMA-II; Ginsburg & Baroody, 1990) to children and adults with WS (age range: 10-38 years). This comprises a series of numerical questions, standardised for ages 2 to 8 years. Rather than assessing each area independently as separate subtests, the TEMA-II assesses abilities within a single series of questions, with question sequence dictated by the typical development of numerical competences. Given the age group of individuals with WS targeted, assessment began with questions aimed at the level for 4-year-old TD children, and it was simply assumed that the questions preceding this would have all been correctly answered. However, given that individuals with neurodevelopmental disorders are likely to follow atypical developmental trajectories in numerical development (Ansari & Karmiloff-Smith, 2002), following the TEMA-II for individuals developing atypically assumes an even profile of abilities measured by items of sequentially increasing difficulty. Although it is possible that success with questions aimed at TD 4-year-olds is preceded by success with all classes of questions aimed at a younger age group, it is also possible that some classes of questions pose more difficulty than others and might not have been answered successfully by someone with a neurodevelopmental disorder, had they been administered.

The O'Hearn and Landau study showed that the WS group had similar overall TEMA-II performance to that of the 6-year-old TD controls. However, verbal and nonverbal composite scores yielded divergent profiles. Verbal items included counting, reading and writing numerals, whereas nonverbal items included items that assessed the mental number line, adding objects and the concept of 'more'. As with some of the other studies reported earlier, the items included in each composite were based on the authors' knowledge of typical development, but may well be subjective when applied to an atypical group. One solution would have been to report correlational analyses between performance on the verbal and nonverbal subtests of the Kaufman Brief Intelligence Test (Kaufman & Kaufman, 1990) and TEMA-II verbal and nonverbal composite scores, respectively. Nevertheless, the results yielded no group differences on the verbal composite but relatively weaker performance on the nonverbal composite in the WS group compared with TD controls. This is consistent with the strong influence of verbal ability on TEMA performance reported in young children with WS (mean age: 6 years) in Chapter 18. This study therefore adds further evidence to the findings reported earlier that the approximate-number system is impaired in WS. It does not, however, speak to the developmental origins of this deficit or to the impact of these origins on subsequent development.

In summary, some of the number studies reviewed in this chapter do not take the neuro-constructivist, developmental approach at all and focus solely on either a snapshot in childhood or on the phenotypic end state. Yet, developmental interactions between brain, environment and behaviour strongly influence the cognitive mechanisms that drive performance. As such, tasks purported to call on verbal or nonverbal skills in TD groups might not be driven by verbal or nonverbal mechanisms, respectively, in an atypical group.

Ansari and colleagues (2003) took this more neuroconstructivist approach in their exploration of the cardinality principle in WS. The cardinality principle refers to the ability to know that the total number of objects in a set is the same as the last number produced in a number sequence when counting those objects. When children are presented with a 'How many?' task (Gelman & Gallistel, 1978; Wynn, 1990), they do one of two things: they either use the cardinality principle and say the last number enumerated or, when they are younger and do not understand cardinality, they count the objects sequentially, but when asked 'So, how many?', they simply recount the objects all over again. 'How many?' generates a counting procedure that, at the younger age, is not underpinned by an understanding that the final number represents the cardinality of the set. Karen Wynn devised a nice study for TD children to bring out this difference. In her 'give-a-number' task (Wynn, 1990, 1992), she presented children with a bowl of marbles and asked them to give her four marbles, six marbles and so on. In other words, instead of asking 'How many?' her task encouraged children to reveal whether they understood the function of counting, that is, she differentiated between those who could count (a little like a sequential poem) and those who knew what counting was for. Her results showed that when asked to get a given number of marbles, children below 3.5 years of age merely gathered together a handful of objects (they were 'grabbers'), whereas older children counted out the number requested ('counters'), thus demonstrating a conceptual shift at about 3 years, at which time children make a link between counting and cardinality (Wynn, 1990).

Ansari and colleagues (2003) used two tasks, one of which was Wynn's give-a-number task, to examine whether children with WS who could count actually had the cardinality principle. The WS participants (age range: 6-11 years) were compared with TD children (age range: 2-5 years). The first task asked children to help a puppet who did not know how to count. They were presented with two to six animals stuck to a board and asked: 'Tell the puppet how many animals there are'. The second task replicated Wynn's design described earlier. For both tasks, there was no group difference in the number of correct responses given, and in the give-a-number task, both groups were more accurate (made fewer errors) when giving the puppet between one and three marbles (small numbers) than when giving the puppet between four and six marbles (large numbers). However, this lack of group difference changed when the WS group was split into a high-language group and a low-language group (visuospatial ability was equivalent between the two subgroups). While the high-language group performed consistently at or close to ceiling, the low-language group was significantly worse at giving both small and large numbers of marbles to the puppet, with chance performance for large numbers. Thus, the language abilities of the participants with WS seem to be associated with differential performance on these number tasks. This was supported by correlational analyses that demonstrated an association between verbal abilities and give-a-number performance in the children with WS but not in TD children, and between visuospatial abilities and performance in TD children but not in those with WS. Thus, even though as a group the WS and TD groups exhibited similar overt performance, it is only through measuring the contributions of verbal and visuospatial abilities to performance that one can start to uncover the differing developmental trajectories, that is, the fact that the WS group's performance is driven by different cognitive mechanisms from the TD group, indicative of an atypical number trajectory in WS. This indicates that in WS development, poor visuospatial skills may be compensated for by better language abilities. However, Ansari and colleagues note that verbal ability does not offer complete compensation, because the WS group was still performing below the level expected of their verbal mental age. The capacity for language to compensate is therefore still constrained by the visuospatial deficits of the individual and by the visuospatial demands of the task.

In a subsequent study, Ansari et al. (2007) asked children (mean CA: 10 years) and adults (mean CA: 29 years) with WS and four TD groups (4-5 years, 6-7 years, 9-10 years, adults) to estimate as quickly as possible how many dots were in a visual display. The number of dots presented was 2, 3, 5, 7, 9 or 11. To stop participants from counting the dots, displays were presented for 250 ms and participants were told not to count but to guess, with the emphasis on speed rather than accuracy. Numbers up to 3 were identified with 100% accuracy by all groups. However, larger numbers elicited less accurate responses, thus providing evidence for differences in how large and small numbers are processed in the TD and WS groups. The successful results with small numbers indicate either that individuals with WS are able to subitise (see also O'Hearn et al., 2011), that is, they have the ability to say how many items are in a display without needing to count them, or they are linked to abilities to track individual objects, provided in both cases that the number does not exceed 4. Absolute accuracy in the WS group as a whole was 20%, with approximate accuracy (responses within ±1) at 35.5% for the children and 49% for the adults with WS. This is comparable with the TD children aged 4-5 years, who displayed 15% absolute accuracy and 43% approximate accuracy, but is substantially lower than the performance of the TD children aged 6-7 years (absolute accuracy: 27%, approximate accuracy: 64.5%). The authors note the limited developmental progression in estimation accuracy from childhood to adulthood in individuals with WS, who had a mean difference in CA of nearly 20 years but only showed the equivalent of 2 years of developmental progression (i.e. the difference in accuracy between TD children aged 4-5 years and those aged 6-7 years).

Ansari and colleagues (2007) suggested that this relative lack of developmental progression indicates that the ability to represent magnitude and link these representations with symbols (i.e. numbers) does not develop over time in WS to nearly the same extent as it does in typical development. The authors speculate that in TD development, magnitude representations become 'more discrete' (Ansari et al., 2007), that is, less overlapping, facilitating more accurate representations and links to numerical symbols. However, they argue that if this does not occur in WS, then it would account for both the low accuracy rates for larger numbers and the slow developmental progression in the WS group.

Conclusions

If scientists allowed the adult end state to determine their assumptions about earlier developmental points, our knowledge of WS and other neurodevelopmental disorders would, by definition, be restricted to the phenotypic profile seen in adulthood and constitute a static view of neurodevelopmental disorders. By contrast, the neuroconstructivist framework of studying the dynamics of the developmental trajectories over time from infancy through to adulthood makes it possible to better understand the developmental process itself and to examine cross-domain relations that may not be obvious in the adult end state.

In summary, the characteristic visuospatial weakness in WS (see Chapter 12) constrains numerical cognition in this population, with evidence for impaired performance on tasks that draw on the approximate-number system, such as large-number discrimination in infancy (Van Herwegen et al., 2008), and magnitude comparison and estimation tasks later in ontogeny (Ansari et al., 2007; Paterson et al., 2006; Krajcsi et al., 2009). Development of this system also seems to follow an atypical developmental trajectory. Ansari and colleagues have demonstrated that performance on counting tasks typically associated with visuospatial competence are driven by verbal abilities in WS (Ansari et al., 2003), pointing to compensatory mechanisms that impact positively, albeit in a limited way, on performance.

In addition, estimation of magnitude shows very limited developmental progression in WS, which is also indicative of qualitative differences in how magnitude is processed in this group. A clue to why individuals with WS do more poorly than those with DS in magnitude estimation comes from recent work examining eye tracking of numerical displays. As mentioned earlier, infants with DS tend to scan the entire array, whereas those with WS tend to stay focused on a few nearby items (Karmiloff-Smith et al., submitted). This would suggest than scanning may allow participants either to focus on quantities, as the DS scanning patterns reveal, or on individual items, as the WS scanning patterns reveal. This has implications for training number in WS. Rather than focus on number intervention in school-age children, when number deficits reveal themselves, Karmiloff-Smith (2009) suggests that it should occur very early in infancy and perhaps not focus on number per se but on the scanning patterns that underlie numerical processing. This is consistent with evidence from TD populations suggesting that numerical development initially involves a network of interacting systems, including those involved in attention, memory and visuospatial cognition (Rivera et al., 2005).

Evidently, there is still much to learn about number development in WS, and several of the few existing studies on atypical number cognition—while providing useful data—are limited because they are not truly developmental in the spirit of neuroconstructivism. For example, studies that do not consider the effects of atypical development on the nature of task performance (Krajcsi et al., 2009; O'Hearn & Landau, 2007) make it difficult to interpret any reported behavioural deviations. Future studies, both longitudinal studies and those building task-specific cross-sectional trajectories, should examine cross-domain interactions across developmental time. It is also critical to make cross-syndrome comparisons so that we can determine what is syndrome-general by virtue of having a neurodevelopmental disorder and what is syndrome-specific to impairments in numerical cognition.

Editor commentary (Emily K. Farran & Annette Karmiloff-Smith)

Numerical processing is fundamental to human infants, children and adults and to numerous other species, so when it is impaired, as in many neurodevelopmental syndromes, it poses a serious problem to developmental outcomes. The authors take a neuroconstructivist stance by seeking the infancy precursors to number development, trying to elucidate how contributions from different domain-general processes impact on the emerging domain-specific numerical outcome.

With WS taken as the model disorder, they showed how attention and eye movement scanning of arrays can either focus the infant on individual objects, as in WS, or on approximate quantities, as in DS. These early differences were shown to impact on the differing developmental trajectories of these two syndromes, giving rise to better ultimate numerical abilities in DS (albeit still impaired in comparison with controls) than in WS. So, a small difference early on simply in the way that infants look at the environment can have cascading effects on the phenotypic outcome, with individuals with WS repeatedly showing deficits in the approximate-number system.

Finally, this chapter emphasised the importance of focusing on differences across syndromes in error patterns—as opposed to final levels of performance, where cross-domain relations may no longer be obvious—to clarify why behavioural outcomes that can seem superficially similar are in fact based on very different underlying cognitive processes.

Interestingly, cross-domain interactions differ as development proceeds, with language levels predicting cardinality abilities in WS but visuospatial abilities being related to cardinality in typical development. Comparisons in this chapter between WS and DS emphasise that exploration of associations and dissociations across syndrome groups that show impaired number and mathematical processing, such as developmental dyscalculia, fragile X syndrome and specific language impairment, are important for our understanding of developmental timing of the emergence of number and its precursors, developmental cross-domain interactions and developmental trajectories that lead to phenotypic profiles.

References

Ansari, D. (2010). Neurocognitive approaches to developmental disorders of numerical and mathematical cognition: The perils of neglecting the role of development. *Learning and Individual Differences*, 20, 123–29.

Ansari, D., & Dhital, B. (2006). Age-related changes in the activation of the intraparietal sulcus during nonsymbolic magnitude processing: an event-related functional magnetic resonance imaging study. *Journal of Cognitive Neuroscience*, 18, 1820–28.

Ansari, D., Donlan, C., & Karmiloff-Smith, A. (2007). Typical and atypical development of visual estimation abilities. *Cortex*, 43, 758–68.

Ansari, D., Donlan, C., Thomas, M.S., Ewing, S.A., Peen, T., & Karmiloff-Smith, A. (2003). What makes counting count? Verbal and visuo-spatial contributions to typical and atypical number development. *J Exp Child Psychol*, 85, 50–62.

Ansari, D., Garcia, N., Lucas, E., Hamon, K., & Dhital, B. (2005). Neural correlates of symbolic number processing in children and adults. *NeuroReport*, 16, 1769–73.

Ansari, D., & Karmiloff-Smith, A. (2002). Atypical trajectories of number development: a neuroconstructivist perspective. *Trends in Cognitive Sciences, 6,* 511–16.

Brown, J.H., Johnson, M.H., Paterson, S.J., Gilmore, R., Longhi, E., & Karmiloff-Smith, A. (2003). Spatial representation and attention in toddlers with Williams syndrome and Down syndrome. *Neuropsychologia, 41,* 1037–46.

Cantlon, J.F., Libertus, M.E., Pinel, P., Dehaene, S., Brannon, E.M., & Pelphrey, K.A. (2009). The neural development of an abstract concept of number. *Journal of Cognitive Neuroscience, 21,* 2217–29.

Carey, S. (2001). Cognitive foundations of arithmetic: evolution and ontogenisis. *Mind & Language, 16,* 37–55.

Corbetta, M., Kincade, J.M., Ollinger, J.M., McAvoy, M.P., & Shulman, G.L. (2000). Voluntary orienting is dissociated from target detection in human posterior parietal cortex. *Nature neuroscience, 3,* 292–97.

Dehaene, S., Molko, N., Cohen, L., & Wilson, A.J. (2004). Arithmetic and the brain. *Current Opinion in Neurobiology, 14,* 218–24.

Dehaene, S., Piazza, M., Pinel, P., & Cohen, L. (2003). Three parietal circuits for number processing. *Cognitive Neuropsychology, 20,* 487–506.

Farran, E.K., Jarrold, C., & Gathercole, S.E. (2001). Block design performance in the williams syndrome phenotype: a problem with mental imagery? *Journal of Child Psychology and Psychiatry, 42,* 719–28.

Feigenson, L., Dehaene, S., & Spelke, E. (2004). Core systems of number. *Trends in Cognitive Sciences, 8,* 307–314.

Gelman, R., & Gallistel, C.R. (1978). *The Child's Understanding of Number.* Cambridge, MA: Harvard University Press.

Ginsburg, H., & Baroody, A. (1990). *Test of Early Mathematics Ability Second Edition.* Austin, TX: Pro-Ed.

Holloway, I.D., & Ansari, D. (2010). Developmental specialization in the right intraparietal sulcus for the abstract representation of numerical magnitude. *Journal of Cognitive Neuroscience, 22,* 2627–37.

Howlin, P., Davies, M., & Udwin, O. (1998). Syndrome specific characteristics in Williams syndrome: to what extent do early behavioural patterns persist into adult life? *Journal of Applied Research in Intellectual Disabilities, 11,* 207–226.

Isaacs, E.B., Edmonds, C.J., Lucas, A., & Gadian, D.G. (2001). Calculation difficulties in children of very low birthweight. *Brain, 124,* 1701–1707.

Karmiloff-Smith, A. (1998). Development itself is the key to understanding developmental disorders. *Trends in Cognitive Sciences, 2,* 389–98.

Karmiloff-Smith, A. (2009). Nativism versus neuroconstructivism: rethinking the study of developmental disorders. *Developmental Psychology, 45,* 56–63.

Karmiloff-Smith, A. (2011). Static snapshots versus dynamic approaches to genes, brain, cognition and behaviour in neurodevelopmental disorders. *International Review of Research on Developmental Disabilities, 40,* 1–16.

Karmiloff-Smith, A., D'Souza, D., Van Herwegen, J., Dekker, T., Rodic, M., Xu, F., et al. (submitted). Adult neuropsychology models: Inappropriate for neurodevelopmental genetic syndromes.

Kaufman, A.S., & Kaufman, N.L. (1990). *Kaufman Brief Intelligence Test First Edition.* Circle Pines, MN: American Guidance Service.

Krajcsi, A., Lukács, Á., Igács, J., Racsmány, M., & Pléh, C. (2009). Numerical abilities in Williams syndrome: dissociating the analogue magnitude system and verbal retrieval. *Journal of Clinical and Experimental Neuropsychology, 31,* 439–46.

Le Corre, M., & Carey, S. (2007). One, two, three, four, nothing more: an investigation of the conceptual sources of the verbal counting principles. *Cognition, 105,* 395–438.

Meyer-Lindenberg, A., Kohn, P., Mervis, C.B., Kippenhan, J.S., Olsen, R.K., Morris, C.A., et al. (2004). Neural basis of genetically determined visuospatial construction deficit in Williams syndrome. *Neuron, 43,* 623–31.

Moyer, R.S., & Landauer, T.K. (1967). Time required for judgements of numerical inequality. *Nature*, **215**, 1519–20.

Moyer, R.S., & Landauer, T.K. (1973). Determinants of reaction time for digit inequality judgments. *Bulletin of the Psychonomic Society*, **1**, 167–68.

O'Hearn, K., Hoffman, J., & Landau, B. (2011). Small subitizing range in people with Williams syndrome. *Visual Cognition*, **19**, 289–312.

O'Hearn, K., & Landau, B. (2007). Mathematical skill in individuals with Williams syndrome: evidence from a standardized mathematics battery. *Brain and Cognition*, **64**, 238–46.

Paterson, S.J., Brown, J.H., Gsodl, M.K., Johnson, M.H., & Karmiloff-Smith, A. (1999). Cognitive modularity and genetic disorders. *Science*, **286**, 2355–58.

Paterson, S.J., Girelli, L., Butterworth, B., & Karmiloff-Smith, A. (2006). Are numerical impairments syndrome specific? Evidence from Williams syndrome and Down's syndrome. *Journal of Child Psychology and Psychiatry*, **47**, 190–204.

Rivera, S.M., Reiss, A.L., Eckert, M.A., & Menon, V. (2005). Developmental changes in mental arithmetic: evidence for increased functional specialization in the left inferior parietal cortex. *Cerebral Cortex*, **15**, 1779–90.

Simon, T.J. (1997). Reconceptualizing the origins of number knowledge: a "non-numerical" account. *Cognitive Development*, **12**, 349–72.

Stanescu-Cosson, R., Pinel, P., van de Moortele, P.-F., Le Bihan, D., Cohen, L., & Dehaene, S. (2000). Understanding dissociations in dyscalculia. *Brain*, **123**, 2240–55.

Udwin, O., Yule, W., & Martin, N. (1987). Cognitive abilities and behavioural characteristics of children with idiopathic infantile hypercalcaemia. *Journal of Child Psychology and Psychiatry*, **28**, 297–309.

Uller, C., Carey, S., Huntley-Fenner, G., & Klatt, L. (1999). What representations might underlie infant numerical knowledge?'. *Cognitive Development*, **14**, 1–36.

Van Herwegen, J., Ansari, D., Xu, F., & Karmiloff-Smith, A. (2008). Small and large number processing in infants and toddlers with Williams syndrome. *Developmental Science*, **11**, 637–43.

Wechsler, D. (1976). *Wechsler Intelligence Scale for Children—Revised*. Windsor: NFER-Nelson.

Wechsler, D. (1986). *Wechsler Adult Intelligence Scale—Revised UK*. London: The Psychological Association.

Wynn, K. (1990). Children's understanding of counting. *Cognition*, **36**, 155–93.

Wynn, K. (1992). Children's acquisition of the number words and the counting system. *Cognitive Psychology*, **24**, 220–51.

Xu, F., & Arriaga, R.I. (2007). Number discrimination in 10-month-old infants. *British Journal of Developmental Psychology*, **25**, 103–108.

Xu, F., & Spelke, E.S. (2000). Large number discrimination in 6-month-old infants. *Cognition*, **74**, B1–B11.

Xu, F., Spelke, E.S., & Goddard, S. (2005). Number sense in human infants. *Developmental Science*, **8**, 88–101.

Chapter 17

Literacy

Yvonne M. Griffiths

Introduction

There has been a dearth of research investigating reading development in children with general learning difficulties (Saunders, 2007). Williams syndrome (WS) is no exception, with a handful of published studies on literacy development over the past 20 years for this neurodevelopmental disorder across three different languages (English: Howlin et al., 1998; Laing et al., 2001; Levy et al., 2003; Udwin et al., 1987; Udwin et al., 1996; Italian: Menghini et al., 2004; Spanish: Garayzabal & Cuetos, 2008).

A strong foundation in spoken-language skills is essential for reading development, with phonological skills (i.e. speech processing) the main driver of early word reading in typically developing (TD) children. Higher oral language skills (e.g. vocabulary, semantics and grammar skills), coupled with a solid foundation in word reading skill, are essential for skilled reading comprehension (for a review see Snowling & Hulme, 2006). Since verbal language skills (including phonological coding skills) are reported as a characteristic strength in the WS phenotypic profile (see Chapter 11), it would be reasonable to predict that reading might be a relative area of strength for the syndrome.

Evidence from recent reviews of the literature on reading development in WS has revealed severe, persisting word reading difficulties, with end-state reading levels for adults falling within the range of TD children aged 6-9 years (Howlin et al., 1998). However, similar to other learning difficulties, there is wide individual variation in reported levels of word reading ability and reading comprehension is typically weaker than word reading ability in WS (for reviews see Laing, 2002; Mervis, 2009; Snowling & Hulme, 2005).

Theoretical explanations for the reading difficulties and variation in reading outcomes in WS are limited by the absence of evidence from longitudinal studies and intervention research. This chapter will review the evidence on reading development in WS and two other genetically based neurodevelopmental disorders of language: dyslexia, a specific learning difficulty, and Down syndrome (DS), which is characterised by general learning difficulties. Dyslexia is the most common and comprehensively studied learning disability (Shaywitz et al., 2008) with evidence from a large body of research investigating the dyslexic phenotypic profile of reading and cognitive-linguistic skills across the lifespan (for reviews see Hulme & Snowling, 2009; Vellutino et al., 2004), with phonological processing deficits at its core. This research has led to effective theoretically based reading interventions for dyslexia (for reviews see Duff & Clarke, 2010; Griffiths & Stuart, 2011). DS involves a general learning difficulty with a contrasting cognitive-linguistic profile to WS and there is a larger body of literature on reading development than in WS, including some evidence from longitudinal and intervention studies (Byrne et al., 2002; Cupples & Iacono, 2000; Goetz et al., 2008; Kay-Raining Bird et al., 2000; Laws & Gunn, 2002; Lemons & Fuchs, 2010; for reviews see Ehri & Snowling, 2004; Snowling et al., 2008). Specifically, this chapter will focus on evidence from research examining early word reading development and the role of phonological and higher oral language (particularly vocabulary and semantics) as predictors of individual differences in reading development in WS.

By taking a developmental approach to the study of reading in WS and other learning difficulties, this chapter will begin with a short review of the literature on typical reading development, with a focus on the role of phonological and higher oral language in early word reading development. This will provide a theoretical framework to consider how and why the processes involved in typical reading development may be impaired in children with learning difficulties. An examination of the similarities and differences in phenotypic reading and cognitive-linguistic profiles across WS, DS and dyslexia will identify possible syndrome-specific or general cognitive-linguistic factors contributing to variation in the severity of reading difficulties and outcomes. Finally, I will consider practical implications for reading intervention for individuals with WS.

Typical reading development

There is a large body of evidence demonstrating that a strong foundation in spoken-language skills is essential for reading development (Snowling & Hulme, 2006; for a review see Bowey, 2005). However, many factors contribute to reading development and its difficulties, including genetic, cognitive and linguistic factors and variation in the environments that individuals experience as learners.

The goal of reading is to extract meaning from print, and children need to gain competence in two components of reading comprehension to become a skilled reader: word recognition (converting printed words to spoken words) and linguistic comprehension (understanding the meaning carried by spoken language). According to the 'simple view of reading' (Hoover & Gough, 1990), reading comprehension is the product of these two necessary components. Evidence from studies of typical development and reading disorders indicates that both skills are interdependent, but rely on different spoken-language foundation skills as well as other cognitive processes (for a review see Stuart et al., 2008). Word recognition depends on a strong foundation in phonological skills (speech processing skills), whereas linguistic comprehension depends on a solid foundation in broader oral language skills (vocabulary, semantics, grammar; e.g. Muter et al., 2004; Nation et al., 2010).

Most children acquire competence in both skills and become good readers. Others have difficulties with both skills and have general reading difficulties. However, some children have specific difficulties acquiring one of these skills but not the other. Dyslexia is the profile of reading difficulty where children struggle to acquire word recognition, but typically have much less difficulty with reading comprehension (for a review see Hulme & Snowling, 2009). A 'poor comprehender' profile is the reading difficulty where children acquire competence in word recognition skills, but show poor linguistic (reading and listening) comprehension (for a review see Nation, 2005). However, 'pure' dissociations are rare in development (Bishop, 1997) and children's profiles of reading difficulties will be influenced by continuous variation in the severity of difficulty associated with each dimension (Bishop & Snowling, 2004; Pennington & Bishop, 2009).

A framework for word reading development

Ehri's phase theory (for a review see Ehri, 2005) is an influential model of how TD children progress from being a nonreader to a skilled word reader. It describes how different word reading strategies emerge during reading development, as their knowledge of the writing system develops and relations are formed between spoken and written language.

There are various ways to read words. Children need to be able to read words they have not seen before, but they also need to read familiar words with ease and automaticity (Ehri, 2005). Phonological decoding is an important strategy for reading new words, involving the ability to decipher printed words and translate pronunciations by learning that most letters map on to speech sounds in a systematic way. It requires the identification of the sounds of individual letters (or clusters of letters), holding them in mind and blending them into pronunciations that are recognised as real words. Children who are able to use phonological decoding are described as having mastered the 'alphabetic principle' (Byrne, 1998).

There is also a reciprocal relationship between a child's developing phoneme awareness and their early phonological reading skills, including letter knowledge (Burgess & Lonigan, 1998). Phonological-awareness skill is the ability to identify and manipulate units of sounds in spoken words, such as large units (rime and syllable) or small units (phonemes) of sounds. Phonological-awareness development usually proceeds from awareness of large to small units, e.g. the spoken word 'pin' can either be segmented into the large onset–rime unit/p-In/or into small phonemic units, as in/p-I-n/(Carroll et al., 2003; Goswami & Bryant, 1990). Phoneme awareness skills can be assessed by tasks such as phoneme blending or segmentation. Tasks involving the deletion or transposition of sounds are harder than those requiring comparison or identification, with the segmentation of initial sounds being easier than that of final or medial sounds within spoken words (e.g. Johnston et al., 1996; Yopp, 1988).

Phonological decoding skills are typically measured by assessing a child's ability to read aloud lists of unfamiliar letter strings (e.g. 'prab', 'hin', 'stansert') that obey the phonotactics of their native language. This involves segmentation and blending of letter sound mappings. A nonword reading difficulty is a strong behavioural marker of dyslexia (e.g. van Ijzendoorn & Bus, 1994), with phonological processing skills a concurrent predictor of individual variation in nonword reading (Griffiths & Snowling, 2002).

By contrast, sight word reading (or orthographic learning) refers to a strategy involving memory to automatically read words that have been read before, where 'sight of the word activates its spelling, pronunciation and meaning immediately in memory' (Ehri & Snowling, 2004). According to Ehri's theory, sight word reading is a process dependent on alphabetic knowledge. Initially, children use a partial alphabetic strategy, where they establish partial connections in memory on the basis of the letter sounds they know; for example, they may be able to decode the initial and final letter sounds, but not the medial vowels. Experience of reading new words using a decoding strategy and increased familiarity with the mappings between letters and sounds will establish whole-word-specific orthographic representations in memory, expanding the child's sight word vocabulary (for a review of the self-teaching hypothesis see Share, 2008).

Sight word reading is a faster, more automatic process than a phonological decoding strategy. It is also a more effective strategy for reading irregular words in English, which have inconsistent mappings between letters and sounds. Once children have mastered the mechanics of context-free word reading, this frees up cognitive processing resources when reading connected text, and linguistic comprehension becomes a more important influence on the developing reading system than it used to be earlier in development.

However, the acquisition of accurate and fluent word reading is not the same as being a skilled reader. For some poor readers who master the alphabetic principle and acquire a sight word vocabulary, their reading comprehension of text may still be weak (i.e. poor comprehenders) owing to limited comprehension strategies (e.g. inferencing; Cain et al., 2004) or weak nonphonological oral language skills (Nation et al., 2010).

Phonological skills as predictors of word reading

There is strong evidence supporting the view that phoneme awareness skills are strong longitudinal predictors of typical word reading development (e.g. Muter et al., 2004; Wagner et al., 1994) and better longitudinal predictors of early word reading progress than rime awareness (Muter et al., 2004; Savage & Carless, 2005). Letter knowledge has also been found to be a strong predictor of early word reading (Byrne, 1998; Muter et al., 2004). Both skills co-determine the acquisition of the alphabetic principle (Bowey, 2005).

The predictive role of phoneme awareness for word reading development is stronger in English than in transparent alphabetic orthographies (i.e. writing systems) such as Italian, where phoneme awareness predicts only very early growth in word reading ability (for a review see Seymour, 2005). In transparent orthographies, mappings between letters and sounds are highly regular and alphabetic knowledge is mastered earlier than in English. Performance in rapid automatised naming (RAN) is also an independent predictor of variation in early word reading development in English (for a review see Bowey, 2005). RAN tasks are another measure of phonological processing and require the individual to name visually presented arrays of familiar items (e.g. letters, digits, colours, objects) as quickly as possible. Alphanumeric RAN (letter or digit naming), in particular, is a stronger independent predictor of word reading growth than phonological awareness in transparent orthographies (e.g. Lervag et al., 2009), particularly reading fluency.

Other measures of phonological processing, such as verbal-memory span, are also longitudinal predictors of word reading in typical development, with visual span being a weaker predictor of early word reading development than verbal span (e.g. Caravolas et al., 2001).

Oral language skills in word reading development

Although there is agreement that phonological processing skills are essential for phonological decoding skills, which in turn are important for the acquisition of a sight word vocabulary (e.g. Share, 2008), the role of semantic and other oral language skills in context-free early word reading (i.e. orthographic learning) is a controversial issue (e.g. Laing & Hulme, 1999; Nation & Cocksey, 2009). Ehri's phase model is silent as to the role of semantic processes in context-free word recognition. However, her phase model recognises the role of semantic and syntactic contextual cues to support word recognition for the reader still developing their phonological decoding skills (the partial alphabetic phase), or when trying to read unfamiliar irregular words in text (Ehri & Snowling, 2004). The use of this 'prediction from context' strategy presupposes strengths in higher oral language skills (e.g. Frith & Snowling, 1983). Connectionist frameworks have proved useful for conceptualising the role of phonological and semantic knowledge in developmental theories, such as Ehri's, that see word reading as a highly interactive process in typical development (Snowling & Hulme, 2006). According to Plaut et al.'s (1996) triangle model, during the early stages of word reading, resources are committed to establishing mappings between orthographic and phonological representations (the phonological pathway). In the later stages, activation from semantic information via the semantic pathway (orthography to phonology via semantics) is also involved in the process of reading, providing additional support to the phonological pathway. This has the effect of the semantic pathway supporting the reading of irregular words, which cannot be read by solely relying on the phonological pathway. With training, the two routes eventually become more specialised to deal with different types of words (for a review see Nation & Cocksey, 2009).

Several studies have reported a strong association between irregular word reading and receptive (Bowey & Rutherford, 2007; Goff et al., 2005) or expressive vocabulary (Ouellette, 2006; Ricketts et al., 2007), providing support for the triangle model. Furthermore, recent evidence supports the view that semantic knowledge may be important in the later stages of context-free word reading development (Plaut et al., 1996), and lexical phonology (familiarity with the phonological forms of words), not semantic knowledge, is associated with early word reading development (Nation & Cocksey, 2009).

Finally, social factors are also known to influence early literacy development (Phillips & Lonigan, 2005). These include socioeconomic status, preschool experiences and home literacy environment. The home literacy environment has been shown to have at least a modest effect on phonological processing skills, letter knowledge and oral language in typical development (Burgess et al., 2002) and a factor associated with variation in word reading profiles in dyslexia (Jiménez et al., 2009). Possible home literacy environment factors include the frequency of shared reading, parental values of reading and parental expectations of reading potential.

In summary, current theory and evidence on typical reading development supports the view that phonological skill is the main driver of early word reading development, with semantic and broader oral language skills playing an increasing role in the later stages of reading development (Plaut et al., 1996).

Reading development in Williams syndrome

The typical range of IQ for children with WS (between 50 and 65) is similar to that for DS, with nonverbal skills seriously impaired and language skills a relative strength, a pattern that is the opposite to DS. However, as discussed in Chapters 10 and 11, language skills in WS are not necessarily typical. Although there is very little research investigating early and later phonological development in WS, relatively stronger phonological short-term memory (STM) than visuospatial STM has been reported (see Chapter 8).

A review of the small body of literature on reading development in WS (Mervis, 2009) revealed that of the eight published studies spanning three decades, the majority targeted reading development in older children and adults with WS and only one (Udwin et al., 1996) was longitudinal. A comparison across studies is difficult, given methodological differences.

The following questions will be considered. What is the typical level of reading ability achieved by adults with WS? Can individuals with WS use a phonological reading strategy (indexed by nonword reading skill)? Does their phonological system play a crucial role in driving early word reading development? Do reading and reading-related cognitive-linguistic skills follow a typical, albeit delayed, path of development in WS or is the process of reading development qualitatively different from typical development? And finally, is higher oral language a strong predictor of word reading in WS (as it is in DS; Boudreau, 2002; Cardoso-Martins et al., 2009; Laws & Gunn, 2002)?

Typical end-state word reading attainments in Williams syndrome

The current evidence suggests individuals with WS typically have severe reading difficulties, consistent with other neurodevelopmental disorders of language (Snowling & Hulme, 2005). Similar to DS, there is much variability in reading ability within WS groups that is unrelated to age (DS: Ehri & Snowling, 2004; WS: Mervis, 2009; both syndromes: Snowling & Hulme, 2005), and as in DS there is some evidence that word reading ability is relatively stronger than reading comprehension (DS: Byrne et al., 2002; Groen et al., 2006; WS: Howlin et al., 1998; Laing et al., 2001). This is the opposite profile to dyslexia, where word level reading is typically more severely impaired than reading comprehension skill (Catts et al., 2006; Frith & Snowling, 1983; Shaywitz et al., 1999; Snowling & Hulme, 2005). In a UK study of 62 adults with WS (Howlin et al., 1998), with IQs between 50 and 69, the average level of word reading ability was equivalent to a reading age (RA) of 8 years 8 months (range: 6 years to 18 years) and average reading comprehension was equivalent to 7 years 2 months (range: 6 years 3 months to 12 years 6 months). A quarter of the sample was unable to obtain a basal score on the test of single-word reading (RA below 6 years), and yet some individuals were at 'ceiling' on the test (RA 18 years). This suggests a relatively higher level of reading ability for adults with WS than for adults with DS, since the average RA equivalent in the follow-up of Laws and Gunn's (2002) group of adolescents (15-17 years) with DS was 6 years 9 months (range: 5 years 3 months to 11 years 3 months).

Two English-language studies have investigated reading-related cognitive skills in WS (Laing et al., 2001; Levy et al., 2003). Laing et al. (2001) targeted a group of children and adults with WS with a mean age of 15 years 1 month (range: 9 years to 27 years 7 months), and compared their reading profiles with a younger group of TD children (age range: 5-9 years) matched on verbal mental age (MA) and word level RA. The WS group obtained an average RA equivalent of 6 years 10 months on a standardised test of single-word reading, indicating very rudimentary levels of word reading skills for the sample as a whole. The discrepancy between word reading and reading comprehension skills reported by Howlin et al. (1998) was replicated in this study. Similar to the dyslexia phenotype (Stanovich & Siegal, 1994), listening comprehension skills were relatively stronger than reading comprehension skills in this WS group and on a par with their level of verbal ability.

A slightly older sample (mean age: 16 years 5 months) of individuals with WS was studied by Levy et al. (2003); word reading skills were also stronger than in the WS group in the Laing et al. (2001) study, reaching an average level of word reading equivalent to 8 years 6 months. The wide variation in reading attainments within the group and the association between higher IQ and stronger reading ability were in line with other studies of WS and DS (WS: Howlin et al., 1998; Laing et al., 2001; Udwin et al., 1987; DS: Cardoso-Martins & Frith, 2001; Mervis, 2009). By contrast, the IQ is typically a weaker predictor of the severity of reading difficulty in dyslexia (see Hulme & Snowling, 2009).

Garayzabal and Cuetos (2008) included a group of native Spanish children and adolescents with WS, younger in chronological age (CA; range: 8-15 years) than Laing et al.'s (2001) and Levy et al.'s (2003) groups. Their word reading profiles were compared with a younger verbal-MA-matched group of TD children (CA range: 6-9 years). The WS group's reading profiles in Menghini et al.'s (2004) study of native Italian adolescents and adults (mean CA: 17 years 7 months) were also compared with a younger verbal-MA-matched group (CA range: 6-8 years). However, as noted previously, the writing system within which a child learns to read will place constraints on the development of reading and reading-related skills. In particular, phoneme awareness is a predictor of early but not later word reading in transparent orthographies (e.g. Spanish, Italian, Norwegian, Finnish or Czech), with RAN being a stronger predictor of reading development and difficulties (for reviews see Seymour, 2005, and Caravolas, 2005). Since reading accuracy is expected to be high for such groups, nonstandardised measures of reading fluency are used. Standardised tests were not used in these two studies, but the next section will report the WS groups' levels of performance on experimental reading measures relative to the younger verbal-MA-matched control groups.

Can individuals with Williams syndrome use a phonological reading strategy?

Laing et al. (2001) reported evidence for the use of a phonological reading strategy in WS, as indicated by the observation that levels of nonword reading ability were in line with word reading ability (although there was a trend for the WS group to read fewer non-words correctly than the control group; WS: 4.87/20 [24%] correct nonwords; TD: 9.73/20 [49%] correct nonwords). The average level of nonword reading obtained for the slightly older WS group in the Levy et al. (2003) study was equivalent to an RA of 8 years

2 months, with much individual variation in nonword reading ability. Although the majority had a marked nonword reading impairment (falling at the 10th centile), three of the 20 participants achieved nonword reading scores falling within the average range at the 40th centile for their age in the general population. All three participants were within the subgroup with the highest overall IQ (>68) in the sample, but presented relatively weaker word reading skills (falling at the 10th centile). All other individuals with WS were reported to have nonword reading scores that fell below the 10th centile. As a group, after removing three 'non-readers' (excluded because they were unable to reach basal levels on the nonword reading test and were struggling to name the letters included at the start of the word reading test), there was a trend for word reading skills to be relatively stronger than nonword reading abilities word reading standard score: 77, RA equivalent: 9 years 6 months; nonword reading standard score: 75, RA equivalent: 8 years 2 months), similar to the profile commonly observed in dyslexia (e.g. Griffiths & Snowling, 2002; van Ijzendoorn & Bus, 1994). When the three non-readers were left in the group, the average group word recognition standard score fell to 68 (RA equivalent: 8 years 6 months). Hence, the gap disappears when nonreaders are included in the sample. The results demonstrate that WS children learn to read by relying on a phonological reading strategy, and emphasise the need to be cautious when interpreting results from samples including non-readers.

In the Garayzabal and Cuetos (2008) study, although the WS group had weaker levels of word reading accuracy than the TD controls, their levels of nonword reading accuracy were comparable. This indicates a marked word reading difficulty because, as mentioned previously, dyslexic reading difficulties in transparent orthographies typically manifest in slow reading times, with good levels of accuracy. However, a nonword reading deficit (accuracy) was observed for Menghini et al.'s (2004) WS group relative to their verbal-MA-matched control group, but with no group differences in reading times. Groups did not differ in their word reading accuracy or fluency. In the absence of standard scores, it is difficult to interpret the relative differences in results across the two transparent languages (both are shallow orthographies with simple syllables). Garayzabal and Cuetos (2008) suggest the differences in results may reflect Menghini et al.'s (2004) older sample of predominantly adults, who may have developed compensatory strategies in word reading, or this may reflect instructional methods emphasising a 'look-and-say' sight word strategy.

Both English WS studies reported associations between word and nonword reading for the WS groups (Laing et al., 2001; Levy et al., 2003), similar to the pattern observed in typical development. This result provides evidence supporting the view that WS children depend on phonological processes when learning to read, in a similar way to TD children.

Component word reading skills have been examined more closely in DS than in WS groups. Evidence from studies with adults with DS indicates that severe nonword reading deficits persist into adulthood (Fowler et al., 1995), but much individual variability in levels of attainment is reported, from being able to decode two or fewer nonwords (described as novice readers) to being able to decode 11-29 nonwords (developing readers). In contrast to WS, a severe difficulty using a phonological reading strategy in DS has been reported across studies, with relatively stronger whole-word reading skills than nonword decoding abilities (e.g. Boudreau, 2002; Byrne et al., 2002; Cardoso-Martins et al., 2009; Kay-Raining Bird, Cleave & McConnell, 2000; Roch & Jarrold, 2008). This is the opposite profile to the one just reported in WS and dyslexia. Similarly, Cardoso-Martins et al. (2009) reported differences in component word reading skill profiles for a native English DS group and an RA-matched dyslexic group, with a smaller 'regularity effect' observed for the DS group. In typical development and dyslexia, a regularity effect is where there is an advantage in reading accuracy for regular words over irregular words, which has been argued to reflect a reader's reliance on a phonological strategy (Metsala et al., 1998). Cardoso-Martins et al. (2009) suggest that a reduced reliance on a phonological strategy when reading irregular words may have led to fewer 'regularisation' errors in the DS group (e.g. reading 'was' as/wass/or 'pint' as/pInt/). However, differences in instructional methods may also account for the result. Until recently, the predominant method for teaching reading to children with DS or other intellectual disabilities was nonphonics-based (e.g. look-and-say method; see Conners, 1992). Children learn to associate whole printed words with their spoken forms, but this approach does not allow readers to acquire the strategies to read new words, giving rise to difficulties using a decoding strategy for reading nonwords (Cupples & Iacono, 2002; Groen et al., 2006; Snowling et al., 2008). Hence, it is important to know the method of reading instruction used when examining profiles of component word reading skills in neurodevelopmental disorders.

Does phonology play an important role in driving early word reading development in Williams syndrome?

The next section will examine whether or not the same foundation cognitive-linguistic skills known to predict individual variation in typical word reading development also predict word reading development in WS.

Phonological-awareness skills

Both Laing et al. (2001) and Levy et al. (2003) included concurrent measures of phonemic and rime awareness skills. A weak level of phonological-awareness skills was observed for the individuals with WS in the Laing study across five measures: rime detection, rime production, spoonerisms, identification and phoneme deletion. Although there was a trend for phonological-awareness skills to be weaker in WS than in the younger group matched for verbal MA (and word reading), the difference was only reliable for scores on the phoneme deletion tasks. Rime awareness skills were not reported to differ from WS phoneme awareness skills. This result implies that phoneme and rime awareness skills on the whole are a relative strength for WS (with the exception of the phoneme deletion task), on a par with their verbal MA and current level of word reading.

Levy et al. (2003) also reported phoneme awareness skills to be a relative strength for the individuals with WS in their study, with the average standard scores across three different phonemic awareness tasks from the Comprehensive Test of Phonological Processing (CTOPP; Wagner et al., 1999) falling within the 'borderline to low average range' on the test. When the results for the full sample including the three nonreaders were considered, the strongest standard score of 82 was for the segmenting words test (a phoneme blending task, forming a real word), followed by the segmenting nonword test (a phoneme blending task, forming a nonsense word) with a standard score of 77; the weakest score for the group was on the Elision task from CTOPP (a phoneme deletion test), with an average standard score of 71. Slightly stronger standard scores (84, 81, 73 for the three tests, respectively) were achieved when removing the three nonreaders. This may reflect the relatively stronger word reading skills for this older sample of individuals with WS than for the Laing et al.'s (2001) sample. A measure of implicit rime awareness was used in the study, but both groups were at ceiling on this task.

Phoneme awareness measures were not included in Garayzabal and Cuetos (2008) and Menghini et al.'s (2004) studies, only measures of syllable and rime awareness. An important result to note from Menghini et al.'s (2004) study was the observation of ceiling effects for some of the syllable and rime awareness tasks, indicating strong phonological awareness for larger units of sound. If syllable and rime awareness is stronger than phoneme awareness in WS, this pattern is similar to that observed in young TD children and dyslexic children, who also find phoneme awareness more challenging than syllable or rime awareness (Griffiths & Snowling, 2002; Swan & Goswami, 1997). By contrast, DS children typically only acquire a rudimentary level of phoneme awareness and show an atypical pattern of phonological-awareness development, with greater difficulties for rime awareness than for phoneme awareness (Cardoso-Martins et al., 2002). Further studies are needed to examine the early development of phonological-awareness skills in WS.

Letter knowledge

As noted earlier, letter knowledge and phoneme awareness skills in typical development are co-determinants of early word reading development. A delay in learning letter knowledge is also one of the earliest risk markers for dyslexia (Gallagher et al., 2000; Pennington & Lefly, 2001). Although a measure of letter knowledge was administered in the Laing et al. (2001) WS study, group mean scores were not reported. As noted earlier, the standardised test of word reading used in Levy et al.'s (2003) study assesses letter and word identification, but only an overall naming score is reported.

Rapid automatised reading and other phonological processing skills

Laing et al. (2001) and Levy et al. (2003) included additional measures of phonological processing skills, such as RAN tasks, verbal STM and nonword repetition. Not only are these skills known to be predictors of word reading in typical development, but they are also reliable markers of cognitive deficits in dyslexia (Rose, 2009; for a review see Bowey, 2005). Laing et al.'s (2001) WS group performed at the level expected for their verbal MA and RA on a RAN task (composite score for picture and digit naming times), verbal STM and nonword repetition, indicating that phonological processing skills are not differentially impaired as they are in dyslexia.

Levy et al. (2003) observed severe RAN difficulties in their older WS group, using an object naming task, with the average naming time for the group reported to be at 'floor' on the standardised CTOPP. Garayzabal & Cuetos (2008) also reported severe RAN deficits for their group of WS children, with reliably slower naming times in the WS group than in a younger verbal-MA-matched group of TD children across all three RAN tasks used in their study, particularly for the letter RAN task. Evidence from typical development has suggested that the letter RAN task may be a marker of ease of letter learning or automaticity in letter recognition (Bowey, 2005), indicating that this would be a weakness in WS.

Interestingly, nonword repetition skills were observed to be a relative strength in Garayzabal and Cuetos' (2008) WS group, with a high level of accuracy for the group as a whole (words: 11.75/12 correct, nonwords: 11.33/12 correct). This contrasts with the profile commonly observed for dyslexia with a specific nonword repetition weakness (e.g. Marshall et al., 2001). Hence, these results suggest phonological processing skills to be a relative strength for WS, with the exception of RAN (see Powell et al., 2007, for similar profiles of children with a specific RAN deficit but without a general intellectual disability).

Concurrent predictors of word reading in Williams syndrome

Phoneme awareness and letter knowledge were concurrent predictors of individual differences in WS word reading in Laing et al.'s (2001) study, but these associations were not independent of age and IQ. The correlations between phoneme awareness skills and word reading were also reported to be weaker in the WS group ($r=0.66$) than in the TD group ($r=0.86$). A similar pattern has been observed in dyslexia, where correlations between concurrent measures of phoneme awareness and word reading for dyslexic children ($r=0.37$) were weaker than those for the younger RA-matched control group ($r=0.64$; the corresponding correlation coefficients for the association between phoneme awareness and nonword reading were 0.48 and 0.71, respectively; Griffiths & Snowling, 2002). This difference in profiles for TD children and poor readers is consistent with the view that orthographic skills must proceed, to some extent, independently of the normal foundation in phonological skills (e.g. Griffiths & Snowling, 2002). Sight word reading skills may be able to draw on additional sources of activation, such as semantic representations (Frith & Snowling, 1983; Nation & Snowling, 1998), which are not available for nonword reading. However, it is important to note that the relationship between phoneme awareness and reading observed in typical development and dyslexia is independent of IQ. In the Levy et al. (2003) study, only one of the three phoneme awareness tasks, the Elision task, reliably correlated with word reading and nonword reading in the WS sample, after controlling for nonverbal IQ.

Interestingly, letter name knowledge, but not letter sound knowledge, has been observed as a concurrent (Boudreau, 2002; Snowling et al., 2002) and longitudinal (Laws & Gunn, 2002) predictor of word reading in DS. Snowling and Hulme (2005) suggest that this may reflect a difficulty in DS in applying their phoneme awareness knowledge to reading. In order to acquire an alphabetic reading strategy, children need to understand the principle of phoneme invariance (i.e. that two phonemes are the same in some respects across differing phonetic contexts; Byrne, 1998; Carroll, 2004). However, the individuals with DS in the Snowling et al. (2002) study were unable to identify final phonemes in spoken words; they could only identify initial ones. Snowling and Hulme (2005) suggest that the ability to learn letter names may be an index of the ability of individuals with DS to learn associations between visual symbols and their names. On the one hand, the relatively stronger phoneme awareness skills observed in WS would predict fewer difficulties with learning letter sounds. Unfortunately, the letter knowledge task used in the WS group reported by Laing et al. (2001) did not differentiate between letter name knowledge and letter sound knowledge. Studies are needed that begin to follow phonological and oral language development in children with WS and DS before they receive formal literacy instruction, to establish precursors of word reading development in these syndromes.

Turning to RAN and reading, RAN was the only concurrent predictor of reading in Laing et al.'s (2001) WS group, with slower naming times associated with poorer word reading accuracy after controlling for age and IQ. Correlations between RAN and reading were not reported in the other studies or in any of the DS group studies (but see the case profile of KS, a girl with DS, in the next section).

In summary, the results indicate that word reading skills in WS are weak, which is perhaps unsurprising given their language impairments, but there is much individual variation in end-state levels of word reading attainment and in the acquisition of foundation literacy skills, similar to the situation in dyslexia and DS. The evidence suggests that WS readers rely on a phonological reading strategy, with word reading development associated with phonological processing skills and IQ. With the exception of a relative impairment in RAN, their phonological processing skills are on a par with their verbal MA. Although the range of reading scores across samples indicates that a small number of individuals with WS were able to acquire age-appropriate word level reading skills, the lack of evidence from longitudinal studies limits any conclusions at present about possible risk and protective factors influencing reading outcomes in WS.

Oral language skills as a concurrent predictor of reading attainment in Williams syndrome

There is very limited evidence from WS reading research to address the role of wider oral language in their reading development. Variability in receptive-vocabulary scores was also observed in Howlin et al.'s (1998) adult sample (mean RA: 10 years, range: 4-18 years, with 18 years being the test ceiling), but correlations with reading were not reported. In the Levy et al. (2003) study, receptive-vocabulary skills did not correlate with word reading in the WS group, but the subgroup of individuals defined as readers in the group also had stronger verbal skills than the rest of the sample.

Recent research has indicated that oral language skills may be a stronger predictor of word reading development in DS than phonological skills (Byrne et al., 2002; Cardoso-Martins et al., 2009; Snowling & Hulme, 2005). In DS, readers perform better than nonreaders on measures of oral language (Cardoso-Martins et al., 2009; Laws & Gunn, 2002). Cardoso-Martins et al. (2009) reported the readers in their DS sample to have oral language skills on a par with their MA, whereas the nonreaders showed the typical DS profile of weaker verbal than nonverbal ability. Furthermore, receptive language correlates concurrently and longitudinally with reading in DS (Boudreau, 2002; Cardoso-Martins et al., 2009; Laws & Gunn, 2002). Interestingly, several other language measures (including expressive vocabulary and receptive grammar skills) were also correlated strongly with word reading and spelling in Cardoso-Martins et al.'s (2009) DS group, and were better predictors of reading than visuospatial cognitive skills. This is in contrast to evidence for a strong concurrent association between visual perceptual skills and word reading in DS (Fidler et al., 2005). However, measures of oral language or phoneme awareness skills were not included in Fidler et al.'s (2005) analyses and the DS group included individuals with relatively stronger verbal abilities than typically observed for the syndrome. The issue of individual differences is particularly critical in groups with neurodevelopmental disorders. The role in WS of wider oral language abilities and/or visual perceptual deficits (see Chapters 12 and 13) in reading and spelling development is under-researched. Given the results from Cardoso-Martins et al.'s (2009) DS study, it would be fruitful to consider these factors in WS.

Longitudinal research following children before they receive formal reading instruction is required to establish the direction of causality between reading and oral language development. It is not known whether having relatively spared oral language skills is an important precursor to early word reading acquisition or whether gains in vocabulary and morphosyntactic skills are a consequence of having acquired some reading skills (Cardoso-Martins et al., 2009). Readers with the strongest oral language skills may be able to support their partial alphabetic knowledge in reading words, particularly when reading irregular words (Nation & Snowling, 1998). Some evidence for an association between more positive word reading outcomes and strengths in oral language has been reported in longitudinal studies of children with a family risk of dyslexia (Snowling et al., 2007) and studies of 'compensated' dyslexic university students (e.g. Hatcher et al., 2002). There is also some evidence supporting a neural basis for the two different reading outcomes of compensation and persistence in dyslexia (Shaywitz et al., 2003).

Nonetheless, evidence from case studies of individuals with a hyperlexic reading profile (i.e. who read at a higher level than predicted by their MA) demonstrate that it is possible to acquire strong word recognition skills in the context of strong phonemic and grapho-phonemic skills but low general cognitive abilities (for reviews see Ehri & Snowling, 2004; Nation, 1999) and comprehension skills. Similarly, evidence from a recent case study of an 8-year-old girl (KS) with DS shows that some children with intellectual impairments can acquire phonological reading skills (nonword reading accuracy) and fluency in word reading in the context of severe impairments in nonverbal domains and oral language (grammar and vocabulary) (Groen et al., 2006). Possible protective factors associated with KS's strong word reading development included an enriched preschool home literacy environment and a profile of strengths in speech processing skills (phoneme awareness, RAN, speech rate), verbal STM and visual STM. Very little is known about the influence of the preschool home literacy environment of children with WS.

It would be inaccurate to suggest that KS is a skilled reader for her age. She had weak reading comprehension skills, which is unsurprising given her reported weaknesses in broader oral language skills. Close inspection of her reading comprehension strategies revealed that she was able to retain literal information when reading but struggled to use knowledge-based inferences in reading.

It is interesting that RAN would seem to be a protective factor for KS's word reading development. The absence of a RAN deficit in the context of language impairment has been reported to be a possible protective factor from associated word reading difficulties for children with developmental language impairment (Bishop et al., 2009). RAN has not been investigated in any other published studies of reading in DS, but letter RAN is also a known concurrent predictor of word and nonword reading for adults with mild general learning difficulties, independent of their verbal IQ (Saunders & DeFulio, 2007). Hence, it would be interesting to further explore RAN as a longitudinal predictor of word reading development in WS, to establish whether strengths in RAN are a protective factor against the most severe word reading difficulties for this syndrome, too.

Semantic skills in early word reading acquisition in Williams syndrome

Only one study has investigated the role of phonological and semantic skills underlying sight word reading development in WS (Laing et al., 2001) using a word learning task. Previous studies had demonstrated that preschool TD children who could use phonetic cues in a word learning task were stronger readers than peers who relied on visual cues (Ehri & Wilce, 1985; Rack et al., 1994). Laing and Hulme (1999) extended this work demonstrating that TD young children showed sensitivity to cues differing in their phonetic similarity as well as in the imageability (i.e. semantics) of sight words to be learnt, with word learning stronger for highly imageable words than those with low imageability (see also Vellutino et al., 1995). The phonetic cue readers also retained many of the words when their verbal recall of the taught items was tested 1 week later.

When Laing et al. (2001) examined word learning for a WS group, a benefit from the phonetic cues to learn to read sight words was observed, but in contrast to the findings with TD children, word learning in the WS group was not influenced by the imageability of the word. Unfortunately, the long-term retention of the cues learnt by the children with WS was not assessed. These findings are in line with other studies reporting that individuals with WS rely less on semantics than on phonology in their decoding skills on verbal-STM tasks (e.g. Grant et al., 1997; Thomas et al., 2001; but see Brock, 2007). The WS group also learnt fewer cues than the TD children, which the authors interpret as indicating that their learning strategy when reading new words is not only different but also less effective than that of TD children—an important issue to be further explored in future research.

Given the reported relative strengths of phonological coding over semantic processing in WS, a natural prediction would be for WS children to show a reduced semantic boost when reading irregular words, with a greater reliance on a phonological reading strategy than a sight word strategy. This would be the opposite profile to the one observed for dyslexic children (without co-occurring oral language deficits) (Nation & Snowling, 1998). Another prediction would be a difficulty using contextual cues to support partial decoding of unfamiliar regular words in text (partial alphabetic phase). However, as noted previously, the role of semantics in early word reading development for typical populations is itself controversial (Nation & Cocksey,2009), but further experimental and longitudinal research investigating the role of phonology and semantics in typical and atypical reading development is needed.

Finally, as discussed earlier, the home literacy environment is known to be an important influence on TD children's early oral language development and their phonological and reading development (Phillips & Lonigan, 2005). Similar to TD children, there is expected to be wide variation in the environments that children with learning difficulties experience, at home and at school, which will contribute to their reading outcomes (Snowling et al., 2008), and yet there is only a small body of research on home literacy environment and reading development in neurodevelopmental disorders. There is some evidence for variations in home literacy environments to be one of the contributing factors to reading outcomes in DS (Trenholm & Mirenda, 2006; van Bysterveldt et al., 2010) and other general learning difficulties (van der Schuit et al., 2009). Other evidence for environmental influences on reading development comes from studies demonstrating that children with DS have stronger reading and language skills when taught in mainstream schools, as opposed to special schools (Buckley et al., 2006; Laws et al., 2000). Further research from cross-syndrome comparisons using longitudinal studies following DS and WS children prior to the onset of formal literacy instruction is required to better understand the role of environmental factors on reading development for children with intellectual disabilities.

Summary

In summary, the relatively strong phoneme awareness skills reported by Levy et al. (2003) for the readers in their sample indicate that phoneme awareness skills are a relative strength, certainly in older children with WS, in contrast to the profile observed in DS. Good levels of nonword repetition in WS are a further index of strengths in phonological processing, consistent with previous studies (e.g. Grant et al., 1997). The current evidence is silent as to the early development of phonological-awareness skills (phonemic and rime awareness) and letter learning in WS and the role that these skills play as predictors of individual variation in early and later reading growth, because there is no longitudinal evidence from studies following the early acquisition of phoneme and rime awareness. Further research needs to investigate the RAN deficits associated with WS (Garayzabal & Cuetos, 2008; Laing et al., 2001; Levy et al., 2003) and establish whether naming speed is a longitudinal predictor of reading in this syndrome, as it is in dyslexia.

Current evidence suggests that children with WS rely quite heavily on the phonological pathway when learning to read, with less use of their semantic pathway—opposite to the profile reported in the literature of the dyslexic reader, with strengths in oral language but weaknesses in phonology. However, there is clearly evidence of wider variation in phonological and oral language skills for children with WS and DS than originally thought, as is the case for dyslexia when it co-occurs with developmental language impairment (Bishop & Snowling, 2004). Methods that recognise the continuous variation in cognitive and linguistic skills in neurodevelopmental disorders, and that approach reading as an interactive process, are better placed to understand the mechanisms and processes underlying the variation in reading development for children with general learning difficulties. The adoption of this approach in recent research has significantly advanced theories in the field of dyslexia, which could be applied profitably to studies of WS and other neurodevelopmental disorders.

Reading intervention

There is a strong body of evidence from research indicating that—with appropriate, well-implemented and theoretically based phonological interventions—attaining alphabetic reading is in reach of the majority of children with reading difficulties (Ehri & Snowling, 2004; Hulme & Snowling, 2009; Rose, 2009), including those with moderate learning difficulties (e.g. Hatcher & Hulme, 1999). At present, there are no evaluations of reading intervention programmes for poor readers with WS that use randomised controlled or quasi-experimental controlled designs. However, on the basis of their language profiles and evidence from studies reporting effective intervention for other language-based disorders, it would be reasonable to predict that some individuals with WS would benefit from combined oral-language-based and phonology-based reading interventions. Although effective reading interventions have been implemented for both children with dyslexia and individuals with DS, not all individuals made gains in reading skill (dyslexia: for a review see Duff, 2008; DS: Goetz et al., 2008; Lemons & Fuchs, 2010). Unsurprisingly, phonological and oral language skills are known to predict response to intervention in dyslexia (Duff, 2008). Intervention programmes targeting oral language skills can boost the word reading for these 'nonresponders' (e.g. Duff et al., 2009) and also improve language and reading comprehension skills for children identified with specific reading comprehension difficulties (Clarke et al., 2010). Environmental factors known to influence the response to intervention include the quality of the initial reading instruction, the presence or absence of fidelity checks on implementation, the adequacy of intensity and duration, and the appropriateness of the content for the profile of reading difficulty (for reviews see Carroll et al., 2011; Rose, 2009).

Dyslexic children who show poor levels of response to reading intervention are also more likely to be rated by their teachers as inattentive in class (e.g. Hatcher et al., 2006). Limited concentration is a reported characteristic of WS (see Chapter 18), with an increased risk of attention deficit hyperactivity disorder in WS as indicated by an epidemiological study (Leyfer et al., 2006) and with an increased risk of attention deficit hyperactivity disorder more generally for individuals with intellectual disabilities (Hastings et al., 2005). Concentration and attention skills, therefore, are another factor to take into account when considering WS reading intervention. The use of behaviour rating scales is useful as a screener, but developmentally appropriate and sensitive measures of attention control are required to examine relationships with reading in future research (Gooch et al., 2011; Shaywitz & Shaywitz, 2008).

Conclusions and future directions for reading research in Williams syndrome

Current evidence suggests that the reading outcomes for some individuals with dyslexia are more favourable than those for children with general learning difficulties as in DS and WS. Indeed, the severity of the reading difficulties for each syndrome is largely consistent with the degree of oral language impairment (Snowling & Hulme, 2005), but the role of environmental factors (e.g. parental input and school experiences) need to be explored in future research.

There is an urgent need for an evidence base to inform practitioners of effective reading intervention for children with WS. Future research investigating the predictors of longitudinal growth in reading from preschool is recommended, with the developmental trajectory approach (see Chapter 1) well suited to explore the interactive role of phonological and semantic knowledge and processes in early and later reading development in atypically developing populations. Controlled research studies evaluating the efficacy of theoretically based reading intervention are required, with instruction targeting phonological and oral language skills. Identifying the factors predicting variation in response to reading intervention in WS, including cognitive-linguistic, attention and environmental factors (e.g. home literacy environments, instructional methods), would inform both theory and practice. Research investigating spelling development in WS is also needed, to examine the role of phonology, oral language and visuospatial processing weaknesses in orthographic development.

Editor commentary (Emily K. Farran & Annette Karmiloff-Smith)

Adults with WS have an average RA of 8 years 8 months. Despite this substantial impairment, relatively little is known about the development of reading ability in WS. This chapter considered reading ability in WS within the context of the much broader body of knowledge of reading ability in other neurodevelopmental syndromes, such as DS and dyslexia.

In typical development, phonological skills are the predominant predictors of early word reading, whereas oral language skills such as vocabulary, semantics and grammatical skills are predictive of reading comprehension. In this chapter, we learnt that word reading is stronger than reading comprehension in WS, a pattern that is also observed in DS. However, despite this cross-syndrome association, individuals with WS show strong phonological awareness and rely on a phonological reading strategy, whereas individuals with DS who show comparatively poor phonological awareness and are more reliant on a sight word reading strategy. This is indicative of qualitatively different developmental trajectories for reading in these two groups. Although there are no published studies that indicate the level of letter knowledge in WS, the chapter suggested that letter knowledge, mediated by impaired RAN, might represent a constraint on the development of reading in WS. Environmental effects such as home literacy environments and type of reading instruction as contributing factors to reading outcomes should also be taken into account.

For example, Mervis and John (2010) report that although a phonics reading approach is preferable to a whole-word approach for children with WS, less than half of their sample were being taught to read using a phonics approach. A neuroconstructivist approach to the development of reading, therefore, has strong implications for the potential effectiveness of reading instruction and intervention.

References

Bishop, D.V.M. (1997). Cognitive neuropsychology and developmental disorders: uncomfortable bedfellows. *Quarterly Journal of Experimental Psychology, Section A-Human Experimental Psychology*, 50, 4, 899–923.

Bishop, D.V.M., McDonald, D., Bird, S., & Hayiou-Thomas, M.E. (2009). Children who read words accurately despite language impairment: who are they and how do they do it? *Child Development*, 80, 2, 593–605.

Bishop, D.V.M., & Snowling, M.J. (2004). Developmental dyslexia and specific language impairment: same or different? *Psychological Bulletin*, 130, 858–88.

Boudreau, D. (2002). Literacy skills in children and adolescents with Down syndrome. *Reading and Writing*, 15, 497–525.

Bowey, J. (2005). Predicting individual differences in learning to read. In M.J. Snowling & C. Hulme (Eds), *The Science of Reading: A Handbook* (pp. 155–172). Oxford: Blackwell.

Bowey, J., & Rutherford, J. (2007). Imbalanced word reading profiles in eighth-graders. *Journal of Experimental Child Psychology*, 96, 169–96.

Brock, J. (2007). Language abilities in Williams syndrome: a critical review. *Development and Psychopathology*, 19, 97–127.

Buckley, S., Bird, G., Sacks, B., & Archer, T. (2006). A comparison of mainstream and special education for teenagers with Down syndrome: implications for parents and teachers. *Down Syndrome Research and Practice*, 9, 54–67.

Burgess, S.R., Hecht, S.A, & Lonigan, C.J. (2002). Relations of home literacy environment to the development of reading-related abilities: a one-year longitudinal study. *Reading Research Quarterly*, 37, 408–26.

Burgess, S.R., & Lonigan, C.J. (1998). Bi-directional relations of phonological sensitivity and pre-reading abilities: evidence from a preschool sample. *Journal of Experimental Child Psychology*, 70, 117–41.

Byrne, B. (1998). *The Foundation of Literacy: The Child's Acquisition of the Alphabetic Principle*. Hove: Psychology Press.

Byrne, A., MacDonald, J., & Buckley, S. (2002). Reading, language and memory skills: a comparative longitudinal study of children with Down syndrome and their mainstream peers. *British Journal of Educational Psychology*, 72, 513–52.

van Bysterveldt, A., Gillon, G., & Foster-Cohen, S. (2010). Literacy environments for children with Downs syndrome. What's happening at home? *Down Syndrome Research and Practice*, 12, 98–102.

Cain, K., Oakhill, J., & Bryant, P.E. (2004). Children's reading comprehension ability: concurrent prediction by working memory, verbal ability, and component skills. *Journal of Educational Psychology*, 96, 31–42.

Caravolas, M. (2005). The nature and causes of Dyslexia in different languages. In M.J. Snowling & C. Hulme (Eds). *The Science of Reading: A Handbook* (pp. 336–55). Oxford: Blackwell.

Caravolas, M., Hulme, C., & Snowling, M.J. (2001). The foundations of spelling ability: evidence from a 3-year longitudinal study. *Journal of Memory and Language*, 45, 751–74.

Cardoso-Martins, C., & Frith, U. (2001). Can individuals with Down syndrome acquire alphabetic literacy skills in the absence of phoneme awareness? *Reading and Writing*, 14, 361–75.

Cardoso-Martins, C., Michalick, M.F., & Pollo, T.C. (2002). Is sensitivity to rhyme a developmental precursor to sensitivity to phoneme? Evidence from individuals with Down syndrome. *Reading and Writing*, **15**, 439–54.

Cardoso-Martins, C., Peterson, R., Olson, R., & Pennington, B. (2009). Component reading skills in Down syndrome. *Reading and Writing*, **22**, 277–92.

Carroll, J.M. (2004). Letter knowledge precipitates phoneme segmentation, but not phoneme invariance. *Journal of Research in Reading*, **27**, 212–25.

Carroll, J.M., Bowyer-Crane, C., Duff, F., Hulme, C., & Snowling, M.J. (2011). *Effective Intervention for Language and Literacy in the Early Years*. Oxford: Wiley-Blackwell.

Carroll, J.M., Snowling, M.J., Hulme, C., & Stevenson, J. (2003). The development of phonological awareness in pre-school children. *Developmental Psychology*, **39**, 913–23.

Catts, H.W., Adlof, S.M., & Weismer, S.E. (2006). Language deficits in poor comprehenders: a case for the simple view of reading. *Journal of Speech, Language and Hearing Research*, **49**, 278–93.

Clarke, P.J., Snowling, M.J., Truelove, E., & Hulme, C. (2010). Ameliorating children's reading comprehension difficulties: a randomised controlled trial. *Psychological Science*, **21**, 8, 1106–1116.

Conners, F.A. (1992). Reading instruction for students with moderate mental retardation: review and analysis of research. *American Journal of Mental Retardation*, **96**, 577–97.

Cupples, L., & Iacono, T. (2000). Phonological awareness and oral reading skill in children with Down syndrome. *Journal of Speech, Language and Hearing Research*, **43**, 595–608.

Cupples, L., & Iacono, T. (2002). The efficacy of 'whole word' versus 'analytic' reading instruction for children with Down syndrome. *Reading and Writing*, **15**, 549–74.

Duff, F.J. (2008). Defining reading disorders and evaluating reading interventions: perspectives from the Response to Intervention model. *Educational and Child Psychology*, **25**, 31–36.

Duff, F.J., & Clarke, P.J. (2010). Practitioner review: reading disorders: what are the effective interventions and how should they be implemented and evaluated? *Journal of Child Psychology and Psychiatry*, **52**, 3–12.

Duff, FJ., Fieldsend, E., Bowyer-Crane, C., Hulme, C., Smith, G., Gibbs, S., et al. (2009). Reading with vocabulary intervention: evaluation of an instruction for treatment non-responders. *Journal of Research in Reading*, **31**, 319–36.

Ehri, L.C. (2005). Learning to read words: theory, findings, and issues. *Scientific Studies of Reading*, **9**, 167–88.

Ehri, L., & Snowling, M.J. (2004). Developmental variation in word recognition. In C. Addison Stone, E.R. Silliman, B.J. Ehren, & K. Apel (Eds), *Handbook of Language and Literacy: Developmental Disorders* (pp. 433–60). New York, NY: Guildford Press.

Ehri, L.C., & Wilce, L.S. (1985). Movement into reading: is the first stage of printed word learning visual or phonetic? *Reading Research Quarterly*, **20**, 163–79.

Fidler, D.J., Most, D.E, & Guiberson, M.M. (2005). Neuropsychological correlates of word identification in Down syndrome. *Research in Developmental Disabilities*, **26**, 487–501.

Fowler, A.E., Doherty, B.J., & Boynton, L. (1995). The basis of reading skill in young adults with Down syndrome. In D. Rosenthal & L. Nadel (Eds), *Down Syndrome: Living and Learning in the Community* (pp. 182–96). New York, NY: Wiley-Liss.

Frith, U., & Snowling, M, J. (1983). Reading for meaning and reading for sound in autistic and Dyslexic children. *British Journal of Developmental Psychology*, **1**, 329–42.

Gallagher, A., Frith, U., & Snowling, M.J. (2000). Precursors of literacy-delay among children at genetic risk of Dyslexia. *Journal of Child Psychology and Psychiatry*, **41**, 203–213.

Garayzabal, E., & Cuetos, F. (2008). Learning to read in children with Williams syndrome [article in Spanish]. *Psicotherma*, **20**, 672–77.

Goetz, K., Hulme, C., Brigstocke, S., Carroll, J., Nasir, L., & Snowling, M.J. (2008). Training reading and phoneme awareness skills in children with Down syndrome. *Reading and Writing*, 21, 395–412.

Goff, D.A., Pratt, C., & Ong, B. (2005). The relations between children's reading comprehension, working memory, language skills and components of reading decoding in a normal sample. *Reading and Writing*, 18, 583–616.

Gooch, D., Snowling, M.J., & Hulme, C. (2011). Time perception, executive function and phonological skills in children with Dyslexia and/or ADHD symptoms. *Journal of Child Psychology and Psychiatry*, 52, 2, 195–203.

Goswami, U., & Bryant, P.E. (1990). *Phonological Skills and Learning to Read*. London: Lawrence Erlbaum.

Grant, J., Karmiloff-Smith, A., Gathercole, S., Paterson, S., Howlin, P., Davies, M., et al. (1997). Phonological short-term memory and its relationship to language in Williams syndrome. *Cognitive Neuropsychiatry*, 2, 81–99.

Griffiths, Y.M., & Snowling, M.J. (2002). Predictors of exception word and nonword reading in Dyslexic children: The severity hypothesis. *Journal of Educational Psychology*, 94, 1, 34–43.

Griffiths, Y.M., & Stuart, M. (2011). Reviewing evidence-based practice for pupils with dyslexia and literacy difficulties. *Journal of Research in Reading*. [Epub ahead of print 18 May 2011].

Groen, M., Laws, G., Nation, K., & Bishop, D. (2006). A case of exceptional reading accuracy in a child with Down syndrome: underlying skills and the relation to reading comprehension. *Cognitive Neuropsychology*, 23,1190–1214.

Hastings, R.P., Beck, A., Daley, D., & Hill, C. (2005). Symptoms of ADHD and their correlates in children with intellectual disabilities. *Research in Developmental Disabilities*, 26, 456–68.

Hatcher, J., Snowling, M.J., & Griffiths, Y.M. (2002). Cognitive assessment of Dyslexic students in higher education. *British Journal of Educational Psychology*, 72, 119–33.

Hatcher, P., & Hulme, C. (1999). Phonemes, rhymes and intelligence as predictors of children's responsiveness to remedial instruction: evidence from a longitudinal intervention study. *Journal of Experimental Child Psychology*, 72, 130–53.

Hatcher, P.J., Hulme, C., Miles, J.N.V., Carroll, J.M., Hatcher, J., Gibbs, S., et al. (2006). Efficacy of small group reading intervention for beginning readers with reading-delay: a randomized controlled trial. *Journal of Child Psychology and Psychiatry*, 47, 820–27.

Hoover, W.A., & Gough, P.B. (1990). The simple view of reading. *Reading and Writing*, 2, 127–60.

Howlin, P., Davies, M., & Udwin, O. (1998). Cognitive functioning in adults with Williams syndrome, *Journal of Child Psychology and Psychiatry*, 39, 183–89.

Hulme, C., & Snowling, M.J. (2009). *Developmental Disorders of Language, Learning and Cognition*. Oxford: Wiley-Blackwell.

van Ijzendoorn, M.H., & Bus, A.G. (1994). Meta-analytic confirmation of the nonword reading deficit in developmental Dyslexia. *Reading Research Quarterly*, 29, 266–75.

Jiménez, J.E., Rodriguez, C., & Ramirez, G. (2009). Spanish developmental dyslexia: prevalence, cognitive profile and home literacy experiences. *Journal of Experimental Child Psychology*, 103, 165–85.

Johnston, R.S., Anderson, M., & Holligan, C. (1996). Knowledge of the alphabet and explicit awareness of phonemes in pre-readers. *Reading and Writing*, 8, 217–34.

Kay-Raining Bird, E., Cleave, P.L., & McConnell, L. (2000). Reading and phonological awareness in children with Down syndrome: a longitudinal study. *American Journal of Speech-Language Pathology*, 9, 319–30.

Laing, E., & Hulme, C. (1999). Phonological and semantic processes influence beginning readers' ability to learn to read words. *Journal of Experimental Child Psychology*, 73, 183–207.

Laing, E.C., Hulme, C., Grant, J., & Karmiloff-Smith, A. (2001). Learning to read in Williams syndrome: looking beneath the surface of atypical reading development. *Journal of Child Psychology and Psychiatry*, **42**, 729–39.

Laing, E.C. (2002). Investigating reading development in atypical populations: the case of Williams syndrome. *Reading and Writing: An Interdisciplinary Journal*, **15**, 575–87.

Laws, G., Byrne, A., & Buckley, S. (2000). Language and memory development in children with Down syndrome at mainstream schools and special schools: a comparison. *Educational Psychology*, **20**, 447–57.

Laws, G., & Gunn, D. (2002). Relationship between reading, phonological skills and language development in individuals with Down syndrome: a five year follow-up study. *Reading and Writing*, **15**, 527–48.

Lemons, C.J., & Fuchs, D. (2010). Modeling response to reading intervention in children with Down syndrome: an examination of predictors of differential growth. *Reading Research Quarterly*, **45**, 134–68.

Lervag, A., Braten, I., & Hulme, C. (2009). The cognitive and linguistic foundations of early reading development: a Norwegian latent variable longitudinal study. *Developmental Psychology*, **45**, 764–81.

Levy, Y., Smith, J., & Tager-Flusberg, H. (2003). Word reading and reading-related skills in adolescents with Williams syndrome. *Journal of Child Psychology and Psychiatry*, **44**, 576–87.

Leyfer, O.T., Woodruff-Borden, J., Klein-Tasmen, B.P., Fricke, J.S., & Mervis, C.B. (2006). Prevalence of psychiatric disorders in 4-16 year olds with Williams syndrome. *American Journal of Medical Genetics Part B: Neuropsychiatric Genetics*, **141B**, 615–22.

Marshall, C.M., Snowling, M.J., & Bailey, P.J. (2001). Rapid auditory processing and phonological processing in normal readers and readers with dyslexia. *Journal of Speech, Hearing and Language Research*, **44**, 925–40.

Menghini, D., Verucci, L., & Vicari, S. (2004). Reading and phonological awareness in Williams syndrome. *Neuropsychology*, **18**, 29–37.

Metsala, J.L., Stanovich, K.E., & Brown, G.D.A. (1998). Regularity effects and the phonological deficit model of reading disabilities: a meta-analytic review. *Journal of Experimental Psychology*, **90**, 279–93.

Mervis, C.B. (2009). Language and literacy development of children with Williams syndrome. *Topics in Language Disorders*, **29**, 149–69.

Mervis, C.B., & John, A.E. (2010). Cognitive and behavioral characteristics of children with Williams syndrome: implications for intervention approaches. *American Journal of Medical Genetics Part C: Seminars in Medical Genetics,* **154C**, 229–48.

Muter, V., Hulme, C., Snowling, M.J., & Stevenson, J. (2004). Phonemes, rimes, vocabulary and grammatical skills as foundations of early reading development: evidence from a longitudinal study. *Developmental Psychology*, **40**, 665–81.

Nation, K., & Snowling, M.J. (1998). Individual differences in contextual facilitation: evidence from dyslexia and poor reading comprehension. *Child Development*, **69**, 996–1001.

Nation, K. (1999). Reading skills in hyperlexia: a developmental perspective. *Psychological Bulletin*, **125**, 338–55.

Nation, K. (2005). Children's reading comprehension difficulties. In M.J. Snowling & C. Hulme (Eds), *The Science of Reading* (pp. 248–65). Oxford: Blackwell.

Nation, K., & Cocksey, J. (2009). The relationship between knowing a word and reading it aloud in children's word reading development. *Journal of Experimental Child Psychology*, **103**, 296–308.

Nation, K., Cocksey, J., Taylor, J.S.H., & Bishop, D.V.M. (2010). A longitudinal investigation of early reading and language skills in children with poor reading comprehension. *Journal of Child Psychology and Psychiatry*, **51**, 1031–1039.

Ouellette, G.P. (2006). What's meaning got to do with it: The role of vocabulary in word reading and reading comprehension. *Journal of Educational Psychology*, **98**, 554–66.

Pennington, B.F., & Bishop, D.V.M. (2009). Relations among speech, language and reading disorders. *Annual Review of Psychology*, **60**, 283–306.

Pennington, B.F., & Lefly, D.L. (2001). Early reading development in children at family risk for Dyslexia. *Child Development*, **72**, 816–33.

Phillips, B.M., & Lonigan, C.J. (2005). Social correlates of emerging literacy. In M.J. Snowling & C. Hulme (Eds), *The Science of Reading* (pp. 173–87). Oxford: Blackwell.

Plaut, D.C., McClelland, J.L., Seidenberg, M.S., & Patterson, K. (1996). Understanding normal and impaired word reading: computational principles in quasi-regular domains. *Psychological Review*, **103**, 56–115.

Powell, D., Stainthorp, R., Stuart, M., Garwood, H., & Quinlan, P. (2007). An experimental comparison between rival theories of rapid automatised naming performance and its relationship to reading. *Journal of Experimental Child Psychology*, **98**, 46–68.

Rack, J., Hulme, C., Snowling, M.J., & Wightman, J. (1994). The role of phonology in young children learning to read words: The direct mapping hypothesis. *Journal of Experimental Child Psychology*, **57**, 42–71.

Ricketts, J., Nation, K., & Bishop, D.V.M. (2007). Vocabulary is important for some, but not all reading skills. *Scientific Studies of Reading*, **11**, 235–57.

Roch, M., & Jarrold, C. (2008). A comparison between word and nonword reading in Down syndrome: The role of phonological awareness. *Journal of Communication Disorders*, **41**, 305–18.

Rose, J. (2009). *Identifying and Teaching Children and Young People with Dyslexia and Literacy Difficulties*. Nottingham: DCSF Publications.

Saunders, K.J. (2007). Word attack skills in individuals with mental retardation. *Mental Retardation and Developmental Disabilities Research Reviews*, **13**, 78–84.

Saunders, K.J., & DeFulio, A. (2007). Phonological awareness and rapid naming predict word attack and word identification in adults with mild mental retardation. *American Journal on Mental Retardation*, **112**, 155–66.

Savage, R.S., & Carless, S. (2005). Phoneme manipulation not onset-rime manipulation ability is a unique predictor of early reading. *Journal of Child Psychology and Psychiatry*, **46**, 1297–1308.

van der Schuit, M., Peeters, M., Segers, E., van Balkom, H., & Verhoeven, L. (2009). Home literacy environment of pre-school children with intellectual disabilities. *Journal of Intellectual Disability Research*, **53**, 1024–1037.

Seymour, P.K. (2005). Early reading development in European orthographies. In M.J. Snowling & C. Hulme (Eds), *The Science of Reading: A Handbook* (pp. 296–315). Oxford: Blackwell.

Share, D.L. (2008). Orthographic learning, phonology and the self-teaching hypothesis. In R. Kail (Ed.), *Advances in Child Development and Behavior*, vol 36 (pp. 31–82). Amsterdam: Elsevier.

Shaywitz, S.E., Fletcher, J.M., Holahan, J.M. Schneider, A.E., Marchione, K.E., Stuebing, K.K., et al. (1999). Persistence of dyslexia: The Connecticut longitudinal study at adolescence. *Pediatrics*, **104**, 1351–59.

Shaywitz, S.E., Morris, R., & Shaywitz, B.A. (2008). The education of Dyslexic children from childhood to adulthood. *Annual Review of Psychology*, **59**, 451–75.

Shaywitz, S.E., & Shaywitz, B.A. (2008). Paying attention to reading: The neurobiology of reading and Dyslexia. *Development and Psychopathology*, **20**, 1329–49.

Shaywitz, S.E., Shaywitz, B.A., Fulbright, R.K., Skudlarski, P., Mencl, W.E., Constable, R.T., et al. (2003). Neural systems for compensation and persistence: young adult outcome of childhood reading disability. *Biological Psychiatry*, **54**, 1, 25–33.

Snowling, M.J., & Hulme, C. (2005). Learning to read with a language impairment. In M.J. Snowling & C. Hulme (Eds), *The Science of Reading: A Handbook* (pp. 397–412). Oxford: Blackwell.

Snowling, M.J., & Hulme, C. (2006). Language skills, learning to read and reading intervention. *London Review of Education*, **4**, 63–76.

Snowling, M.J., Hulme, C., & Mercer, R. (2002). A deficit in rime awareness in children with Down syndrome. *Reading and Writing*, **15**, 471–95.

Snowling, M.J., Muter, V., & Carroll, J.M. (2007). Children at family risk of dyslexia: a follow-up in adolescence. *Journal of Child Psychology and Psychiatry*, **48**, 609–618.

Snowling, M.J., Nash, H.M., & Henderson, L.M. (2008). The development of literacy skills in children with down syndrome: implications for intervention. *Down Syndrome Research and Practice*.

Stanovich, K.E., & Siegal, L.S. (1994). The phenotypic performance profile of reading disabled children: a regression-based test of the phonological core variable-difference model. *Journal of Educational Psychology*, **86**, 24–53.

Stuart, M, Stainthorp, R., & Snowling, M. (2008). Literacy as a complex activity: deconstructing the simple view of reading. *Literacy*, **42**, 59–66.

Swan, D., & Goswami, U. (1997). Phonological awareness deficits in developmental Dyslexia and the phonological representations hypothesis. *Journal of Experimental Child Psychology*, **66**, 18–41.

Thomas, M.S.C., Grant, J., Gsödl, M., Laing, E., Barham, Z., Lakusta, L., Tyler, L.K., et al. (2001). Can atypical phenotypes be used to fractionate the language system? The case of Williams syndrome. *Language and Cognitive Processes*, **16**, 143–76.

Trenholm, B., & Mirenda, P. (2006). Home and community literacy experiences of individuals with Down syndrome. *Down Syndrome Research and Practice*, **10**, 30–40.

Udwin, O., Davies, M., & Howlin, P. (1996). A longitudinal study of cognitive abilities and educational attainment in Williams syndrome. *Developmental Medicine and Child Neurology*, **38**, 1020–29.

Udwin, O., Yule, W., & Martin, N. (1987). Cognitive abilities and behavioral characteristics of children with idiopathic infantile hypercalcaemia. *Journal of Child Psychology and Psychiatry*, **28**, 297–309.

Vellutino, F.R., Fletcher, J.M., Snowling, M.J., & Scanlon, D.M. (2004). Specific reading disability (dyslexia): what have we learned in the past four decades? *Journal of Child Psychology and Psychiatry*, **45**, 2–40.

Vellutino, F.R., Scanlon, D., & Spearing, D. (1995). Semantic and phonological coding in poor and normal readers. *Journal of Experimental Child Psychology*, **59**, 76–123.

Wagner, R.K., Torgesen, J.K., & Rashotte, C.A. (1994). Development of reading-related phonological processing abilities: evidence of bi-directional causality from a latent variable longitudinal study. *Developmental Psychology*, **30**, 73–87.

Wagner, R.K., Torgesen, J.K., & Rashotte, C.A. (1999). *The Comprehensive Test of Phonological Processing*. Austin, RX: Pro-Ed.

Yopp, H.K., (1988). The validity and reliability of phonemic awareness tests. *Reading Research Quarterly*, **23**, 159–77.

The Neuroconstructivist Approach to Domain-General and Domain-Specific Processes

Chapter 18

Integrating domain-general and domain-specific developmental processes: Cross-syndrome, cross-domain dynamics

Ann Steele, Janice Brown and Gaia Scerif

Introduction

Earlier chapters reviewed strengths and weaknesses in specific domains of cognitive functioning in Williams syndrome (WS), including the latest findings on early language (Chapter 10), as well as later visuospatial cognition (Chapters 12 and 13), numeracy (Chapter 16) and literacy (Chapter 17). These in-depth investigations of domain-specific outcomes are a necessary starting point to understand the WS cognitive profile. But how do domains interact dynamically over developmental time? It is to this question that we now turn. As a case in example, the current chapter discusses the role of a specific set of domain-general skills (attentional abilities) in constraining the development of domain-specific processes for infants and young children with WS, because not only can functioning in individual domains be atypical, but it may also differ in its relationships with domain-general processes.

Indeed, attention represents an area of weakness in adults, children and infants with WS (see Chapter 6) and this is likely to present a barrier to learning across domains. Precisely how do these influences operate? As multiple processes fall under the umbrella term of attention, the detailed profile of relative attentional strengths and weaknesses over the lifespan may differentially impact on learning in individuals with WS at distinct time points compared with individuals with other neurodevelopmental disorders or with typical development. Here, we ask novel questions of old and new data, aiming to elucidate the relationships between attention, language and number early in the development of people with WS. In order to better understand whether these cross-domain relations are specific to WS, we raise these questions with respect to infants with WS, and compare them with infants with Down syndrome (DS) and with typically developing (TD) children. We also ask how attentional processes relate to precursors of literacy and numeracy in older children with WS or DS and in TD children, to assess potentially changing relationships across domain-general and domain-specific processes over developmental time.

In addition, we contrast the attentional profile of WS to that of another neurodevelopmental disorder of known genetic origin, fragile X syndrome, to illustrate insights that can be gained from cross-syndrome comparisons. Fragile X syndrome is associated with the silencing of a single gene on the X chromosome and is the most common genetically inherited cause of learning disability (for an overview see Hagerman & Hagerman, 2002). Intriguingly, although WS and fragile X syndrome have rarely been compared directly in attentional terms, the two disorders have both been argued to be characterised by dorsal-stream deficit (e.g. Atkinson et al., 2003; Kogan et al., 2004a, 2004b) and yet have a rather distinct profile in other domain-specific processes, such as social cognition and vocabulary in late childhood and adulthood: whereas the former are areas of relative strength (despite their atypical trajectories and underlying neural processes) in WS (see Chapters 11 and 15), on average in fragile X syndrome they represent areas of weakness (Cornish et al., 2005; Grant et al., 2007; Roberts et al., 2001). It is therefore of interest to us, in the context of cross-domain dynamics and cross-syndrome comparisons, to investigate how detailed attentional profiles may differ across infants and young children with WS and those with fragile X syndrome, and speculate on how in turn these differences may be linked to differences in domain-specific development for the two groups (Scerif & Steele, 2011).

These are of course exploratory questions and preliminary answers. We aim to spur further studies and truly believe that the field is now ripe to bridge the domain-specific and domain-general aspects of developing cognition in people with WS, and capitalise further on cross-syndrome comparisons.

Existing evidence of interactions across domains

Let us begin with a foray into the literature on cross-domain dynamics. A growing literature, discussed in detail in other chapters in this volume, very clearly demonstrates how in an atypically developing cognitive system, relative strengths and weaknesses interact and potentially do so differentially over developmental time. For example, Jarrold and colleagues have long argued that visuospatial weaknesses in WS clearly interact with aspects of spatial language (e.g. Phillips et al., 2004) and visual working memory (e.g. Jarrold et al., 1999). Furthermore, work on cardinality understanding in children with WS indicates that this is bootstrapped by language abilities, whereas visuospatial skills underpin individual differences in this ability for TD children (Ansari et al., 2003). Chapter 12 also details how complex interactions across processes may account for the poor visuoconstruction abilities so often reported in WS: difficulties in using mental imagery when performing visuoconstruction tasks may put a strain on already limited visual working memory abilities in individuals with WS (Farran et al., 2001; Stinton et al., 2008) and these cascading effects could be driven by atypical dorsal-stream development. Consistent with this suggestion, Chapter 13 discusses how the interaction between prefrontal systems, dedicated to action selection, and dorsal stream, implicated in visuospatial control deficits, result in evident difficulties in inhibiting inappropriate responses in the motor/visuospatial domain, but less evident difficulties in the verbal domain. However, further interactions across areas of strength and weakness in WS make it highly unlikely that the weaknesses demonstrated by people with WS can be fully characterised solely as 'dorsal-stream-deficient'. For example, Chapter 12 highlights how increased interest in social stimuli (faces, people) might drive individuals with WS to experience these stimuli to a much greater degree than do other groups that are also characterised by dorsal-stream deficits (e.g. autistic spectrum disorder and fragile X syndrome). In turn, these increased interactions with social stimuli may be at the core of the relatively good processing of biological motion displayed by people with WS (Jordan et al., 2002), albeit supported by atypical neural pathways (Sarpal et al., 2008). This growing literature demonstrates how interactions across domain-specific processes over developmental time shape the cognitive landscape of individuals with WS as a whole, rather than resulting in selectively intact or impaired processes (for discussion see Karmiloff-Smith, 1998, 2007, 2009).

In the more specific context of the constraints placed by attentional processes on domain-specific learning, by contrast, the review of existing evidence will be brief by necessity, because the impact of distinct attentional constructs on domain-specific aspects of cognition over infancy, the preschool and the early school years is a surprisingly under-studied area of research. This is despite the fact that theories of adult attention posit a key role for attentional processes as a gateway to learning and memory (Posner & Rothbart, 2005), and this is therefore likely to also apply to children. For example, although it is clear that letter and vocabulary knowledge, together with phonological skills, are strong predictors of later reading and language (Carroll et al., 2003; Muter et al., 1997b; 2004; Nation & Snowling, 2004), their relations to specific attentional processes, if any, have not been investigated. This is because studies that have assessed relationships between early literacy (such as single-word reading) and attention have primarily measured attention in terms of classroom behaviours rather than in terms of the cognitive constructs (e.g. Adams & Snowling, 2001; Adams, Snowling, Hennessy, & Kind, 1999; Fuchs et al., 2005). Noteworthy is the fact that although some evidence points to some domain-general attentional processes such as executive control as predictors of reading success over the school years (e.g. Gathercole & Pickering, 2000), studies of younger children have not focused on whether—and if so, which—specific cognitive or behavioural attentional markers predict early literacy. Similarly, although executive control processes distinguish low and high mathematics ability in school-aged children (e.g. (Bull & Scerif, 2001), findings in this area have primarily focused on the school years, rather than earlier in childhood (c.f. Bull et al., 2008). Furthermore, although executive attention constitutes one component aspect of attention, it is not the only candidate as a gateway for learning (see Posner & Rothbart, 2005): sustained and selective attentional processes may be just as critical. Indeed, in a recent longitudinal study of TD children aged between 3 and 6 years (Steele et al., in press), we discovered that distinct attentional processes were concurrently related to skills known to act as precursors to later literacy and numeracy and, 1 year later, to reading and basic numeracy themselves.

These examples underscore the need to study whether—and if so, precisely how—attentional processes relate to critical domain-specific outcomes, even in TD children.

To our knowledge, these questions have not hitherto been posed of cross-domain dynamics between attention, language and number in infants and young children with WS.

Attention and domain-specific development in infancy: language and number

Given the difficulties in recruiting sufficiently large samples of very young children with WS, few studies have been able to assess their domain-specific abilities and even fewer have targeted their attention profiles. We capitalised on two previously published studies asking these questions of infants and toddlers with WS (Brown et al., 2003; Paterson et al., 1999). Paterson and colleagues assessed comprehension of single words and discrimination of simple numerosities through a preferential looking paradigm designed for young infants, and found that the relative strengths in vocabulary reported for older children and adults with WS did not characterise infants with WS, whereas early numerosity discrimination abilities were in line with their developmental level, a finding at odds with their later greater numerical difficulties than expected given their overall level of cognitive functioning. Brown and colleagues instead targeted sustained-attention and attention-orienting abilities in the same group of infants with WS, and found relative strengths in sustaining attention but weaknesses in attention orienting. As a whole, the findings underscored the need to map domain-specific and domain-general strengths or weaknesses from infancy, rather than assuming a priori similar cognitive profiles to those encountered later in development.

In total, 14 infants and toddlers with WS, 19 with DS and 16 TD children, recruited via the Williams Syndrome Foundation and the Down Syndrome Association, had contributed to those studies. Infants and toddlers across these groups were of comparable general ability using the Bayley Scales of Infant Development Second Edition (BSID-II; Bayley, 1993; see Table 18.1). We complemented the original data with previously unexplored variables gathered from the same infants. For the first time, we asked whether attentional profiles related to domain-specific skills in infancy.

Attention measures

Children were assessed on a variety of attentional measures. A sustained attention task presented each child with three toys for 45 seconds each and children's responses were coded from videotape (Ruff & Lawson, 1991) to measure the duration of sustained attention and the number of periods of sustained attention. Orienting of attention was measured through a double-step saccade task (Gilmore & Johnson, 1997) that examined the ability to use information to update spatial representations and plan eye movements. A computer screen was used to display trials in which two targets were briefly and sequentially presented after fixation had been established. Measures reported here are accurate looks to target 1, representing 'simple orienting' ability, and accurate looks to target 2 (after a successful look to target 1), representing the ability to incorporate previous information into the orienting of eye movements (here labelled 'updated orienting'). A measure of familiarisation time was taken from a face-processing task and reflects the amount of looking time at familiarisation stimuli over four familiarisation trials of 30 seconds each. We selected it here as a broad measure of attention, in that it may relate to habituation. Moreover, we speculated that three items from an infant temperament measure, the Infant Behaviour Questionnaire (Rothbart, 1981), would relate to attention: Distress and Latency to Approach Sudden or Novel Stimuli (here labelled 'Distress to Novel Stimuli' for brevity) and Distress to Limitations both load onto frustration/irritability (which predicts low attentional focusing in later childhood), and Duration of Orienting, which may be indicative of sustained or casual attention (Rothbart, 1999).

Domain-specific skills

Receptive vocabulary was assessed through a parental report questionnaire—the MacArthur Communicative Development Inventories (Fenson et al., 1993). Receptive-vocabulary scores are used here as a broad measure of verbal mental age (VMA).

In addition, single-word comprehension was measured using a preferential looking task in which pairs of picture stimuli were presented accompanied by a verbal label for one of the images (Paterson et al., 1999). This yielded measures of looking times to pictures matching and nonmatching the verbal label, plus a difference score (obtained by subtracting looking times to nonmatching stimuli from looking times to matching stimuli). One would predict longer looking times to pictures matching labels that infants comprehended.

The ability to detect number was assessed by familiarising participants to exemplars of numbers and then measuring looking times to familiar or novel numbers or exemplars (Paterson et al., 1999). This yielded measures of looking time to the novel or familiar numerosity, plus a difference score (calculated by subtracting looking times for the familiar numerosity from looking times to the novel numerosity), with greater looking towards the novel stimuli indexing greater dishabituation (i.e. recognition of the difference) to the novel stimuli.

Group profiles in individual domains

We first asked about how the attention, language and number profiles of infants with WS differed from those of infants with DS or TD children (see Table 18.1). Chronological age differed between the groups, with the TD infants and toddlers being younger than the other children, but all three groups were of comparable mental age (as measured on the BSID-II) and VMA.

The experimental attention orienting task suggested difficulties for infants with WS, compared with the other two groups, both in terms of simple orienting of attention and in terms of orienting of attention that requires updating with recent spatial information. By contrast, the pattern of results from the experimental attention tasks indicated that infants with DS, but not those with WS, displayed deficits in sustained attention, a pattern supported by parental reports: infants with DS scored higher than the other two groups on Distress to Novel Stimuli. Furthermore, longer looking times during familiarisation for infants with DS were consistent with previous findings (e.g. Rothbart

Table 18.1 Attention, language and numeracy profiles in infants (Brown et al., 2003; Paterson et al., 1999; unpublished data)

Attention measure	WS (n=14) [a]	DS (n=19)[a]	TD (n=16)[a]	Group difference (p value)	Bonferroni post-hoc tests[b]
Sample characteristics					
Chronological age (months)	28.98 (4.50)	29.11 (4.70)	15.21 (2.51)	<.001	WS=DS>TD
Cognitive ability, BSID II (raw score)[c]	100.99 (9.76)	100.89 (9.96)	99.44 (10.81)	ns	
Receptive vocabulary (score)	39.54 (24.03)	38.56 (12.52)	30.97 (21.50)	ns	
Experimental attention measures					
Sustained attention					
Total duration (seconds)	61.80 (30.32)	33.57 (22.91)	51.45 (30.78)	.018	WS=TD>DS
Number of sustained-attention periods	4.46 (1.69)	3.32 (1.29)	5.06 (2.41)	.022	TD>DS
Orienting of attention (% correct looks)					
Simple orienting	27.19 (8.33)	49.49 (12.99)	43.63 (12.34)	<.001	WS<TD=DS
Updated orienting	20.50 (16.93)	47.71 (13.85)	51.04 (10.17)	<.001	WS<TD=DS
Looking time (seconds)					
Total familiarisation time	60.19 (6.34)	72.43 (10.45)	56.91 (9.21)	<.001	WS=TD<DS
Parent-report attention measures					
IBQ (scores)[d]					
Distress to Novel Stimuli	2.54 (0.77)	3.45 (0.51)	2.75 (0.38)	<.001	WS=TD<DS
Distress to Limitations	3.84 (0.73)	3.51 (0.67)	3.69 (0.62)	ns	
Duration of Orienting	4.06 (1.33)	4.58 (0.88)	3.45 (0.89)	.022	TD<DS
Language and number measures					
Vocabulary (looking time in seconds)					
Looking to matching stimuli	2.41 (0.35)	2.40 (0.53)	2.69 (0.55)	ns	
Looking time to nonmatching stimuli	1.57 (0.37)	1.84 (0.40)	1.59 (0.41)	ns	
Difference score	0.84 (0.45)	0.56 (0.80)	1.10 (0.83)	ns	

(Continued)

Table 18.1 (Cont'd.)

Attention measure	WS (n=14) [a]	DS (n=19)[a]	TD (n=16)[a]	Group difference (p value)	Bonferroni post-hoc tests[b]
Numerosity (looking time in seconds)					
Looking to familiar numerosity	0.77 (0.31)	2.27 (0.84)	1.35 (1.03)	<.001	WS=TD<DS
Looking to novel numerosity	1.87 (0.50)	2.16 (1.16)	1.59 (0.98)	ns	
Difference score	1.10 (0.57)	−0.11 (1.62)	0.24 (1.24)	.032	WS>DS, WS=TD

Abbreviations: BSID II = Bayley Scales of Infant Development II (Bayley, 1993); DS = Down syndrome; IBQ = Infant Behaviour Questionnaire (Rothbart, 1981); TD = typical development; WS = Williams syndrome.

[a]The data are provided as mean (standard deviation).

[b]All group differences remained as reported here when differences in verbal mental age were controlled for.

[c]Scores were too low in the WS and DS groups to calculate a Mental Development Index (the standardised score); therefore raw scores are reported here.

[d]The response rates were somewhat higher for the WS (86%, n=12) and TD (88%, n=14) groups than for the DS group (58%, n=11).

and Hanson, 1983; Miranda and Fantz, 1973) and with parental reports of longer Duration of Orienting.

Broadly speaking, these results extend those reported by Brown and colleagues (2003) and indicate that in very early childhood, children with WS have deficits in attention orienting, but sustained-attention abilities that are at least in line with their lower developmental level (although questions still remain about their ability to disengage attention and about whether 'simply delayed' sustained attention may be underpinned by the same cognitive factors—a point to which we return), a profile that is distinct from children with DS. On the language measures, there were no differences between the groups on vocabulary (as previously reported in Paterson et al., 1999), indicating that the verbal advantage often reported in older children and adults with WS is not present in infancy. Similarly, the number difficulties reported in older individuals with WS were not found here, with infants with WS being as capable of discriminating simple numerosity as TD infants were, whereas the infants with DS performed more poorly primarily because they looked at the familiar numerosity for longer than any of the other groups, a pattern that is consistent with their longer familiarisation times across tasks.

Relationships between attention and domain-specific skills across groups

Partial correlation analysis controlling for age allowed us to investigate the relationships between performance on the experimental attention tasks and the parent-report attention measures and between performance on the number and language tasks within each of the groups (for full details see Table 18.2). Although this approach is somewhat exploratory rather than being hypothesis-driven, we feel this is justified in the context of these early forays into cross-domain dynamics. However, we also acknowledge the limitations of this approach and the possibility that other (unmeasured) factors may influence the results. Therefore, where possible we highlight deviations from or consistency with a priori predictions we had in mind when embarking on this exercise.

Let us begin with relationships for TD children, to get a sense for what the expected pattern of intercorrelations may be in this young age group. There were relationships between aspects of sustained attention and number discrimination, in that a greater number of sustained attention episodes related to a smaller difference between looking at familiar and novel numerosities. This relationship may seem counter-intuitive, except that more sustained attention episodes were also associated with longer looking to the familiar numerosity, a pattern that could be driven by individual differences in familiarisation time: individual infants who sustained attention for longer may have required a longer time to familiarise themselves with the stimuli and this would have resulted in smaller differentiation between the familiar and novel numerosities. This finding reiterates the point highlighted with regard to 'adequate' sustained attention in infants with WS: more sustained attention episodes do not necessarily index adaptive behaviour; they may index either a greater need to process stimuli or a tendency to remain fixated on/ return to certain stimuli more than other infants. There were also relationships between sustained attention and simple word comprehension whereby fewer periods of sustained attention correlated with longer looking to the object that did not match a verbal label, that is, poorer comprehension. It is therefore clear that the extent to which relationships exist between attentional measures and domain-specific measures across domains could be driven by a common factor (e.g. familiarisation time or interest in visual detail). This remains an intriguing question even in TD infants.

Of note, for infants with WS, the only correlation between attentional measures and domain-specific measures that even approached significance was a negative correlation between the 'updated orienting' measure and duration of looks to familiar numerosities. Thus, poorer orienting of attention that required updating about spatial information related to greater looking at familiar numerosities (i.e. poorer numerosity discrimination).

By contrast, infants with DS demonstrated a pattern of relations that was more similar to the typical one. For example, shorter duration of sustained attention related to longer looking at stimuli that did not match the verbal label in the word comprehension task. Further similarities to the typical pattern for infants with DS were found in relation to the parent report of attention (the Infant Behaviour Questionnaire) in that both groups had negative correlations between parent-report measures associated with low attentional focusing in later childhood and numerosity discrimination. For infants with DS, this was represented by a significant negative correlation between Distress to Novel Stimuli and looks to new numerosities, whereas for the TD group the negative correlation between Distress to Limitations and looks to new numerosities approached significance. Furthermore, in infants with DS, longer looking time during familiarisation tended to relate to greater looks towards the novel numerosity. While this might seem counter-intuitive, several studies have indicated that children with DS need more time to process information, which may be reflected in this relationship.

Table 18.2 Correlations coefficients for the associations between attention, numeracy and literacy measures in infants (controlled for chronological age) (Brown et al., 2003; Paterson et al., 1999; unpublished data)

Attention measure	WS (n=14)						DS (n=19)						TD (n=16)					
	Number			Language			Number			Language			Number			Language		
	New	Fam	Diff	Match	Nonmatch	Diff	New	Fam	Diff	Match	Nonmatch	Diff	New	Fam	Diff	Match	Nonmatch	Diff
Experimental attention measures																		
Sustained attention																		
Duration	0.095	−0.096	0.137	−0.070	0.143	−0.169	−0.205	0.070	−0.182	0.043	**−0.584***	0.333	0.038	0.364	−0.268	0.142	−0.433	0.304
Number	0.262	0.121	0.159	−0.203	0.181	−0.302	0.029	−0.186	0.118	0.096	−0.079	0.103	−0.234	0.430	**−0.526***	0.129	**−0.549***	0.351
Orienting attention																		
Simple	−0.281	0.135	−0.321	−0.178	−0.326	0.127	0.086	−0.270	0.202	0.188	−0.208	0.230	0.289	0.490	−0.182	0.055	−0.441	0.250
Updated	0.022	−0.499	0.302	0.111	−0.394	0.403	−0.294	0.061	−0.240	−0.007	−0.073	0.034	0.403	0.165	0.168	−0.251	−0.157	−0.092
Looking time	0.202	−0.227	0.305	−0.007	−0.139	0.107	0.433	−0.152	0.386	0.031	−0.088	0.066	0.436	−0.056	0.373	0.393	−0.232	0.374
Parent-report attention measures																		
IBQ																		
Distress to Novel Stimuli	−0.070	−0.231	0.382	0.245	0.054	0.250	0.018	−0.331	0.186	0.317	−0.314	0.369	−0.444	−0.031	−0.309	−0.279	0.144	−0.256
Distress to Limitations	0.299	0.413	0.025	−0.289	0.308	−0.060	**−0.476***	−0.260	−0.201	−0.266	0.176	−0.263	0.007	−0.171	0.145	−0.227	0.018	−0.161
Duration of Orienting	0.042	−0.077	0.080	−0.150		−0.101	0.270	−0.109	0.249	0.397	−0.135	0.327	0.149	−0.151	0.236	0.328	0.019	0.210

Abbreviations: Diff = difference; DS = Down syndrome; Fam = familiar; IBQ = Infant Behaviour Questionnaire (Rothbart, 1981); TD = typical development; WS = Williams syndrome

* p<.05

In summary, then, profiles in individual domains for infants with WS depict sustained attention, language and number abilities that are in line with developmental level (but see below for caution in interpreting performance at the level of much younger TD children), whereas there are relative weaknesses in the orienting of attention. Going beyond comparisons across groups and instead looking at within-group relationships across domains for infants with WS (and in contrast to the TD and DS children), these poorer orienting skills tend to relate to numerosity discrimination, indicating that weaknesses in disengaging attention across individuals with WS may constrain number abilities that at the group level seem equivalent to those of younger TD infants, that is, 'simply delayed' (for discussion of MA-level performance and interpretations of 'delay' see Karmiloff-Smith et al., 2003).

One potential account for this preliminary relationship is that difficulties in disengaging/reorienting visual attention in infants with WS gate difficulties in disengaging from visual stimuli in general, but affect these children differentially when stimuli are presented in competition with multiple or complex items, as when judgements of numerosity of this kind are required (Van Herwegen et al., 2008). This suggestion could be studied empirically relatively easily by assessing changes in the ability to disengage/reorient from stimuli in number discrimination tasks when stimuli are manipulated in terms of their number or complexity. In addition, and more importantly, it would be critical to know whether these early disengagement differences predict number abilities, such as magnitude comparisons or judgements, longitudinally. Of note, for TD infants and those with DS, much stronger emerging relationships were apparent between sustained attention and both language and number skills, and between parent-report measures of attention and numerosity, whereas similar relationships were not found for infants with WS. The question remains, however, whether and how these aspects of attention matter to domain-specific skills later in development for children with WS.

Attention and domain-specific development in early childhood: literacy and numeracy

We asked parallel questions of an independent dataset on young primary-school-aged children with WS (Steele et al., in preparation) in order to examine how the patterns presented in the previous section may change with development. In total, 27 children with WS, 26 children with DS and 63 TD children were recruited via the Williams Syndrome Foundation, Down Syndrome Education International and local primary schools and nurseries (see Table 18.3). Their vocabulary knowledge was assessed using the British Picture Vocabulary Scale Second Edition (BPVS-II; Dunn et al., 1997), yielding a measure of VMA, whereas nonverbal mental age was measured through the Pattern Construction subscale of the British Ability Scales Second Edition (BAS-II; Elliott et al., 1996).

Attention measures

The Continuous Performance Test (CPT) was used to measure children's ability to sustain attention for a prolonged period without being distracted. Children were instructed to press a button every time they saw an animal on the screen. Distracter items were everyday objects and were randomly intermixed. The task began with extensive and slow practice, but during the experimental run stimuli were presented on the screen for 300 ms, followed by a blank screen for 1250 ms. A correct 'hit' to a target stimulus resulted in a 'woohoo' reward sound, or nothing for a 'miss' response. Incorrect responses following distracter stimuli resulted in an incorrect sound tone. The task comprised 100 trials, of which 20% presented targets (animals), and completion time was approximately 4 minutes. Our measures of interest were number of missed targets (number of omission errors), mean reaction time per hit and number of responses to nontargets (number of commission errors).

A visual search task was used to measure the ability to select relevant stimuli (targets) while ignoring irrelevant distracters (nontargets). Children were presented with two search displays on a touch screen. Each display contained 90 randomly arranged items made up of 20 targets (animals) and 70 nontargets (objects). A successful touch ('hit') on an animal resulted in the appearance of a star, which remained on screen for the remainder of the task, whereas a touch on a distracter resulted in no feedback. There was no time limit; however, the task ended automatically when a total of 18 correct responses were reached or 40 responses were made overall. We recorded mean search speed (mean reaction time between touches), mean distance between successive touches and number of errors across the two runs.

Domain-specific skills

Letter knowledge was assessed following the protocol set out by the Phonological Abilities Test (Muter et al., 1997a). Children were presented with all 26 lower-case letters from the alphabet in random order and asked to give the name or sound associated with each letter. In addition, rhyme awareness and phoneme awareness were measures with two tasks designed for children as young as 3 years of age, in which they were asked to match an object/animal picture with one of two others either rhyming with it or sharing a phoneme of onset (Carroll et al., 2003). Early word reading was tested using an unstandardised (but frequently used) list of 42 words commonly included in the first stages of reading schemes, the Early Word Reading test (Hatcher et al., 1994).

Cardinality understanding was measured extending the 'give-a-number' protocol (Wynn, 1990). Children were asked to give the experimenter small (one, two or three) and large (seven, eight and nine) numbers of counting cubes, three times for each numerosity, attaining a point for every correct response. The Test of Early Mathematics Ability Third Edition (TEMA-III; Ginsburg & Baroody, 2003) was used to assess basic numerical abilities.

Group profiles in individual domains

Differences across the three groups are reported in Table 18.3. Nonverbal mental age did not differ between groups, and VMA did not differ for children with DS and TD children but was significantly higher for children with WS, highlighting the relative strength in receptive vocabulary often reported in older people with WS. Combined with the data on receptive vocabulary from younger children in the earlier part of this chapter, this indicates that the relative language strength begins to emerge at some point between toddlerhood and the school years. So, in considering group differences, we checked whether these were driven by differential VMA.

Differences between the groups in performance on the experimental attention measures were also evident, with children with WS making fewer omission errors on the CPT than the other two groups, even after controlling for their greater verbal abilities. However, when VMA was controlled for, children with WS made a greater number of commission errors than did either the DS of the TD groups. These findings point to a relative strength in sustained attention in children with WS (as measured by the lower frequency of omissions) but a greater propensity for impulsive or uninhibited responses (as measured by the higher frequency of commissions). The latter, as an index of executive difficulties, is consistent with the executive-function problems reported for older individuals with WS (Chapter 8). Of note, a smaller number of omissions does not necessarily index better sustained attention overall: as an extreme example, responding perseveratively on every trial would result in no omissions and many commissions. At a minimum, nonetheless, we can say that children with WS did not miss as many targets as children with DS or as younger TD children.

On the visual search task, children with DS were slower than the other children, perhaps as a result of generally slower motor processing. Children with DS made more errors on this task than the other groups; however, when taking into account their higher verbal ability, children with WS also made significantly more errors than the TD group but not than the DS group. TD children exhibited shorter distances between touches, a finding to which we return later.

Literacy skills, such as recognising letters and reading words, tend to develop rapidly following some form of instruction. Therefore, comparing school-aged children with WS or DS with a group of TD 3-year-olds would not be appropriate in this instance. In order to overcome this issue, we also compared our participants with a second group of TD children aged 3-5 years for literacy measures. Logistic regressions indicated that group membership did not matter to the likelihood of displaying rhyme awareness, whereas VMA did, indicating that the chances of having rhyme awareness increased with increasing VMA. In the context of phoneme awareness, membership of the WS group contributed variance to the model, indicating that children with WS were more likely to have phoneme awareness than the other two groups, an intriguing finding because it appeared in the context of single-word reading scores that were no different from the other children. This distinction between acoustic (Majerus et al., 2010) or phonological strengths that do not necessarily associate with good reading is interesting and consistent with studies of older readers with WS (e.g. Laing, 2002; Laing et al., 2001). Indeed, Majerus and colleagues (2010) go as far as suggesting that higher sensitivity to sometimes irrelevant acoustic discriminations for both speech and nonspeech sounds may in fact thwart the process of reading acquisition over development, by hindering unambiguous mappings between phonemes and graphemes. VMA also contributed to phoneme awareness, again showing that phoneme awareness improved with increasing VMA. The three groups did not differ in letter knowledge and word reading. However, when verbal ability was controlled

Table 18.3 Attention, literacy and numeracy profiles in young children (unpublished data)

Attention measure	WS (n=27)[a]	DS (n=26)[a]	TD (n=22)[a,b]	Group difference	Bonferroni post-hoc tests	Controlling for VMA
Sample characteristics						
Age (months)	78.48 (11.25)	82.58 (14.13)	40.59 (3.25)	<.001	WS=DS>TD	WS<DS=TD
Verbal MA[c] (months)	60.70 (20.50)	40.25 (9.56)	47.18 (10.74)	<.001	WS>DS=TD	
Nonverbal MA[d] (months)	38.22 (6.67)	38.50 (8.49)	43.14 (9.28)	ns		
Experimental attention measures						
Sustained attention/Continuous Performance Test						
No. of omission errors[e]	8.12 (5.25)	12.67 (4.73)	13.32 (5.87)	<.001[f]	WS<DS=TD	WS<DS=TD
Mean RT per hit (ms)	789.63 (185.56)	830.62 (209.78)	886.57 (229.77)	ns		
No. of commission errors	17.19 (19.24)	13.17 (13.40)	6.14 (6.46)	ns[f]		WS>DS=TD
Selective attention/visual search task						
Mean RT between touches (ms)	2494.12 (770.68)	4508.99 (2926.05)	2612.80 (1182.72)	<.001[f]	WS=TD<DS	WS=TD<DS
Mean distance between touches (pxls)	227.11 (58.54)	209.78 (69.56)	83.84 (27.01)	<.001[f]	TD<WS=DS	TD<WS=DS
Number of errors	15.73 (14.08)	30.48 (20.83)	7.98 (8.59)	<.001[f]	WS=TD<DS	WS=DS>TD

(Continued)

Table 18.3 (Cont'd.)

Literacy and numeracy measures

Attention measure	WS (n=27)[a]	DS (n=26)[a]	TD (n=22)[a,b]	Group difference	Bonferroni post-hoc tests	Controlling for VMA
Literacy tasks[g]						
Rhyme awareness[h]	15 (56%)	4 (15%)	38 (60%)			
Phoneme awareness[h]	17 (63%)	4 (15%)	26 (41%)			
Mean letter knowledge[i]	15.96 (8.74)	16.36 (8.90)	11.62 (10.92)	ns[f]		WS=TD<DS
Mean word reading[j]	8.37 (13.63)	10.48 (14.44)	6.57 (12.75)	ns[f]		WS=TD<DS
Numeracy tasks						
Cardinality[k]	11.48 (5.95)	7.92 (5.88)	8.86 (4.09)	ns		
TEMA-III (raw score)	13.30 (9.29)	8.48 (8.04)	7.36 (7.09)	.030	WS=DS WS>TD	

Abbreviations: DS = Down syndrome; MA = mental age; ns = not significant; No. = number; pxls = pixels; RT = reaction time; TD = typical development; TEMA-III = Test of Early Mathematics Ability, third edition (Ginsburg & Baroody, 2003); VMA = verbal mental age; WS = Williams syndrome.

[a] The data are provided as mean (standard deviation) unless indicated otherwise; [b] n=63 for literacy; [c] Assessed using the British Picture Vocabulary Scale II (Dunn et al., 1997); [d] Pattern Construction subscale of the British Ability Scales (Elliott et al., 1996); [e] Total number of targets = 20; [f] When controlling for VMA; [g] The age range of children in the TD group for comparison on literacy measures is 3–5 years to allow for the impact of formal schooling on literacy skills; [h] The data are provided as number of passes (percentage); dichotomous variables are not suitable for multivariate linear regression, so logistic regression analysis was performed; the full model of rhyme awareness was statistically significant (χ^2 [3,116]=49.36, p<.001) as a whole, explained between 35.1% (Cox and Snell R square) and 46.9% (Nagelkerke R square) of the variance in rhyme awareness and correctly classified 78.1% of cases; the full model of phoneme awareness was also significant (χ^2 [3,116]=67.19, p<.001), explained between 44.5% and 60% of the variance in phoneme awareness and correctly classified 82.5% of cases; [i] Total number of letters presented = 26; [j] Total number of words presented = 42; [k] Give-a-number task involving three small and three large numerosities, with three trials each, for a total number of trials of 18.

for, significant differences between the groups did emerge, with children with DS performing better than the other groups on both of these measures. This finding indicates that although on the surface literacy skills across these groups seem comparable, taking into account the poor language skills of the children with DS indicates that their literacy skills are in fact relatively better than those of the other groups. Again, there were no differences between the groups on their cardinality performance, but children with WS scored higher on the TEMA-III than did the other two groups. However, this difference was eliminated by taking into account verbal ability, implying that better TEMA-III scores were supported by better language skills in the WS group.

Relationships between attention and domain-specific skills

In order to explore cross-domain relationships, partial correlations controlling for chronological age differences were conducted between performance on the experimental attention tasks and performance on the numeracy and literacy tasks within each of the groups (see Table 18.4 for full details).

In TD children, omission errors on the CPT (an index of sustained attention) correlated negatively with cardinality and TEMA-III, indicating that poorer sustained attention may impact on the acquisition of numeracy skills. In children aged 3-5 years (to allow for some school exposure to literacy tuition), the time to respond to hits on the CPT (perhaps indexing less impulsive responding) correlated positively with letter knowledge, whereas the number of CPT commission errors correlated negatively with letter knowledge, perhaps indicating a link between slower, more accurate, less impulsive responding and early literacy skills. Word reading was positively correlated with the distance measure from the visual search task, indicating that greater distances between touches bore some relation to better reading skills. Such a finding might seem counter-intuitive if we interpret shorter search distance as representative of absolute search efficiency. However, we have good reasons to believe that, with this particular visual search task (requiring participants to search a large display and rely on their categorical knowledge of animals), longer distances might indicate a qualitatively different and perhaps more sophisticated semantic-based search strategy (e.g. search iteratively for all cats, then all dogs, etc.), rather than a simpler space-based systematic search.

For children with WS, a significant negative correlation was found between cardinality and number of omission errors on the CPT, indicating that better sustained attention in children with WS may relate to better cardinality understanding. Further relationships with cardinality were also found with distance between touches and number of errors on the visual search task, with a greater distance correlating again with better cardinality, a finding that is in line with longer distances relating to better performance in TD children. The negative correlation between cardinality understanding and number of errors on the visual search task is straightforward and indicates that children with WS who made fewer errors on this task were more likely to have better understanding of the cardinality principle. Similar to the situation for children with WS, negative correlations between cardinality score, number of errors on the visual search task and number of commission errors on

Table 18.4 Correlation coefficients for the associations between attention, numeracy and literacy measures in young children (controlled for chronological age) (unpublished data)

	WS (n=27)				DS (n=26)				TD (n=22)				TD (n=63)	
	Numeracy		Reading		Numeracy		Reading		Numeracy		Reading		Reading	
	Card.	TEMA-III	LK	EWR	Card.	TEMA-III	LK	EWR	Card.	TEMA-III	LK	EWR	LK	EWR
Sustained attention/Continuous Performance Test														
No. of omission errors	**-0.446***	-0.390	-0.375	-0.143	0.168	-0.090	0.016	-0.210	**-0.469***	**-0.602***	-0.238	-	0.051	0.033
Mean RT per hit	-0.117	-0.273	-0.052	-0.132	0.235	0.204	0.285	0.347	0.311	0.435	0.396	-	**0.373***	-0.053
No. of commission errors	-0.090	-0.115	-0.121	-0.124	**-0.563***	**-0.548***	-0.309	**-0.555***	0.359	0.066	-0.153	-	**-0.267***	-0.164
Selective attention/visual search task														
Mean RT between touches (ms)	0.081	0.057	-0.009	0.042	0.160	0.042	0.080	0.257	-0.014	-0.026	-0.021	-	-0.009	0.075
Mean distance between touches (pxls)	**0.451***	0.370	0.179	-0.030	0.344	**0.452***	**0.400***	**0.513***	0.339	0.337	0.116	-	0.183	**0.412******
No. of errors	**-0.471***	-0.329	-0.274	-0.072	**-0.528***	**-0.588***	**-0.462***	**-0.461***	-0.276	-0.156	-0.154	-	-0.122	0.004

Abbreviations: Card. = cardinality; DS = Down syndrome; EWR = early word reading; LK = letter knowledge; pxls = pixels; RT = reaction time; TD = typical development; TEMA-III = Test of Early Mathematics Ability, third edition (Ginsburg & Baroody, 2003); WS = Williams syndrome.

* p<.05; *** p<.001

the CPT emerged for children with DS. These findings further support the proposal that children who are more prone to making errors, perhaps because of a lack of inhibition, are less likely to have good cardinality understanding, regardless of group. This may be related to difficulties concentrating in the classroom in general or more specifically to difficulties in going beyond the counting sequence to grasp the fundamental mapping between number words and cardinality (reported for children with WS by Ansari et al., 2003). Further positive correlations emerged for children with DS between the visual search distance and TEMA-III, letter knowledge and word reading, again suggesting that search distance may not indicate higher or lower search efficiency in absolute terms, but may indicate a qualitatively different search strategy, and one that might relate longer distances to better performance across domains. Negative correlations were found between the number of errors on the visual search and on all of the numeracy and literacy measures for children with DS, again supporting a link between greater accuracy and better scholastic performance. A further negative correlation was shown between word reading and number of commission errors on the sustained attention task, indicating that lower impulsivity is associated with better word reading.

Hierarchical regression analyses were then conducted to establish further whether group membership and attention measures made significant and unique contributions to variance on the numeracy and literacy measures. Age significantly explained variance in cardinality scores, and performance on the attention measures explained a further 17% of variance, although none of the individual attention predictors emerged as a significant unique predictor. Of note, the lack of group effects underscores similar relationships between attention measures and cardinality understanding across groups. Age and group membership also explained 39% of the variance in the TEMA-III score, and performance on the attention measures explained a further 19% of variance. In this model, age, WS group membership, DS group membership and CPT omission errors were all statistically significant predictors of unique variance in TEMA-III performance, indicating that basic numeracy performance was influenced uniquely by group membership and impulsivity in this case. Age significantly explained variance in letter knowledge, and performance on the attention measures explained a further 6% of variance. Only age and mean distance between touches on the visual search were statistically significant predictors of unique variance in this model. Just as with cardinality, the lack of group effects indicates similarities across groups. Finally, age and group membership accounted for 35% of the variance in word reading, and a further 9% of the variance was explained when the attention measures were added to the model. Similarly to letter knowledge, age and mean distance between touches on the visual search task were significant predictors of unique variance in word reading. In addition, however, WS and DS group membership were also significant predictors of word reading, underscoring group differences.

In summary, then, the profile for young children with WS in attention, early literacy and numeracy indicates relatively good ability to remain on task but weaknesses in impulsive responding as well as a tendency to make search errors. This is coupled with strengths in phoneme awareness and with literacy and numeracy skills that are at least in line with developmental level (i.e. not relatively more greatly affected than overall cognitive functioning), although again this actually means poorer reading and numeracy than expected given their age. Again, investigating the profile of individual children across domains was highly informative: correlations existed between the attention measures and numeracy but also literacy measures for TD children and children with DS (indicating attentional effects across domains) but, importantly, not for children with WS. In WS, attention measures, such as omission errors, search distance and search errors, related to cardinality understanding alone. Interestingly, for children with WS (and for children with DS), verbal abilities play a role in these profiles, with for example better basic numeracy in children with WS being driven by their advantage in verbal abilities. Again, longitudinal studies are needed to study in more depth what drives these relationships over developmental time.

Insights from other cross-syndrome comparisons in attentional profiles

Beyond the similarities and differences between infants and children with WS and DS, another cross-syndrome comparison can help us shed further light onto the potential relationships between attentional profiles in WS and their development in other aspects of cognition (as we have argued elsewhere with these and other examples; see Scerif & Steele, 2011). Atypical attentional orienting and executive control of eye movements in infants and toddlers with WS or fragile X syndrome, compared with TD children, have been reported across a variety of studies. In an experiment designed to investigate children's ability to inhibit orienting to a suddenly presented but boring peripheral stimulus and to orient faster towards a more exciting and rewarding visual stimulus, young children with fragile X syndrome showed difficulties inhibiting looks towards the sudden peripheral stimuli (Scerif et al., 2005), an executive failure that is consistent with other findings from young children in this group. By contrast, toddlers with WS tested with the same paradigm struggled to orient peripherally at all and remaining fixated on the central stimulus (Cornish et al., 2007), a pattern that is consistent with the findings by Atkinson et al. (2003) and Brown et al. (2003). Furthermore, even when covert orienting skills were assessed, these two groups of young children differed (Cornish et al., 2007). The experimenters presented toddlers with a modification of Posner's covert orienting of attention paradigm (Posner, 1980), in which an orienting cue preceded the appearance of an interesting visual stimulus, with cue and target stimulus appearing either at the same location (valid cueing) or at different locations, requiring children to disengage from the cued location to orient to the target. Infants and toddlers with WS were significantly slower in deploying this disengagement process than those with fragile X syndrome, indicating subtle differences in both covert and overt orienting of attention.

Of note, the patterns of looks in both the voluntary and covert orienting task fit very neatly with suggestions of sticky fixation in infants and older children with WS, especially because the central fixation stimuli were not simple schematics and contained face-like stimuli (e.g. a rotating clown or teddy bear). As Karmiloff-Smith and colleagues have long proposed (e.g. Karmiloff-Smith, 1998, 2007, 2009), this small early difficulty in disengagement from centrally presented stimuli may impact on how infants with WS forage the visual environment and learn about new information that is critical, for example, to estimate numerosities accurately in infancy (Van Herwegen et al., 2008) and later in childhood (Ansari et al., 2007). A similar argument may well be extended to infants with fragile X syndrome: their difficulties in inhibiting orienting to peripheral stimuli may be a precursor of their later high distractibility in new learning situations. Investigating the long-term effects of these early subtle orienting differences requires longitudinal studies tracking infants into childhood.

Further light is shed on these issues by considering comparisons of slightly older toddlers and young children with WS with a further group of children with attentional difficulties. Scerif and colleagues (2004) examined abilities by toddlers with WS, toddlers with fragile X syndrome and TD toddlers. A visual search task was presented on a touch screen computer and children were instructed to find 'monsters' hidden beneath big circles. The search also contained smaller circles representing distracters, and perceptual similarity (size) of these distracters to the targets was manipulated in 'similar' and 'dissimilar' conditions. It was found that even though the two atypical groups did not differ from TD controls in terms of search speed, both groups made a significantly greater number of errors on the task. Further analyses demonstrated that the WS group made significantly more touches to distracters, whereas the fragile X syndrome children made more perseverative errors, in which they would retouch targets that they had already touched. Therefore, it seemed that young children with fragile X syndrome displayed hallmarks of the executive attention difficulties reported for older children with the condition (e.g. Hooper et al., 2008; Sullivan et al., 2007; Munir et al., 2000; Wilding et al., 2002), whereas toddlers with WS were finding it harder to select targets among distracters differentiated solely by size, and their high number of errors reflected this confusion. This study provided evidence for common deficits in selective attention in children with fragile X syndrome and WS, who produced more errors of all kinds than TD children, but found attentional control and appropriate stimulus selection, respectively, relatively more challenging. Of note, children with fragile X syndrome also produced more distracter errors than TD children, suggesting that their attentional difficulties extend beyond executive difficulties alone and do impact on how efficiently they select relevant stimuli among distracters. The latter finding also argues against a simple view of attentional difficulties across the two disorders, with a double dissociation of some impaired and some intact abilities, and pushes towards the neuroconstructivist approach of thinking more carefully about how multiple, differentially affected, attentional processes all contribute to learning across domains. If challenged in a complex visual environment in which to learn, children with WS or fragile X syndrome would struggle to select relevant information and inhibit some types of responses.

Conclusions: exploring cross-domain dynamics

We began by spurring ourselves to interrogate old and new data afresh and to go beyond profiles of domain-specific strengths and weaknesses in both infants and young children with WS. A developmental, neuroconstructivist perspective on individual domains already pointed us to the importance of studying empirically cognitive profiles over developmental time, and our domain-specific data reinforced that point. For example, while relative strengths in sustained attention were apparent for both infants and young children with WS (even though this construct was measured in very different ways across age groups), it was also clear that the vocabulary advantage reported for WS emerged in our older, but not in our younger, age group. There were also some intriguing and unusual patterns of within-domain profiles, for example comparably delayed single-word reading abilities in children with WS despite relative strengths in phoneme awareness. Critically, however, we also asked how individuals within each group recruit dynamically distinct attentional processes in function of domain-specific tasks. This is a question that would be best addressed by prospective longitudinal designs, mapping the directionality of these relationships over the changing environmental demands and constraints imposed on atypical (and typical) developing systems. Here, we begin with a preliminary but necessary step: to demonstrate not only how, in neurodevelopmental disorders, functioning in individual domains can be atypical, but also how it can differ in its relationships with domain-general processes. Typical relationships, reflected in infants and young children with DS despite their developmental delay, do not hold in the same way for infants and young children with WS.

Overall, our findings—albeit preliminary—highlight the rich and novel insights that derive from complementing in-depth domain-specific investigations with a study of the dynamical interplay between domain-general and -specific functions as they emerge over developmental time. We believe that this exercise is critical, particularly in infancy and early childhood, when subtle attentional changes may have long-term cascading effects on learning. Of course, taking a dynamic approach to cross-domain relations may also have practical implications in that it may highlight ways in which interventions could target not only domain-specific processes but also domain-general processes, such as attentional control and working memory, to impact developmental outcomes (e.g. Holmes et al., 2009). First and foremost, however, cross-domain interactions in typical development and their modifications in neurodevelopmental disorders such as WS pose a real problem for strictly modular theories of cognition. According to these, individual domains/modules would be individually and independently spared or impaired. The current data push us further 'beyond modularity' by highlighting, instead, how domain-specific and domain-general processes interact dynamically with each other over developmental time.

Editor commentary (Emily K. Farran & Annette Karmiloff-Smith)

This chapter takes the reader beyond the profile of phenotypic strengths and weaknesses to explore the impact of domain-general processes, namely attentional abilities, on domain-specific abilities. Here, the specific domains of language and number were explored within the context of domain-general attentional abilities. The authors demonstrated that language and number competencies across different neurodevelopmental syndrome groups can be supported by different attentional mechanisms, even if competencies in these domain-specific abilities seem to be similar. For example, number discrimination for infants with WS is associated with impaired orienting of attention, whereas number in TD and DS groups is associated with sustained attention, a relative weakness in the DS group. Thus, even if they were to have similar number skills in infancy, different relationships between domain-general and domain-specific processes would predict syndrome-specific constraints on subsequent development in WS and DS. This infancy example, and the examples presented later in this chapter between WS, DS and TD school-age children and between toddlers with WS and fragile X syndrome, demonstrated how cross-syndrome comparisons enable additional refinement of our understanding of developmental trajectories. Importantly, the neuroconstructivist exploration of cross-domain relationships early in development not only fosters predictions of domain-specific developmental trajectories, but it also emphasises the potential benefits of early domain-general intervention for any neurodevelopmental disorder on the development of domain-specific processes such as literacy and numeracy.

References

Adams, J.W., & Snowling, M.J. (2001). Executive function and reading impairments in children reported by their teachers as 'hyperactive'. *British Journal of Developmental Psychology*, **19**, 293–306.

Adams, J.W., Snowling, M.J., Hennessy, S.M., & Kind, P. (1999). Problems of behaviour, reading and arithmetic: assessments of comorbidity using the Strengths and Difficulties Questionnaire. *British Journal of Educational Psychology*, **69**, 571–85.

Ansari, D., Donlan, C., & Karmiloff-Smith, A. (2007). Typical and atypical development of visual estimation abilities. *Cortex*, **43**, 758–68.

Ansari, D., Donlan, C., Thomas, M.S.C., Ewing, S.A., Peen, T., & Karmiloff-Smith, A. (2003). What makes counting count? Verbal and visuo-spatial contributions to typical and atypical number development. *Journal of Experimental Child Psychology*, **85**, 50–62.

Atkinson, J., Braddick, O., Anker, S., Curran, W., Andrew, R., Wattam-Bell, J., et al. (2003). Neurobiological models of visuospatial cognition in children with Williams syndrome: measures of dorsal-stream and frontal function. *Developmental Neuropsychology*, **23**, 139–72.

Bayley, N. (1993). *The Bayley Scales of Infant Development—Second Edition*. San Antonio, TX: The Psychological Corporation.

Brown, J.H., Johnson, M.H., Paterson, S.J., Gilmore, R., Longhi, E., & Karmiloff-Smith, A. (2003). Spatial representation and attention in toddlers with Williams syndrome and Down syndrome. *Neuropsychologia*, **41**, 1037–46.

Bull, R., Espy, K.A., & Wiebe, S.A. (2008). Short-term memory, working memory, and executive functioning in preschoolers: longitudinal predictors of mathematical achievement at age 7 years. *Developmental Neuropsychology*, **33**, 205–28.

Bull, R., & Scerif, G. (2001). Executive functioning as a predictor of children's mathematics ability: inhibition, switching, and working memory. *Developmental Neuropsychology*, **19**, 273–93.

Carroll, J.M., Snowling, M.J., Stevenson, J., & Hulme, C. (2003). The development of phonological awareness in preschool children. *Developmental Psychology*, **39**, 913–23.

Cornish, K., Kogan, C., Turk, J., Manly, T., James, N., Mills, A., & et al. (2005). The emerging fragile X premutation phenotype: evidence from the domain of social cognition. *Brain and Cognition*, **57**, 53–60.

Cornish, K., Scerif, G., & Karmiloff-Smith, A. (2007). Tracing syndrome-specific trajectories of attention across the lifespan. *Cortex*, **43**, 672–85.

Dunn, L.M., Dunn, L.M., Whetton, C., & Burley, J. (1997). *British Picture Vocabulary Scale II*. Windsor: NFER-Nelson.

Elliott, C.D., Smith, P., & McCulloch, K. (1996). *The British Ability Scales II*. Windsor: NFER-Nelson.

Farran, E.K., Jarrold, C., & Gathercole, S.E. (2001). Block design performance in the Williams syndrome phenotype: a problem with mental imagery? *Journal of Child Psychology and Psychiatry and Allied Disciplines*, **42**, 719–28.

Fenson, L., Dale, J., Resnick, S., Thal, D., Bates, E., Hartung, J.P., et al. (1993). *MacArthur Communicative Development Inventories: User s Guide and Technical Manual*. San Diego, CA: Singular Publishing Group.

Fuchs, L.S., Compton, D.L., Fuchs, D., Paulsen, K., Bryant, J.D., & Hamlett, C.L. (2005). The prevention, identification, and cognitive determinants of math difficulty. *Journal of Educational Psychology*, **97**, 493–513.

Gathercole, S.E., & Pickering, S.J. (2000). Working memory deficits in children with low achievements in the national curriculum at 7 years of age. *British Journal of Educational Psychology*, **70**, 177–94.

Gilmore, R.O., and Johnson, M.H. (1997). Body-centered representations for visually-guided action emerge during early infancy. *Cognition*, **65**, B1–B9.

Ginsburg, H.P., & Baroody, A.J. (2003). *The Test of Early Mathematics Ability—Third Edition*. Austin, TX: Pro-Ed.

Grant, C.M., Apperly, I., & Oliver, C. (2007). Is theory of mind understanding impaired in males with fragile X syndrome? *Journal of Abnormal Child Psychology*, **35**, 17–28.

Hagerman, R.J., & Hagerman, P.J. (2002). *Fragile X Syndrome: Diagnosis, Treatment, and Research*, 3rd edn. Baltimore, MD: Johns Hopkins University Press.

Hatcher, P.J., Hulme, C., & Ellis, A.W. (1994). Ameliorating early reading failure by integrating the teaching of reading and phonological skills: the phonological linkage hypothesis. *Child Development*, **65**, 41–57.

Holmes, J., Gathercole, S.E., & Dunning, D.L. (2009). Adaptive training leads to sustained enhancement of poor working memory in children. *Developmental Science*, **12**, F9–F15.

Hooper, S.R., Hatton, D., Sideris, J., Sullivan, K., Hammer, J., Schaaf, J., et al. (2008). Executive functions in young males fragile X syndrome in comparison to mental age-matched with controls: baseline findings from a longitudinal study. *Neuropsychology*, **22**, 36–47.

Jarrold, C., Baddeley, A.D., & Hewes, A.K. (1999). Genetically dissociated components of working memory: evidence from Down's and Williams syndrome. *Neuropsychologia*, **37**, 637–51.

Jordan, H., Reiss, J.E., Hoffman, J.E., & Landau, B. (2002). Intact perception of biological motion in the face of profound spatial deficits: Williams syndrome. *Psychological Science*, **13**, 162–67.

Karmiloff-Smith, A. (1998). Development itself is the key to understanding developmental disorders. *Trends in Cognitive Sciences*, **2**, 389–98.

Karmiloff-Smith, A. (2007). Williams syndrome. *Current Biology*, **17**, R1035–36.

Karmiloff-Smith, A. (2009). Nativism versus neuroconstructivism: rethinking the study of developmental disorders. *Developmental Psychology*, **45**, 56–63.

Karmiloff-Smith, A., Scerif, G., & Ansari, D. (2003). Double dissociations in developmental disorders? Theoretically misconceived, empirically dubious. *Cortex*, **39**, 161–63.

Kogan, C.S., Bertone, A., Cornish, K., Boutet, I., Der Kaloustian, V.M., Andermann, E., et al. (2004a). Integrative cortical dysfunction and pervasive motion perception deficit in fragile X syndrome. *Neurology*, **63**, 1634–39.

Kogan, C.S., Boutet, I., Cornish, K., Zangenehpour, S., Mullen, K.T., Holden, J.J., et al. (2004b). Differential impact of the FMR1 gene on visual processing in fragile X syndrome. *Brain*, **127**, 591–601.

Laing, E. (2002). Investigating reading development in atypical populations: The case of Williams syndrome. *Reading and Writing*, **15**, 575–87.

Laing, E., Hulme, C., Grant, J., & Karmiloff-Smith, A. (2001). Learning to read in Williams syndrome: looking beneath the surface of atypical reading development. *The Journal of Child Psychology and Psychiatry and Allied Disciplines*, **42**, 729–39.

Majerus, S., Poncelet, M., Berault, A., Audrey, S., Zesiger, P., Serniclaes, W., et al. (2010). Evidence for atypical categorical speech perception in Williams syndrome. *Journal of Neurolinguistics*, **24**, 249–67.

Miranda, S.B., and Fantz, R.L. (1973). Visual preferences of Down's syndrome and normal infants. *Child Development*, **44**, 555–61.

Munir, F., Cornish, K.M., & Wilding, J. (2000). A neuropsychological profile of attention deficits in young males with fragile X syndrome. *Neuropsychologia*, **38**, 1261–70.

Muter, V., Hulme, C., & Snowling, M. (1997a). *Phonological Abilities Test (PAT)*. London: Psychological Corporation.

Muter, V., Hulme, C., Snowling, M.J., & Stevenson, J. (2004). Phonemes, rimes, vocabulary, and grammatical skills as foundations of early reading development: evidence from a longitudinal study. *Developmental Psychology*, **40**, 665–81.

Muter, V., Hulme, C., Snowling, M., & Taylor, S. (1997b). Segmentation, not rhyming, predicts early progress in learning to read. *Journal of Experimental Child Psychology*, **65**, 370–96.

Nation, K., & Snowling, M.J. (2004). Beyond phonological skills: broader language skills contribute to the development of reading. *Journal of Research in Reading*, **27**, 342–56.

Paterson, S.J., Brown, J.H., Gsödl, M.K., Johnson, M.H., & Karmiloff-Smith, A. (1999). Cognitive modularity and genetic disorders. *Science*, **286**, 2355–58.

Phillips, C.E., Jarrold, C., Baddeley, A.D., Grant, J., & Karmiloff-Smith, A. (2004). Comprehension of spatial language terms in Williams syndrome: evidence for an interaction between domains of strength and weakness. *Cortex*, **40**, 85–101.

Posner, M.I. (1980). Orienting of attention. *Quarterly Journal of Experimental Psychology* **32**, 3–25.

Posner, M.I., & Rothbart, M.K. (2005). Influencing brain networks: implications for education. *Trends in Cognitive Sciences*, **9**, 99–103.

Roberts, J.E., Mirrett, P., & Burchinal, M. (2001). Receptive and expressive communication development of young males with fragile X syndrome. *American Journal on Mental Retardation,* **106**, 216–30.

Rothbart, M.K. (1981). Measurement of temperament in infancy. *Child Development*, **52**, 569–78.

Rothbart, M.K. (1999). *Developing a Model for the Study of Temperament*. Presented at a meeting of the Society for Research in Child Development, Albuquerque, NM.

Rothbart, M.K., & Hanson, M.J. (1983). A caregiver report comparison of temperamental characteristics of Down syndrome and normal infants. *Developmental Psychology*, **19**, 766–69.

Ruff, H.A., & Lawson, K.R. (1991). Assessment of infants' attention during play with objects. In C.E. Schaefer, K. Critlin & A. Sandgrund (Eds), *Play Diagnosis and Assessment* (pp. 115–29). New York, NY: John Wiley and Sons.

Sarpal, D., Buchsbaum, B.R., Kohn, P.D., Kippenhan, J.S., Mervis, C.B., Morris, C.A., et al. (2008). A genetic model for understanding higher order visual processing: functional interactions of the ventral visual stream in Williams syndrome. *Cerebral Cortex*, **18**, 2402–2409.

Scerif, G., Cornish, K., Wilding, J., Driver, J., & Karmiloff-Smith, A. (2004). Visual search in typically developing toddlers and toddlers with fragile X or Williams syndrome. *Developmental Science*, **7**, 116–30.

Scerif, G., Karmiloff-Smith, A., Campos, R., Elsabbagh, M., Driver, J., & Cornish, K. (2005). To look or not to look? Typical and atypical development of oculomotor control. *Journal of Cognitive Neuroscience*, **17**, 591–604.

Scerif, G., & Steele, A. (2011). Neurocognitive development of attention across genetic syndromes: inspecting a disorder's dynamics through the lens of others. *Progress in Brain Research*, **189**, 285–301.

Steele, A., Karmiloff-Smith, A., Cornish, K.M., & Scerif, G. (in preparation). Atypical routes to numeracy and literacy: attentional processes as gateways.

Steele, A., Karmiloff-Smith, A., Cornish, K.M., & Scerif, G. (in press). The multiple sub-functions of attention: a developmental gateway to literacy and numeracy. *Child Development*.

Stinton, C., Farran, E.K., & Courbois, Y. (2008). Mental rotation in Williams syndrome: an impaired ability. *Developmental Neuropsychology*, **33**, 565–83.

Sullivan, K., Hatton, D.D., Hammer, J., Sideris, J., Hooper, S., Ornstein, P.A., et al. (2007). Sustained attention and response inhibition in boys with fragile X syndrome: measures of continuous performance. *American Journal of Medical Genetics Part B: Neuropsychiatric Genetics*, **144B**, 517–32.

Van Herwegen, J., Ansari, D., Xu, F., & Karmiloff-Smith, A. (2008). Small and large number processing in infants and toddlers with Williams syndrome. *Developmental Science*, **11**, 637–43.

Wilding, J., Cornish, K., & Munir, F. (2002). Further delineation of the executive deficit in males with fragile-X syndrome. *Neuropsychologia*, **40**, 1343–49.

Wynn, K. (1990). Children's understanding of counting. *Cognition*, **36**, 155–93.

Future theoretical and empirical directions within a neuroconstructivist framework

Annette Karmiloff-Smith and Emily K. Farran

Beyond Williams syndrome

In this book, we took Williams syndrome (WS) as a model neurodevelopmental disorder to illustrate how a neuroconstructivist, multilevel analysis could provide a rich and very detailed account of a disorder at the levels of gene expression, behaviour, cognition and brain. We particularly stressed the importance of differentiating between overt behaviour and the cognitive and neural processes that sustain it, as well as highlighting the significance of establishing full developmental trajectories for both typical and atypical development. Indeed, the book placed the neuroconstructivist approach to developmental disorders at its very heart and denounced the fact that almost everything we know about the atypical brain emanates from studies of adult brains, that is, the developed brain rather than the developing brain. Clearly, it remains necessary to trace brain anatomy, brain biochemistry and brain function across developmental time from infancy to adulthood.

To go beyond WS as a model disorder, cross-syndrome comparisons at the levels of gene expression, brain, cognition and behaviour are critical. Indeed, although different syndromes are caused by different gene mutations, it is becoming increasingly clear, particularly where transcription factors are concerned, that even when particular genes are not mutated in a given disorder, they may lie downstream to other genes that are mutated, and therefore their expression may also change, as demonstrated by the overexpression of *MAP1B* lymphoblastoid cell lines from individuals with WS (Antonell et al., 2010a, 2010b). Dynamic gene pathways can give rise to similar developmental outcomes even when different genes are mutated. And the opposite also holds: different outcomes can emerge from similar genetic mutations. So, a focus at all levels on cross-syndrome associations and not merely on cross-syndrome dissociations is crucial. As the book has repeatedly stressed, genes cannot be thought of in terms of static one-to-one mappings between gene function and cognitive outcome because the temporal and spatial expression of genes can change over developmental time.

Numerous examples are given throughout this book to illustrate the same arguments with reference to the development of the brain. For example, in typical development, when processing number, different neural circuits are activated in young children compared with adults (Rivera et al., 2005), and evidence presented in Chapter 6 demonstrates a similar change at the behavioural level, from a two-component system of attention at preschool age to a three-component system at school age. The importance of development is also exemplified in the atypical brain. Here, critical interactions between genes, behaviour, brain and environment affect neural pathways and, in turn, behavioural and cognitive outcome. For example, although individuals with WS show a typical susceptibility to visual illusions, this is accompanied by atypical neural activation (Grice et al., 2003). Furthermore, a comparison between attention deficit hyperactivity disorder and WS demonstrates that similar deficits in response inhibition can be caused by differential activation of neural circuits (Mobbs et al., 2007; Rubia et al., 2005), whereas comparison of autism spectrum disorders (ASDs) and WS reveals an association at the behavioural level for processing faces but a dissociation at the neural level (Grice et al., 2001). Conversely, the book provides numerous examples in which apparently similar abnormalities in brain structure or function are associated with more than one syndrome, yet each has a different syndrome-specific overall cognitive profile. Examples include atypicalities in the corpus callosum (observed in WS, autism, schizophrenia, Tourette syndrome), dorsal-stream abnormality (reported in WS, fragile X syndrome, developmental coordination disorder, autism) and cerebellum abnormalities (observed in WS, fragile X syndrome and fetal alcohol syndrome). This exemplifies, again, that the brain is a developing system and that the brain of an individual with a neuro-developmental disorder is likely to develop in a subtly atypical manner from the outset. Moreover, just as we posited above that genes and behaviour should not be considered in terms of one-to-one mappings, the same argument holds for brain–behaviour relations.

Our neuroconstructivist approach means that it is critical to raise cross-syndrome questions at multiple levels of analysis, such as: is this brain/cognitive/behavioural deficit syndrome-specific or is it syndrome-general, that is, is it characteristic of all atypical development where learning difficulties obtain or unique to a particular syndrome? Do impaired sleep patterns differ from syndrome to syndrome, as discussed in Chapter 7, and do such differences affect the consolidation of learning in the same way across different neurodevelopmental disorders? How do we explain the wide range of individual differences both within syndromes and across syndromes presenting with similar overall IQ scores? Do scores 'in the normal range' necessarily mean that processes are intact or do atypical neural and/or cognitive processes underlie the proficient behaviour? Actually, the very concept of 'intact and impaired modules' is, from a neuroconstructivist stance, theoretically flawed because it ignores the dynamic processes of development over time. Will longitudinal studies of the atypically developing brain, using a convergence of several methodologies, yield insights that cross-sectional studies miss? How does having a neurodevelopmental disorder subtly change the environment in which the atypical infant/child develops? Theoretically driven intervention studies that consider the dynamics of development will become increasingly critical in our future attempts to answer these vital questions.

Domain relevance versus domain specificity

The neuroconstructivist approach also differentiates domain-relevant mechanisms from domain-specific or domain-general ones. Take the discovery of a *FOXP2* mutation in members of a family who have a speech and language deficit (Lai et al., 2003). This initially led to claims that the *FOXP2* gene was a 'gene for language' (Gopnik & Crago, 1991) and that its discovery announced the era of cognitive genetics (Pinker, 2001), as if one could map more or less directly from genes to cognition. It soon became apparent, however, that the *FOXP2* gene was more likely to contribute to subtle differences in very basic-level processes (Fisher & Scharff, 2009) involved, for instance, in the planning of rapid movement sequences and their timing, which is indeed very relevant to human speech but not specific to it (Karmiloff-Smith, 2009). Interestingly, it turns out that in passerine birds that learn their song (e.g. zebra finches, canaries), the *foxp2* gene has greater expression during the period when the chick is learning its song than during subsequent production of the song in the adult (Haesler et al., 2004; see also Bolhuis et al., 2000), indicating that the gene plays a role in learning and plasticity. Other research reveals that in the mouse, the *foxp2* gene is initially expressed in multiple brain areas, but its expression becomes progressively confined to motor circuits, particularly the cerebellum (Lai et al., 2003), highlighting its importance in movement planning.

Because *FOXP2* is a highly conserved gene across species, it has become obvious that *FOXP2* in humans is not a gene specific to speech and language. It is extremely relevant to speech and language because speech is a domain where the planning of rapid movement sequences and their timing is most critical in the human case. However, subsequent research (Vargha-Khadem et al., 1995) showed that the *FOXP2* mutation also leads to deficits in fine motor, nonverbal domains such as the perception and production of simple rhythms and the planning of non-language-related facial movement sequences. So, the effects of the *FOXP2* mutation are much more widespread and subtle than initially thought because the gene contributes to something more basic and general than only speech: the coordination and timing of rapid movement sequences. It is obvious that genes do not act in isolation in a predetermined way. The profiles of downstream genes to which *FOXP2* binds indicate roles in a wide range of general, not domain-specific, functions including morphogenesis, neuronal development, axon guidance, synaptic plasticity and neurotransmission (Teramisu & White, 2006). This differs from theorising at the level of cognitive modules and points to the multilevel complexities of genotype–phenotype relations in understanding human development in any domain.

The function of the *FOXP2* gene constitutes a particularly nice example of domain relevance, whereby the planning of rapid movement sequences is most relevant to human speech but not solely specific to it. Thinking of functions in terms of domain relevance rather than domain specificity also raises a different set of questions. If one considers a gene to contribute solely to a domain-specific process such as vocal communication, then one only targets animal models such as bird song or mouse cries. By contrast, if one considers a process to be domain-relevant, then one can ask what other processes involve, say, the rapid planning of movement sequences and their timing; for example, in the human case that could be the playing of a musical instrument such as the piano or the violin. Moreover, when creating an animal model of the mutation on the *foxp2* gene, the scientist would not only focus on vocal communication (the animal equivalent of human speech) but would also ask a domain-relevant question: which other processes in the animal's repertoire call for the planning of rapid movement sequences and their timing? This is a deeper, neuroconstructivist question.

Note that neuroconstructivism does not rule out domain specificity; it argues that domain specificity cannot be taken for granted when one domain is more impaired than another (Karmiloff-Smith, 1998), because these are relative comparisons and not absolute ones. Rather, full developmental trajectories and cross-domain interactions must always be explored. Unlike the nativist perspective, neuroconstructivism offers a truly developmental approach that focuses on change and emergent outcomes.

Associations versus dissociations

Let us briefly take again the case of WS and autism spectrum disorder (ASD), discussed in several of the book chapters. Never have two syndromes seemed so dissociated at first blush. ASDs are likely to be caused by multiple genes of small effect. Phenotypically, individuals with ASD are aloof, dislike looking at eyes/faces, prefer to interact with objects rather than people and are good at spatial puzzles. WS, as we have seen, is caused by the hemizygous deletion of 28 genes, four of which are likely to be of large effect. In sharp contrast to people with ASD, individuals with WS are phenotypically very friendly, fascinated by eyes/faces, prefer to interact with people rather than objects and are very poor at spatial tasks. Yet, a closer, subtler scrutiny reveals many associations. In early development, individuals with WS and individuals with ASD both have difficulties with rapid eye movement planning, atypical eye gaze following, atypical pointing, atypical triadic attention, hyperacusis, obsessions and atypical sustained and selective attention. In later development, again both have better piecemeal learning than global learning, poor generalisation, heightened sensitivity to sounds, deficits identifying complex emotional expressions, poor judgement of personal space, problems with pragmatics of language, failure on nonword repetition tasks and failure on a number of theory-of-mind tasks. The in-depth phenotyping of the associations between syndromes is likely to lead to deeper understanding of the subtle differences between each individual syndrome. This book presents the reader with many examples of associations across syndromes, but poses just as many questions, such as: if different neural activation is observed for children with attention deficit hyperactivity disorder and WS during response inhibition, how does this compare with other neurodevelopmental disorders who also show impaired response inhibition such as autism, fragile X syndrome and Turner syndrome? If spatial language is impaired in WS and Down syndrome, yet these two disorders show contrasting cognitive profiles, what are the cognitive constraints on the development of spatial language in each group? If individuals with WS and individuals with fragile X syndrome both show deficits in cerebellar function and dorsal-stream processing, what can the associations and dissociations in the cognitive profiles of these groups tell us about these two overlapping brain networks? These questions, and many more, cry out for multilevel, cross-syndrome comparisons.

Taking genotype–phenotype relations in Williams syndrome one step further

Our knowledge of the genetic deletion involved in WS has increased substantially over recent years, with now 28 genes clearly delimited and knowledge of the gene expression of many of them well advanced. However, genotype–phenotype correlations are never straightforward, particularly in the case of rare syndromes. For more common ones, including dyslexia, developmental dyscalculia and ASD, behavioural genetics has made some huge advances in terms of identifying multiple genes of small effect. In WS, one avenue of very promising research has been the study of patients with partial deletions in the WS critical region. Often picked up in cardiology owing to heart murmurs, some patients turn out to have just two of the genes deleted in the WS critical region, namely *ELN* (encoding elastin) and *LIMK1* (encoding LIM domain kinase 1), whereas others have just three, four, five or more of the 28 genes deleted. Such patients, although constituting rare case studies, turn out to be very informative of genotype–phenotype relations if compared by in-depth phenotyping.

However, there are at least two important cautionary notes that need to be borne in mind. First, the researcher has to take account of the single, remaining copy of the genes on the nondeleted chromosome. These may be polymorphic and thus explain some of the individual differences we witness in WS. So, for instance, an initial study of two patients with just *ELN* and *LIMK1* deleted found some indication of facial dysmorphology as well as spatial deficits in the cognitive profile (Frangiskakis et al., 1996). The authors concluded that *ELN* was causal in the facial dysmorphology of WS and that *LIMK1*, expressed in the brain, was responsible for the spatial impairments typical of the syndrome. However, subsequent research (Gray et al., 2006; Karmiloff-Smith et al., 2002) identified patients also with *ELN* and *LIMK1* deleted but who had neither facial dysmorphology nor spatial impairments. Indeed, they had none of the WS cognitive profile, indicating that if *ELN* and *LIMK1* play any role in the outcome, it is attributable to allelic differences on the remaining two genes or to combinations with other genes. More recent studies of patients with more genes deleted but not the full WS deletion point to the four telomeric genes on the WS critical region as the most likely to be contributing to the full WS cognitive and physical profile. This type of in-depth phenotyping of physical and cognitive traits on patients with slightly varying genetic mutations within the WS critical region may help delineate the complexities of genotype–phenotype relations, but with a second proviso.

Our second proviso is that such studies must be truly developmental in nature, both in terms of gene expression over time and in terms of the changing cognitive profile. One longitudinal study of a child with 24 of the 28 WS genes deleted (Karmiloff-Smith et al., in preparation) revealed that at 28 months of age, the child's developmental level was chronological-age-appropriate, leading to the conclusion that the genes deleted played no role in the WS outcome. However, at 9 years of age, her developmental level had pulled away from the typical trajectory and had become significantly closer to the WS trajectory, but was still different from it. In other words, had we taken a snapshot of genotype/phenotype correlations at 28 months, our conclusions would have been very different from those drawn at 9 years of age.

Deeper accounts of syndrome-specific traits: the example of facial dysmorphology

Many neurodevelopmental disorders are first recognised by their facial dysmorphology. This is clearly true of individuals with WS, but also for those with Down syndrome, Angelman syndrome, Prader–Willi syndrome, Cornelia de Lange syndrome, Fabry disease, fragile X syndrome and many others. Yet, these dysmorphologies can differ quite considerably between individuals with the same syndrome and are sometimes very subtle. Moreover, the rarity of certain conditions makes it difficult for clinicians to develop the skills necessary for recognising each set of atypical facial gestalts. Yet, to date, such assessments had been done solely by clinical examination. Again, huge technological advances now offer methodologies that are far more precise than the human clinician's eye. Pioneering work led by Peter Hammond at the Molecular Medicine Unit of the Institute of Child Health in London has created computer programmes that take photographs of a face and analyse its particular morphology. It works by gathering multiple, simultaneous three-dimensional face images of unaffected and affected children, then computing the average faces of each group and calculating the extent to which individual subjects from the group are expected to vary from the group average. Next, pattern recognition algorithms are applied to determine the average rate of success in classifying unseen faces as affected or unaffected. During the development of the early versions of the software, it was tested on a number of genetic conditions in cooperation with clinical geneticists in the UK and USA (Hammond et al., 2004; Hammond, 2007). Since then, Hammond has focused on extending the conditions covered by travelling extensively throughout the world to collect three-dimensional face scans of children and adults with a wide range of different genetic conditions, thereby increasing the power of the analyses (Hammond et al., 2005; Bhuiyan et al., 2006; Cox-Brinkman et al., 2007). Other collaborations led, for instance, to a mouse model of the WS facial dysmorphology (Tassabehji et al., 2005), which has helped to narrow down the genes in the WS critical region that may play a role in altering facial structure during development.

Most interestingly, although most clinicians would claim that ASD yields no facial dysmorphology, Hammond's most recent work indicates that underlying some subgroups there may indeed be a particular facial dysmorphology in autism in terms of differences in symmetry (Hammond et al., 2008). Previously, the heterogeneity of ASDs had confounded attempts to identify causes and pathogenesis. Hammond and his colleagues have now used dense surface-modelling techniques to compare the facial morphology of 72 boys with ASD and 128 first-degree relatives with that of 254 unrelated controls. Pattern-matching algorithms succeeded in discriminating the faces of boys with ASD from those of matched controls and also in discriminating the faces of unaffected mothers of children with ASD from matched female controls. The authors detected significant facial asymmetry in boys with ASD, notably depth-wise in the supra- and periorbital regions anterior to the frontal pole of the right hemisphere of the brain. Unaffected mothers of children with ASD displayed similar significant facial asymmetry, which was more exaggerated than that in matched controls, and in particular they showed vertical asymmetry

of the periorbital region. Unaffected fathers of children with ASD did not show any significant facial asymmetry compared with controls. The authors argued that previously
identified right dominant asymmetry of the frontal poles of boys with ASD could explain
their facial asymmetry through the direct effect of brain growth. The atypical facial asymmetry of unaffected mothers of children with ASD obviously requires further brain studies before the same explanation can be proposed. An alternative but not mutually exclusive
explanation is a simultaneous and parallel effect on face and brain growth by genetic factors.
In this case, diagnosis at birth may not be possible because of the required developmental
time for the genetic differences to impact on the phenotypic outcome. Both possibilities
indicate the need for coordinated face and brain studies on ASD probands and their first-
degree relatives, especially on unaffected mothers, given that their unusual facial asymmetry
suggests an ASD susceptibility arising from maternal genes. Together with clinical assessments, this advance in understanding facial dysmorphology in autism (Hammond et al.,
2008) could contribute to an earlier diagnosis in the not too distant future. Indeed, the study
of very young babies, as we shall see in the final section, holds huge promise for future
neuroconstructivist research on atypical development.

Diagnosing and remediating neurodevelopmental disorders in the very early months of life: a promise for the future

Nowadays, as obstetricians and paediatricians become increasingly aware of the WS traits
such as facial dysmorphology, heart problems and general developmental deficits that alert
to the need for a genetic test, WS is relatively easy to diagnose at birth. Other syndromes,
such as ASDs, dyslexia and developmental dyscalculia, whose diagnosis only occurs after
2 or 3 years or more, are obviously far less noticeable at birth, although the genetic risk in
families with older children already diagnosed with these disorders is worth keeping in
mind in the search for subtle early clues. Given the neuroconstructivist focus on cascading
developmental trajectories and early interdomain relationships that only become domain-
specific over developmental time, should we not now be thinking about intervention in
the first months of life, especially if diagnosis can be done early, instead of waiting for
more obvious problems to become apparent?

The neuroconstructivist approach would search for very low-level impairments in the
neonate profile—at the levels of brain, cognition and behaviour—that might affect gene
expression and have cascading effects on developmental outcomes. Throughout the book we
have seen how processes such as early attention, eye movement planning, eye gaze following,
auditory processing, movement planning and contingent reaction can impact on subsequently developing domains. For instance, the different profiles of early attention in WS
and Down syndrome were shown to impact on the development of number and language in
syndrome-specific ways (Chapter 18). It is thus these basic processes that our intervention
studies should initially target, rather than training in specific domains. Moreover, interventions should be syndrome-specific based on scientific research, they should start as early
as possible in the infant developmental trajectory and measure outcome across several
different domains, at the levels of behaviour, brain, cognition and gene expression. Such

an approach may seem like wishful thinking in a future ideal world; yet, our neuroconstructivist approach argues that they are not optional but essential building blocks for helping children with neurodevelopmental disorders reach their full potential.

References

Antonell, A., Del Campo, M., Magano, L.F., Kaufmann, L., de la Iglesia, J.M., Gallastegui, F., et al. (2010a). Partial 7q11.23 deletions further implicate GTF2I and GTF2IRD1 as the main genes responsible for the Williams–Beuren syndrome neurocognitive profile. *Journal of Medical Genetics*, **47**, 313–20.

Antonell, A., Vilardell, M., & Perez Jurado, L.A. (2010b). Transcriptome profile in Williams–Beuren syndrome lymphoblast cells reveals gene pathways implicated in glucose intolerance and visuospatial construction deficits. *Human Genetics*, **128**, 27–37.

Bhuiyan, Z.A., Klein, M., Hammond, P., van Haeringen, A., Mannens, M.M., Van Berckelaer-Onnes, I., et al. (2006). Phenotype-genotype correlations in Cornelia de Lange syndrome: the Dutch experience. *Journal of Medical Genetics*, **43**, 568–75.

Bolhuis, J.J., Cook, S., & Horn, G. (2000). Getting better all the time: improving preference scores reflect increases in the strength of filial imprinting. *Animal Behaviour*, **59**, 1153–59.

Cox-Brinkman, J., Vedder, A., Hollak, C., Richfield, L., Mehta, A., Orteu, A., et al. (2007). Three-dimensional face shape in Fabry disease. *European Journal of Human Genetics*, **15**, 535–42.

Fisher, S.E., & Scharff, C. (2009). FOXP2 as a molecular window into speech and language. *Trends in Genetics*, **25**, 166–77.

Frangiskakis, J.M., Ewart, A.K., Morris, C.A., Mervis, C.B., Bertrand, J., Robinson, B.F., et al. (1996). LIM-kinase1 hemizygosity implicated in impaired visuospatial constructive cognition. *Cell*, **86**, 59–69.

Gopnik, M., & Crago, M.B. (1991). Familial aggregation of a developmental language disorder. *Cognition*, **39**, 1–30.

Gray, V., Karmiloff-Smith, A., Funnell, E., & Tassabehji, M. (2006). In-depth analysis of spatial cognition in Williams syndrome: a critical assessment of the role of the LIMK1 gene. *Neuropsychologia*, **44**, 679–85.

Grice, S.J., de Haan, M., Halit, H., Johnson, M.H., Csibra, G., Grant, J., et al. (2003). ERP abnormalities of illusory contour perception in Williams syndrome. *NeuroReport*, **14**, 1773–77.

Grice, S., Spratling, M.W., Karmiloff-Smith, A., Halit, H., Csibra, G., de Haan, M., & et al. (2001). Disordered visual processing and oscillatory brain activity in autism and Williams syndrome. *NeuroReport*, **12**, 2697–2700.

Hammond, P. (2007). The use of 3D face shape modelling in dysmorphology. *Archives of Disease in Childhood*, **92**, 1120–26.

Hammond, P., Forster-Gibson, C., Chudley, A.E., Allanson, J.E., Hutton, T.J., Farrell, S.A., et al. (2008). Face–brain asymmetry in autism spectrum disorders, *Molecular Psychiatry*, **13**, 614–23.

Hammond, P., Hutton, T.J., Allanson, J.E., Campbell, L.E., Hennekam, R.C., Holden, S., et al. (2004). 3D analysis of facial morphology. *American Journal of Medical Genetics*, **126**, 339–48.

Hammond, P., Hutton, T.J., Allanson, J.E., Buxton, B., Campbell, L., Clayton-Smith, J., et al. (2005). Discriminating power of localized 3D facial morphology. *American Journal of Human Genetics*, **77**, 999–1010.

Haesler, S., Wada, K., Nshdejan, A., Morrisey, E.E., Lints, T., Jarvis, E.D., et al. (2004). *FoxP2* expression in avian vocal learners and non-learners. *Journal of Neuroscience*, **24**, 3164–75.

Karmiloff-Smith, A. (1998). Development itself is the key to understanding developmental disorders. *Trends in Cognitive Sciences*, **2**, 389–98.

Karmiloff-Smith, A., Farran, E.K., Broadbent, H., Longhi, E., D'Souza, D., & Dubois, S. (in preparation). Spatial cognition in Williams syndrome: separating human and murine models of egocentric navigational space and allocentric object-oriented space.

Karmiloff-Smith, A., Grant, J., Ewing, S., Carette, M.J., Metcalfe, K., Donnai, D., et al. (2002). Using case study comparisons to explore genotype/phenotype correlations in Williams–Beuren syndrome. *Journal of Medical Genetics*, **40**, 136–40.

Karmiloff-Smith, A. (2009). Nativism versus neuroconstructivism: rethinking the study of developmental disorders. *Developmental Psychology*, **45**, 56–63.

Lai, C.S., Gerrelli, D., Monaco, A.P., Fisher, S.E., & Copp, A.J. (2003). FOXP2 expression during brain development coincides with adult sites of pathology in a severe speech and language disorder. *Brain*, **126**, 2455–62.

Mobbs, D., Eckert, M.A., Mills, D., Korenberg, J., Bellugi, U., Galaburda, A.M., et al. (2007). Frontostriatal dysfunction during response inhibition in Williams syndrome. *Biological Psychiatry*, **62**, 256–61.

Pinker, S. (2001). Talk of genetics and vice versa. *Nature*, **413**, 465–66.

Rivera, S.M., Reiss, A.L., Eckert, M.A., & Menon, V. (2005). Developmental changes in mental arithmetic: evidence for increased functional specialization in the left inferior parietal cortex. *Cerebral Cortex*, **15**, 1779–90.

Rubia, K., Smith, A.B., Brammer, M.J., Toone, B., & Taylor, E. (2005). Abnormal brain activation during inhibition and error detection in medication-naïve adolescents with ADHD. *American Journal of Psychiatry*, **162**, 1067–75.

Tassabehji, M., Hammond, P., Karmiloff-Smith, A., Thompson, P., Thorgeirsson, S.S., Durkin, M., et al. (2005). GTF2IRD1 in craniofacial development of humans and mice. *Science*, **310**, 1184–87.

Teramisu, I., & White, S.A. (2006). FoxP2 regulation during undirected singing in adult songbirds. *Journal of Neuroscience*, **26**, 7390–94.

Vargha-Khadem, F., Watkins, K., Alcock, K., Fletcher, P., & Passingham, R. (1995). Praxic and nonverbal cognitive defects in a large family with a genetically transmitted speech and language disorder. *Proceedings of the National Academy of Sciences of the USA*, **92**, 930–33.

Author Index

Adams, J.W. 341
Adamson, L.B. 191
Adolphs, R. 270
Agapitou, P. 136
Aitken, J.A. 280
Akagawa, H. 70
Albano, A.M. 109
Alivisatos, B. 228
Allen Institute for Brain Science 63, 65, 66
Alloway, T.P. 138
Allport, A. 249
Almazan, M. 31, 207, 208
Almeida, Q.J. 174
Andari, E. 282
Andersen, R.A. 172
Andreou, G. 136, 142
Andrus, B.M. 72
Annaz, D. 15, 17, 18, 20, 26, 27, 28, 29, 72,
    93, 137, 139, 140, 141, 144, 214, 268
Ansari, D. 104, 300, 304, 306, 307, 308,
    309, 340, 355, 357
Antonell, A. 237, 363
Arber, S. 65
Ardila, A. 165
Ardinger, R.H., Jr. 88
Arens, R. 93, 139, 140
von Arnim, G. 92, 187, 205
Arnold, R. 93, 104
Arriaga, R.I. 302
Ashburner, J. 159
Ashe, A. 63
Aslin, R. 43
Atkinson, J. 90, 119–20, 123, 124, 126, 128,
    129, 156, 167, 168, 174, 175, 176, 225,
    227, 228, 239, 240, 248, 249, 250,
    251, 252, 253, 254, 257, 340, 356
Atkinson, R.C. 149
Atsumori, H. 42
Attias, J. 90
Aylward, G.P. 120

Babbitt, D.P. 90
Back, E. 269, 271, 281
Backhaus, J. 138
Baddeley, A.D. 149, 150
Baldwin, D.A. 196
Bandettini, P.A. 40
Barisinikov, K. 151
Baron-Cohen, S. 3, 269, 279
Baroody, A.J. 306, 349, 352, 354
Barratt-Boyes, B.G. 103
Bates, E. 195
Baughman, F.D. 30
Baumer, A. 85

Bayarsaihan, D. 66–7, 68
Bayes, M. 85
Bayley, N. 342, 345
Bear, M.F. 74
Becerra, A.M. 2, 189, 190, 191, 192, 197, 215
Bechar, T. 205, 211
Beebe, D. 137
Beglinger, L. 288
Beilin, H. 187
Bellugi, U. 2, 14, 15, 44, 91, 92, 152, 158, 170,
    187, 188, 193, 198, 205, 206, 207, 209, 210,
    211, 226, 230, 252, 255, 265, 266, 270, 280, 281
Bennett, F.C. 205
Bennett, M.K. 65
Benton, A.L. 20, 230, 265
Berg, J.S. 282
Berry-Kravis, E. 74
Berthoz, A. 249
Bertone, A. 230
Bertrand, J. 23, 29, 190, 191, 192
Bess, F.H. 90
Beuren, A.J. 1, 92
Bhuiyan, Z.A. 368
Bihrle, A.M. 92
Billstedt, E. 103
Bilousova, T.V. 74
Bird, L.M. 88
Biro, S. 124
Bishop, D.V.M. 25, 31, 188, 207, 213, 214,
    315, 326, 327
Black, J.A. 88
Blakemore, S.-J. 40, 173
Blunden, S. 136, 137
Boddaert, N. 38, 43, 44, 46, 48, 158
Bódizs, R. 139
Bolhuis, J.J. 5, 365
Bonham Carter, R.E. 88
Booth, R. 170
Born, J. 138
Botta, A. 63, 65, 85
Botting, N. 217
Boudreau, D. 318, 321, 323, 324
Bourgeron, T. 3
Bowdle, B. 21, 28
Bowey, J. 314, 316, 317, 322, 323
Braddick, O.J. 90, 119–20, 228, 248, 249,
    250, 251, 252, 254
Breckenridge, K. 121, 125, 126, 127, 129
Bretherton, I. 196
Brock, J. 29, 104, 105 151, 154, 188, 288, 326
Broder, K. 88
Bromberg, H.S. 208
Bronson, G.W. 248
Brosnan, M.J. 170, 232

Brown, J.H. 46, 123, 125, 126, 128, 129, 192, 301, 342, 344, 345, 347, 356
Brown, R. 195
Bruce, V. 266
Bruno, E. 87
Bryant, P.E. 315
Buckley, S. 327
Bull, R. 341
Bullemer, P. 157
Bullens, J. 234
Burger, C. 72
Burgess, N. 257
Burgess, S.R. 315, 317
Bus, A.G. 315, 320
Butler, M.G. 89
Butterworth, B. 50
Byrne, A. 314, 318, 321, 324
Byrne, B. 315, 316, 323
van Bysterveldt, A. 327

Cabeza, R. 216
Cain, K. 316
Cairo, S. 63
Cambiaso, P. 90
Campbell, L.E. 46, 50, 51, 158, 159
Campbell, R. 229
Campos, R. 281, 283, 284, 287, 288
Cantlon, J.F. 300
Caraveo, G. 68
Caravolas, M. 316, 319
Cardoso-Martins, C. 318, 319, 321, 322, 324, 325
Carey, J.C. 89
Carey, S. 24, 266, 301
Carlesimo, G.A. 154, 155
Carless, S. 316
Carpenter, P.A. 3
Carr, J. 105
Carrasco, X. 173
Carroll, J.M. 315, 323, 328, 341, 349
Casey, B.J. 5, 39
Cashon, C.H. 191
Castellanos, F.X. 50
Catterall, C. 212
Catts, H.W. 318
Cavina-Pratesi, C. 254
Cherniske, E.M. 73, 88, 89, 90, 91, 92, 93, 103, 104, 107, 108
Cherubini, A. 73
Chervin, R.D. 143
Chiang, M.-C. 44, 45, 158
Church, J.A. 40
Clahsen, H. 2, 15, 30, 31, 38, 207, 208, 209
Clark, H.H. 235
Clarke, P.J. 313, 328
Cleave, P.L. 321
Clements, W.A. 287
Cocksey, J. 317, 327
Cohen, L.G. 4
Cole, V.L. 232
Collette, J.C. 69
Collins, R.T. 87
Coltheart, M. 209, 231, 288

Computation Biology Center at Memorial Sloan-Kettering Cancer Center 63
Conners, F.A. 321
Cooper, S.A. 108, 109
Corbetta, M. 173, 300
Cornelissen, P. 253
Cornish, K. 123, 125, 126, 128, 129, 254, 340, 356
Corominas, R. 71
Cortesi, F. 142
Costanzo, F. 156
Cowie, D. 175, 176, 252, 255
Cowley, G. 187
Cox-Brinkman, J. 368
Crackower, M.A. 63
Crago, M.B. 365
Crisco, J.J. 149
Csibra, G. 43
Cuetos, F. 313, 319, 320, 322, 323, 327
Cui, H. 172
Cui, X. 39, 42, 43
Cunniff, C. 107
Cunningham, C. 188
Cupples, L. 314, 321
Curran, W. 233
Cuskelly, M. 126

Dadds, M. 126
Dai, L. 85, 282
Dale, P.S. 195
Danoff, S.K. 63, 66, 67, 68
Datson, N.A. 72
Davies, M. 90, 92, 93, 94, 105, 213
Deconinck, F.J.A. 174
DeFulio, A. 326
Dehaene, S. 299, 300, 303, 306
Del Campo, M. 69
Della Sala, S. 150
Deruelle, C. 231, 236, 266, 267, 284
De Sario, A. 69
Devenny, D.A. 73, 104
Dhital, B. 300
Diamond, A. 176
Diamond, R. 266
Díaz, E. 64
Díez-Itza, E. 208
Dilger, S. 109
Dilks, D.D. 227, 239, 253
Dilts, C.V. 93, 252
Dobbs, D. 187
Dodd, H.F. 109, 270, 286
Doeller, C.F. 234
Doherty-Sneddon, G. 282
Don, A.J. 157
Doyle, J.L. 63
Doyle, T.F. 169
Duchaine, B.C. 266
Duff, F.J. 313, 328
Duncan, J. 123, 130
Dunn, D.M. 188
Dunn, L.M. 17, 22, 24, 27, 124, 152, 188, 348, 352
Dupont, B. 89

Dupont, P. 230
Durston, S. 5
Dutly, F. 85
Dykens, E.M. 93, 108

Eaves, L.C. 103
Eckert, M.A. 43, 46, 158, 236, 237
Edelmann, L. 86
Eden, G.F. 228
Edmonston, N.K. 194
Ehninger, D. 73
Ehri, L.C. 314, 315, 317, 318, 325, 326, 328
Eickhoff, S.B. 40
Eilers, R.E. 190
Einfeld, S.L. 108
Eisenberg, D.P. 44, 45, 46, 47, 48, 50, 158
Elgar, K. 229
Eliez, S. 51
Elison, E. 103, 105, 106, 107, 109, 110
Elison, S. 93, 94
Elliot, C.D. 17, 27, 188, 225, 348, 352
Elliott, D. 165, 173, 176, 255
Elman, J. 5
Emerson, E. 108
Endo, M. 65
Engel, P. 92, 187, 205
Enkhmandakh, B. 66
Enns, J.T. 120
Eronen, M. 87
Erraji-Benchekroun, L. 72
European Bioinformatics Institute & Wellcome
    Trust Sanger Institute 63

Faillenot, I. 230
Fan, J. 120, 159
Fantz, R.L. 345
Farah, M.J. 266, 268
Farran, E.K. 29, 104, 170, 171, 172, 225,
    226, 230, 231, 232, 233, 234, 235, 236,
    238, 239, 240, 257, 301, 340
Farroni, T. 232
Feigenson, L. 301, 302
Fenson, L. 189, 195, 343
Fidler, D.J. 325
Fijalkowska, I. 63, 66–7, 68
Finn, R. 187
Fisch, G.S. 105
Fischer, A. 69
Fisher, S.E. 365
Fodor, J.A. 30, 205
Folstein, M.F. 142
Formby, S.C. 234
Foster-Cohen, S. 327
Fowler, A.E. 320
Frangiskakis, J.M. 65, 85, 237, 367
Fredericks, C.M. 173
Frens, M.A. 225
Frigerio, E. 169, 280
Friston, K.J. 159
Frith, U. 170, 226, 317, 318, 319, 323
Frumin, M. 40
Fryssira, H. 86

Fuchikami, M. 72
Fuchs, D. 314, 328
Fuchs, L.S. 341
Fujiki, R. 69
Fuster, J.M. 165

Gagliardi, C. 85, 269, 270, 281
Gais, S. 138
Galaburda, A. 44, 45, 236, 255, 281
Gallagher, A. 322
Gallagher, M. 169
Gallistel, C.R. 307
Garavan, H. 166
Garayzabal, E. 313, 319, 320, 322–3, 327
Garner, C.C. 73
Garnham, W.A. 287
Gathercole, S.E. 138, 341
Geiger, O. 28
Gelman, R. 307
Gentner D. 21, 28
Gerrans, P. 205
Gerstadt, C.L. 120, 124
Getchell, N. 166
Geuze, R.H. 217
Giannotti, A.G. 91
Giddins, N.G. 87
Giedd, J.N. 48
Gillberg, C. 279
Gillon, G. 327
Gilmore, R.O. 342
Ginsburg, H. 306, 349, 352, 354
Girirajan, S. 71
Glanzer, M. 154
Gleitman, L. 236
Glenn, S. 188
Glucksberg, S. 28
Goetz, K. 314, 328
Goff, D.A. 317
Golarai, G. 46, 49, 268–9
Goldenberg, G. 228
Goldman, S.E. 72, 137, 140
Goldman-Rakic, P.S. 123, 125
Gooch, D. 328
Goodale, M.A. 227, 247, 249, 253
Goodman, J.C. 195
Gopnik, A. 193
Gopnik, M. 365
Gosch, A. 29, 269
Goswami, U. 315, 322
Gothelf, D. 90, 216
Gottlieb, G. 5
Gough, P.B. 314
Gould, J. 288
Gowen, E. 173
Gozal, D. 136
Gräff, J. 69
Grafodatskaya, D. 69
Grant, C.M. 340
Grant, J. 31, 151, 207, 216, 326, 327
Gray, P.A. 63
Gray, V. 238, 367
Greer, M.K. 93, 126

Grice, S.J. 42, 49, 51, 232, 234, 236, 364
Griffiths, Y.M. 313, 315, 320, 322, 323
Groen, M. 318, 321, 325
Gunn, A. 253
Gunn, D. 314, 318, 323, 324

Haas, B.W. 52, 159, 270, 273, 281, 282
Hadenius, A.M. 93
Hadwin, J. 290
Haesler, S. 365
Hagerman, P.J. 340
Hagerman, R.J. 74, 340
Hallidie-Smith, K.A. 87
Hammond, P. 87, 368, 369
Hancock, P.J.B. 271, 272
Hansen, P.C. 228, 253
Hanson, M.J. 345
Harlaar, N. 195
Hastings, R.P. 328
Hatcher, J. 325, 328
Hatcher, P.J. 349
Havy, M. 193
Haworth, C.M. 70
Haxby, J.V. 265
Haywood, K.M. 166
Heller, R. 85
Henderson, S.E. 252
Hennessy, S.M. 341
Henry, L.A. 104
Hermer, L. 235
Hermon, S. 208
Hernandez, D.G. 73
Hick, R. 217
Hill, E.L. 217
Hines, R.J. 45
Hinsley, T.A. 66
Hirai, M. 229
Hirota, H. 85
Hirstein, W. 282
Hitch, G. 149, 150
Ho, H.H. 103
Hobart, H.H. 85
Hobson, P. 280
Hocking, D.R. 173, 174
Hodapp, R.M. 285
Hoeft, F. 47, 158
Hoffman, J.E. 170, 226, 231, 235, 240
Holinger, D.P. 45, 158
Holland, P.C. 169
Hollander, E. 282
Holloway, L.D. 300
Holmes, J. 358
Holtzer, R. 174
Hood, B. 120
Hoogenraad, C.C. 63, 65
Hooper, S.R. 357
Hoover, W.A. 314
Hopyan, T. 93
Hoshi, E. 166
Howald, C. 85
Howlin, P. 92, 103, 104, 105, 106, 109, 110, 187, 280, 290, 304, 313, 318, 319, 324

Huang, Y.-S. 143
Hubel, D.H. 248
Huber, K.M. 173
Hudson, K.D. 170, 171, 172, 226
Hughes, C. 124, 168
Hulme, C. 313, 314, 317, 318, 319, 323, 324, 326, 328, 329
Huppert, T.J. 39, 43
Huttenlocher, P.R. 6, 37

Iacono, T. 314, 321
Iizuka, K. 63
van Ijzendoorn, M.H. 315, 320
Imashuku, S. 90
Innocenti, G.M. 50
Isaacs, E.B. 50, 301

Jackendoff, R. 187
Jackson, T.A. 67
Jacoby, L.L. 156
Jacques, S. 120
Jadayel, D.M. 63
Jan, J.E. 72, 143
Jarrold, C. 29, 105, 152, 160, 172, 206, 211, 225, 226, 230, 231, 235, 236, 239, 240, 321, 340
Jawaid, A. 273, 281
Jeannerod, M. 249
Jernigan, T.L. 44, 158, 255
Jiménez, J.E. 317
Joffe, V. 207
John, A.E. 94, 177, 188, 189, 194, 195, 196, 197, 210, 235, 284, 330
Johns, M.W. 140
Johnson, L.B. 90
Johnson, M.H. 3, 4, 5, 37, 342
Johnson, M.J. 39
Johnson, S.C. 24, 229
Johnston, L.M. 175
Johnston, R.S. 315
Jones, B.L. 120
Jones, W. 38, 43, 45, 173, 198, 213, 270, 280, 281, 284, 286
Jordan, H. 228, 239, 341
Joseph, M.C. 87
Joseph, R.M. 168
Jusczyk, P.W. 191

Kaffman, A. 5
Kalverboer, A.F. 217
Kanwisher, N. 265
Kaplan, P. 88, 252
Karagianni, P. 69
Karas, S. 87
Karmiloff-Smith, A. 2, 3, 4, 5, 6, 14, 25, 29, 30, 31, 38, 39, 40, 42, 46, 49, 85, 92, 122, 144, 151, 192, 193, 206, 207, 208, 214, 267, 269, 279, 283, 287, 300, 301, 303, 306, 309, 341, 348, 357, 365, 366, 367
Karni, A. 138
Kaufman, A.S. 306
Kaufman, N.L. 306
Kawashima, K. 71

Kay-Raining Bird, E. 314, 321
Kelly, T.P. 120
Kempler, D. 26
Kennedy, J.C. 93, 108, 109
Kesler, S.R. 230
Kind, P. 341
Kippenhan, J. 46
Kirkham, N.Z. 120
Kitada, R. 230
Kitagawa, H. 69
Kittler, P. 105
Klein, A.J. 90
Klein, B.P. 105, 150, 252
Kleinke, C.L. 269
Klein-Tasman, B.P. 93, 109, 196, 197, 269,
    280, 287, 288
Knapp, M.L. 269
Kogan, C.S. 254, 340
Koldewyn, K. 228, 229
Konrad, K. 40
Korenberg, J.R. 44, 85
Kovas, Y. 16
Kozuma, S.N. 144
Krajcsi, A. 305, 309
Krause, M. 208
Krinsky-McHale, S.J. 104
Krueger, D.D. 74
Ku, M. 67, 68

Lacroix, A. 213, 215, 270, 281, 284
Lai, C.S. 365
Laing, E.C. 151, 196, 235, 271, 273, 286,
    350, 313, 317, 318, 319, 320, 321, 322,
    323, 324, 326, 327
Lakkakorpi, J. 63
Lakusta, L. 234
Lancioni, G.E. 109
Landau, B. 38, 92, 234, 235, 240, 306, 309
Landauer, T.K. 300, 304
Lawrence, L. 235
Laws, G. 25, 188, 213, 235, 314, 318, 323, 324, 327
Lawson, K.R. 342
Lebold, C.A. 174
Le Corre, M. 301
Leder, H. 266
Lee, A.D. 44
Lee, T.I. 70
Lefly, D.L. 322
Lemons, C.J. 314, 328
Lemos, C. 71
Lervag, A. 316
Leslie, A.M. 2
Levinson, S.C. 236
Levitin, D.J. 90, 93
Levy, F. 120
Levy, Y. 205, 208, 211, 313, 318, 319, 320, 321,
    322, 323, 324, 327
Lewis, T.L. 230
Leyfer, O.T. 72, 93, 108, 165, 328
Li, G. 136
Li, P. 236
Lin, C.C.H. 120

Lincoln, A.J. 196, 197, 279, 287
Lisowski, P. 72
Litchfield Thane, N. 194
Livingstone, M. 248
Lloyd-Fox, S. 43
Loerch, P.M. 72
Logie, R.H. 150
Logothetis, N.K. 40
Lonigan, C.J. 315, 317, 327
Lopez-Rangel, E. 90
Lord, C. 196
Losh, M. 284
Lovegrove, W.J. 228
Lowe, J.B. 103
Luders, E. 45, 158
de Luis, O. 63
Lukács, A. 208, 210
Luna, B. 165

Machery, E. 30, 31, 32
Majerus, S. 151, 350
Makeyev, A.V. 66
Mandolesi, L. 153
Manly, T. 120, 121
Mansuy, I.M. 69
Maquet, P. 138
Marcus, C.L. 142
Marenco, S. 41, 47
Mareschal, D. 289
Mari, M. 175
Marler, J.A. 90
Marriage, J. 94
Marshall, C.M. 323
Marshall, C.R. 91
Martens, M.A. 37, 70, 92, 103, 270,
    273, 280, 281
Martin, N.D.T. 89, 91
Martindale, D.W. 63
Martínez-Castilla, P. 212, 284
Masataka, N. 190
Mason, T.B.A.I. 93
Mason, U.M. 255
Matuga, J.M. 167
May-Benson, T.A. 175
Maylor, E.A. 104
McCarthy, D. 205
McConnell, L. 321
McEwen, B.S. 71
McIntosh, R.D. 228
McKay, K.E. 120
Meaney, M.J. 5
Mechelli, A. 4
Meek, J. 43
Mehler, J. 43
Meltzoff, A. 193
Meng, X. 63
Meng, Y. 65, 66
Menghini, D. 46, 48, 154, 159, 167, 168, 171,
    172, 313, 319, 320, 322
Menon, V. 50
Mercuri, E. 120, 236, 248, 255
Merla, G. 63

Mervis, C.B. 2, 14, 26, 30, 31, 59, 92, 93,
94, 104, 105, 150, 151, 169, 177, 187, 188,
189, 190, 191, 192, 194, 195, 197, 198, 210,
215, 231, 235, 252, 269, 271, 280, 282, 286,
313, 318, 319, 330
Mesulam, M.M. 216
Metcalfe, K.A. 87, 89, 90, 91, 92
Metsala, J.L. 321
Mey, J. 213
Meyer-Lindenberg, A. 14, 43, 45, 46, 47, 48, 49,
74, 158, 159, 194, 216, 229, 234, 236, 253,
257, 268, 270, 282, 301
Miall, R. 173
Miano, S. 142
Micale, L. 63
Mills, D.L. 49, 268
Milne, E. 253
Milner, A.D. 227, 247, 249, 253
Minagawa-Kawai, Y. 43
Ming, X. 141
Minshew, N.J. 273
Miranda, S.B. 345
Mirenda, P. 327
Mirsky, A.F. 120
Mishkin, M. 247
Miyake, A. 165
Mobbs, D. 48, 124, 166, 167, 236, 268,
269, 270, 364
Molko, N. 50
Mondloch, C.J. 266
Monnery, S. 208
Montfoort, I. 129, 234
Mori, T. 63, 66
Morris, C.A. 59, 85, 87, 88, 89, 90,
91, 92, 107
Morris, J.A. 70
Morris, M.E. 174
Morrone, M.C. 248
Moscovitch, C. 155
Moscovitch, M. 265
Moss, S. 109
Mountford, P. 65
Moyer, R.S. 300, 304
Mullen, E.M. 189
Mundy, P. 196
Munir, F. 129, 357
Muñoz, K.E. 109, 282
Musolino, J. 205, 207
Muter, V. 314, 316, 341, 349

Nadel, L. 124, 126, 129
Nakaji, A. 90
Nakamura, K. 71
Nardini, M. 234, 240, 256, 257
Nation, K. 314, 315, 316, 317, 323, 325,
326, 327, 341
National Center for Biotechnology
Information 63
Navon, D. 236
Nazzi, T. 191, 193
Neal, A. 196
Nelson, S.B. 64

Neville, H.J. 49, 216
Newman, C. 255, 256
Newman, R. 190, 191
Nichols, S. 154
Niskar, A.S. 90
Nissen, M.J. 157
Noback, C.R. 64
Nyberg, L. 216

O'Brien, L. 140, 142
Office of National Statistics 107
O'Hearn, K. 92, 228, 239, 306, 308, 309
Okamoto, N. 71
O'Reilly, M.F. 109
Orellana, C. 104
Ortony, A. 21–2
Osborne, L.R. 59, 63, 85
Ouellette, G.P. 317
Owen, A.M. 125
Owens, J.A. 139

Pagon, R.A. 89, 126
Palmer, S.J. 63, 66, 67
Palomares, M. 230, 231, 232, 233, 239, 240
Pani, J.R. 231
Pankau, R. 29, 88, 89, 269
Paperna, T. 63
Paribello, C. 74
Parrott, D. 87
Partsch, C.J. 89, 92
Paterson, S.J. 17, 92, 302, 303, 304, 305, 309,
342, 343, 344, 345, 347
Paul, B.M. 104
Paus, T. 40
Penke, M. 208
Pennington, B.F. 315, 322
Peoples, R.J. 63
Peppé, S. 212
Perenin, M.T. 253
Pérez-Jurado, L.A. 63, 69, 87, 91
Perkins, M. 213
Perner, J. 287
Persico, A.M. 3
Petersen, S.E. 120
Petrides, M. 228
Pezzini, G. 151, 252
Phillips, B.M. 317, 327
Phillips, C.E. 235, 340
Philofsky, A. 213
Piattelli-Palmarini, M. 2, 187
Pickering, S.J. 138, 341
Pierrot-Deseilligny, C. 124
Pinker, S. 2, 14, 187, 208, 365
Plaut, D.C. 317
Pléh, C. 151, 208, 216
Plesa Skwerer, D. 269, 270, 281, 282, 283
Plessen, K.J. 50
Plihal, W. 138
Plissart, L. 90
Plomin, R. 16, 70
Pober, B.R. 59, 73, 88, 89, 90, 91, 107, 252
Poot, R.A. 70

Pope, D.W., Jr. 136
Porter, M.A. 109, 169, 209, 231, 270, 280, 281, 284, 288
Posner, M.I. 120, 341, 356
Powell, D. 323
Pröschel, C. 65
Proulx, E. 63, 67
Pueschel, S.M. 126
Purser, H.R.M. 23, 24, 25
Putman, C.M. 88
Pyers, J.E. 284

Rack, J. 326
Radulescu, E. 41
Rae, C. 49, 74
Rasmussen, P. 279
Raven, J.C. 142, 172
Reilly, J. 212, 213, 279, 284
Reiss, A.L. 43, 44, 46, 48, 52, 158, 159, 236, 270
Reiss, J.E. 228–9, 238, 239
Rhodes, S.M. 48, 169, 171, 172
Riby, D.M. 267, 269, 270, 271, 272, 273, 281
Rice, M.L. 25, 213
Richdale, A. 143, 144
Ricketts, J. 317
Ridder, W.H.I. 253
Riggs, N.R. 165, 169
Riikonen, R. 173
Ring, M. 15
Rivera, S.M. 300, 309, 363
Rizzolatti, G. 249
Robbins, T.W. 123
Roberts, J.E. 340
Robertson, I.H. 120
Robinson, B.F. 151, 188, 194, 198, 216
Roch, M. 321
Rondan, C. 231
Rose, F.E. 267, 281
Rose, J. 322, 328
Rosenbaum, D.A. 255
Rosner, S.R. 173, 211
Ross, E.D. 216
Rossen, M. 209, 210
Rossen, R. 230
Rothbart, M.K. 341, 343, 345
Rowe, J. 129
Rowe, M.L. 196
Rubia, K. 167, 364
Rueda, M.R. 120
Ruff, H.A. 342
Ruffman, T. 287, 288
Rundblad, G. 28, 29
Russell, J. 124, 168
Rutherford, J. 317

Sabes, P.N. 166
Sadato, N. 4
Sadeh, A. 137, 143
Sadler, L.S. 88, 89, 90
Sahyoun, C.P. 53

Sammour, Z.M. 90
Sampaio, A. 45
Sandi, C. 71
Santos, A. 270, 281, 284
Sarimski, K. 139
Sarpal, D. 47, 48, 229, 236, 237, 269, 270, 341
Saunders, K.J. 313, 326
Savage, R.S. 316
Scerif, G. 120, 122, 123, 125, 126, 129, 233, 240, 340, 341, 356, 357
Schacter, D.L. 150
Scharff, C. 365
Schenk, T. 228
Scher, A. 136
Scherer, S.W. 63
Schiller, P.H. 123
Schinzel, A. 85
Schmitt, J.E. 44, 45, 46, 51, 158, 236
Schreck, K.A. 142
van der Schuit, M. 327
Scothorn, D.J. 89
Scott, P. 210
Searcy, Y.M. 104, 187
Selicorni, A. 90
Selvaraj, S. 68
Semel, E.M. 173, 197, 211
Senju, A. 287, 288
Setter, J.E. 104, 212
Seymour, P.K. 316, 319
Sforzini, C. 88, 90
Shah, A. 170, 226
Share, D.L. 316, 317
Shaywitz, B.A. 328
Shaywitz, S.E. 53, 313, 318, 325, 328
Sheih, C.H.P. 89
Shiffrin, R.M. 149
Shott, S.R. 142
Siegal, L.S. 319
Simon, T.J. 51, 301
Sinzig, J. 166, 168
Sirigu, A. 173
Skwerer, D.P. 111
Smith, A.D. 234, 257
Smith, T. 288
Smyth, M.M. 255
Snodgrass, J.G. 156
Snowling, M.J. 313, 314, 315, 317, 318–19, 320–1, 322, 323–4, 325, 326, 327–8, 329, 341
Sober, S.J. 166
Somel, M. 72
Somerville, M.J. 282
Soper, R. 88
Sotillo, M. 283
South, S.T. 71
Southgate, V. 42
Spelke, E.S. 235, 302
Spencer, C.M. 70
Spencer, J.L. 66, 228, 253
Squire, L.R. 149, 150
Stagi, S. 90
Stanescu-Cosson, R. 300

Stanovich, K.E. 319
Stavrakaki, S. 209
Steele, A. 340, 341, 348, 356
Steinbrink, J. 39
Stinton, C. 93, 108, 109, 110, 226, 340
Stoel-Gammon, C. 190
Stojanovik, V. 208, 209, 210, 212
Stromme, P. 1, 85
Stroop, J.R. 168
Stuart, M. 313, 314
Suda, M. 43
Sugden, D.A. 252
Sullivan, K. 25–6, 214, 270, 279, 280, 281,
    283, 284, 357
Sumi, T. 66
Swan, D. 322

Tager-Flusberg, H. 111, 268, 269, 270, 279, 280,
    281, 283, 284, 288
Tanaka, J.W. 266, 268
Tanji, J. 166, 254
Tassabehji, M. 85, 86, 237, 368
Taylor, N.M. 229
Temple, C.M. 2, 38, 210
Teramisu, I. 365
Teramitsu, I. 5
Tew, B. 93
Thomas, M.S.C. 17, 19, 21, 22, 23, 29, 30, 31,
    206, 208, 210, 284, 326
Thomas, N.S. 85
Thompson, P.M. 45, 46, 159, 215, 216
Tomaiuolo, F. 45, 158
Tomasello, M. 196
Tomc, S.A. 280
Tordjman, S. 142
Trenholm, B. 327
Trevarthen, C. 206, 280
Trick, L.M. 120
Tsirempolou, E. 196
Tulving, E. 150
Tümpel, S. 64
Turriziani, P. 157
Tussié-Luna, M.I. 68, 69
Tyler, L.K. 210

Udwin, O. 29, 92, 104, 105, 108,
    139, 150, 169, 190, 211, 213, 304,
    313, 318, 319
Uller, C. 301
Ungerleider, L.G. 40

Valor, L.M. 64
van den Heuvel, O.A. 50
Van der Geest, J.N. 175, 225
Vanderwart, M. 156
Van Essen, D.C. 46, 228
van Ewijk, L. 210
Van Herwegen, J. 29, 303, 309, 348, 357
Van Lancker, D. 26
Vargha-Khadem, F. 365
Varlocosta, S. 207

Vaux, K.K. 89
Velleman, S.L. 190
Vellutino, F.R. 313, 326
Vicari, S. 105, 150, 151, 152, 154, 155,
    156, 157, 171, 194, 195
Vidal, C.N. 50
Vighetto, A. 253
de Villiers, J.G. 284
de Villiers, P.A. 284
Volterra, V. 151, 195, 208, 210
Vosniadou, S. 21–2
de Vrij, F.M. 74

Wagner, R.K. 316, 321
Walker, M.P. 138, 140
Walsh, V. 194
Wang, C.-C. 87
Wang, P.P. 14, 15, 45, 152, 230, 255
Wang, Y.K. 63
Ward, L. 28
Wattam-Bell, J. 249, 251, 252
Webb, S.J. 173
Wechsler, D. 126, 174, 225, 235, 303
Weidenfeld, A. 266
Wen, Y.D. 69
Wessel, A. 87, 88, 107
Westermann, G. 5
Wetmore, D.Z. 73
White, S.A. 5, 365
Wiggs, L. 143, 144
Wilce, L.S. 326
Wilding, J. 125, 357
Williams, C. 236
Williams, J.C.P. 1, 87, 103
Williams, K.T. 194
Williams Syndrome Guideline
    Development Group 107
Wilmut, K. 232, 239
Wing, L. 288
Winter, M. 90
Wishart, J.G. 105
Withers, S. 173
Witkin, H.A. 226
Wollack, J.B. 88
Wolpert, D.M. 173
Wong, A.H. 71
Wong, J. 69
Woodruff-Borden, J. 93
Wynn, K. 307, 349

Xu, F. 302

Yan, Q.J. 74
Yin, R.K. 266
Yonelinas, A.P. 157
Yoon, J.M.D. 229
Yopp, H.K. 315
Yoshimura, K. 69
Young, A.W. 266
Young, E.J. 63, 67
Young, R.A. 70

Ypsilanti, A. 210, 211
Yule, W. 29, 92, 150, 190, 211, 213

Zahn, J.M. 72
Zambello, E. 70

Zelazo, P.D. 120
Zhou, W. 63
Zukowski, A. 208

Subject Index

1-alpha hydroxylase 69
22q syndrome 50–1

acoustic abilities 350
actin dynamics 65
adaptive behaviour 93–4
adenotonsillectomy 136, 137, 143, 144
adult outcomes 103, 111–12
  cognitive and linguistic abilities,
    trajectories of 103–5
  improving outcomes 111
  integration into society 111–12
  mental health 108–9
  physical health 106–7
  provisions for adults 109–11
  social functioning and independence 105–6
    adaptive behaviour 93–4
ageing 72–3, 89, 103, 107
agoraphobia 108
allergies 139
allocentric frames of reference 234, 256–7
alphabetic principle 315, 316
1-alpha hydroxylase 69
amygdala 45, 47, 48, 49
  cross-syndrome comparisons 51
  face processing 270, 273, 274
  hypersociability in amygdala damage 169
  mental state understanding 281–2, 290
  phobias 109
analogy comprehension 21
aneurysms, intracranial 70–1
Angelman syndrome 68, 368
angular gyrus 300
anomalous pulmonary venous return 87–8
anticipatory anxiety 93
anxiety 93
  adulthood 108, 109
  anticipatory 93
  diarrhoea 91
  gene expression 72
  hyperacusis 90
  motor skill deficits 254
  sleep problems 140
  social interaction 289
aortic coarctation 87
aortic stenosis 87
aortic valve, bicuspid 87
apolipoprotein D 72
appearance, physical 86–7
approachability, evaluation of
  face processing 270, 274
  mental state understanding 280, 281, 286
approximate number system/approximate
  magnitude system 301, 302, 303, 304, 305, 306,
    310
arithmetic knowledge, assessment of 304–5
arthritis 89
articulatory loop 149–50, 159
articulatory rehearsal 150
associations versus dissociations 366
asthma 139
atrial septal defect 87
ATRX syndrome 69
attention 119, 122–3, 128–31
  brain 48
  component subsystems in typical
    development 119–21
  control processes 123–5
  domain-general and domain-specific processes,
    integrating 339–42, 358–9
    cross-syndrome comparisons 356–7
    language and number 342–6
    literacy and numeracy 346–56
  dorsal-stream function 229, 249, 254
  Early Childhood Attention Battery 121–2, 126–8
  executive function 169, 171, 172–3
  face processing 270
  inhibition 166, 167
  literacy 328
  motor control and planning in spatial tasks 254
  numeracy 300, 302, 304
  selective *see* selective attention
  sleep 136, 137–8, 140, 143, 145
  spatial cognition and visuomotor
    action 247–8, 254, 257–9
  triadic joint 189, 191–2, 196, 198, 199
  visuospatial construction 226
  see also selective attention; sustained attention
attention deficit hyperactivity disorder (ADHD)
  associations versus dissociations 366
  attention 120
  brain 50, 364
  executive function and motor planning 170, 177
    inhibition 166, 167, 168
  literacy 328
  multilevel analysis 4
  sleep disruption 136, 142–3, 144–5
  in Williams syndrome 93, 108, 165, 328
    sleep disruption 140
auditory cortex 45, 158
auditory selective attention 171
auditory sustained attention 127, 171
Autism Diagnostic Observation Schedule—Generic
  (ADOS-G) 196–7
autistic spectrum disorder (ASD)
  adult outcomes 103
  associations versus dissociations 366
  biological motion tasks 228–9

autistic spectrum disorder (ASD) (*cont.*)
  brain 50, 51, 53, 364
    cerebellar dysfunction 173
    dorsal-stream deficits 228, 229, 230, 253, 254, 259, 341, 364
    cognition 105
      cognitive profile 15–16
      developmental trajectory 18–19
      face recognition 16, 21
      pattern construction 15, 18
      social skills 15
      vocabulary 16, 19
    diagnosis and remediation 369
    face processing 270, 271, 272, 273, 274, 341
    facial dysmorphology 368–9
    gastrointestinal problems 95
    genes 71, 73, 367
      epigenetics 69
    inhibition 166, 168
    interventions 112
    language skills
      grammatical development 195–6
      pragmatics 196–7, 199, 213–14, 217
    mental state understanding and social interaction 279, 281–3, 286–7, 288, 290, 291
    modular versus neuroconstructivist approaches 2–3
    motor planning 170, 173
    orientation coding 230–1
    reaching 175
    sleep problems 95, 141–2, 144–5
    stair descent 175
    visuospatial cognition 226, 236, 240
    in Williams syndrome 197, 287, 288

babble, onset of 189, 190
basal ganglia 45, 46, 51
BAZ1B gene 69–70
Beckwith–Wiedemann syndrome 68
behaviour 92–3
  adaptive 93–4
  adulthood 106, 108, 112
  sleep disruption 136, 137–8, 140, 141, 142, 143
behavioural interventions 109, 111, 112
  sleep hygiene 144
benefits system 110
Benton Judgement of Line Orientation Test (JLOT) 230
Benton Test of Face Recognition 265–6, 269
bicuspid aortic valve 87
binocular vision, suboptimal 90
biochemistry of Williams syndrome brain 49
biological motion tasks 228–9, 237, 239, 341
birds 5, 365
birth weight 89
  low 301
biventricular outflow obstruction 88
bladder capacity 90, 95
bladder diverticulae 90
blind people, visual cortex's recruitment for tactile modality in 4

block construction tasks, interaction between task complexity and performance in 170–1
blood-oxygen-level dependence (BOLD) signal (fMRI) 40
bone density, decreased 107
brain 37, 52–3, 363–4
  ageing 72–3
  attention 119–20, 124–5
  attention deficit hyperactivity disorder 364
  atypical development 37–8
    cross-syndrome comparisons 49–52
    measurement 38–43
    Williams syndrome 43–9
  autistic spectrum disorder 364
  cognitive profile 16
  development 64
  dorsal stream *see* dorsal-stream vulnerability
  face processing 270
  genes 43, 67
    ageing 72
    development of brain 64
  inhibition of irrelevant impulses and stimuli 167
  language skills 198–9, 215–16
  memory 158–9
  mental state understanding 281–2, 290
  numeracy 299–301
  sleep 135, 138
  social skills 48, 216, 216
    cross-syndrome comparisons 50, 51
  ventral stream 227–9, 237, 247, 249–51, 258
    form and motion coherence 249, 251, 252–3, 254
  visual domain 227–30, 247–8
    dorsal-stream vulnerability 252–4, 257–9
    motor control and planning in spatial tasks 254, 255
    visuomotor and visuospatial abilities 248–52
    visuospatial cognition 236–7, 238, 239
  Williams syndrome
    biochemistry 49
    cross-syndrome comparisons 49–52
    electrophysiology 49
    structural and functional atypicalities 43–9
  see also specific parts of the brain
British Ability Scales (BAS) 348
British Picture Vocabulary Scale (BPVS) 188, 348

canaries, *foxp2* gene 365
canonical babble, onset of 189, 190
cardiac problems 87–8, 94, 107
cardinality understanding 307, 310, 349, 353–5, 356
carer support 110–11, 112
carotid artery intima-media thickness 88
cataracts 73, 107
categorisation task (lexical-semantic knowledge) 24, 25
category word fluency task (memory) 155
central nervous system development 64
cerebellum 45, 49, 364
  cross-syndrome comparisons 51
  foxp2 gene (mice) 365
  genes 67

memory 158, 159
    motor control 255, 259
    motor planning 173, 176, 177
cerebrum 52
Children's Communication Checklist 188, 213, 214
Children's Embedded Figures Task (visuospatial
    construction) 226
choline (Cho) 41, 49
chromatin 69
cingulate cortex, dorsal anterior 167
cingulate gyrus 45, 46, 51
Clinical Evaluation of Language Fundamentals
    (CELF) 197
clinical profile 85–6, 94–5
    adaptive behaviour 93–4
    adulthood 106–7, 112
    cardiac problems 87–8
    development 92
    endocrine abnormalities 90–1
    gastrointestinal problems 91–2
    genitourinary abnormalities 89–90
    growth and puberty 89
    hearing and vision 90
    hypercalcaemia 88
    neurological problems 91
    orthopaedic and other connective-tissue
        problems 88–9
    personality and behaviour 92–3
    physical appearance 86–7
    prognosis 94
CLIP2 gene 59, 65, 74
clonazepam 140
coeliac disease 91
cofilin 65, 66
cognition 13–14, 32–3
    adulthood 103–5
    ageing 73
    attention 341, 358
    autistic spectrum disorder 15–16
    brain 51–2
    cognitive profile in Williams syndrome 32, 92
        fractionation 30
        origin 14–17
    developmental trajectories 17–19
        challenges 29–32
        comparing linear 19–21
        figurative language development 21–9
    Down syndrome 15, 16, 105, 142
    fragile X syndrome 105
    genes 70
    language skills 187, 197, 199, 207, 209, 215
    numeracy 301–8
    sleep 136–8, 141, 142, 143, 145
cognitive behavioural interventions 109
Communicative Development Inventory
    (CDI) 189, 190, 194, 195, 196
communicative face skills 269–71
communicative mind 284
componential model of theory of mind 283
Comprehensive Test of Phonological Processing
    (CTOPP) 321–2
conceptual basis for object words 192–3

conceptual/relational and concrete vocabulary
    ability, relationship between 194, 209–10, 216
conceptual thinking 21, 26, 29
concrete- and relational/conceptual
    vocabulary ability, relationship
    between 194, 209–10, 216, 235
connective-tissue problems 88–9, 107
conservation abilities 26
constipation 91
Continuous Performance Test (CPT,
    attention) 348–9, 350, 353, 355
continuous positive airway pressure 144
copying skills 15, 16
copy number variation 71
Cornelia de Lange syndrome 368
coronary artery stenosis 88
corpus callosum 45, 52, 364
    cross-syndrome comparisons 50
    memory 158
cortex 67
cortisol 136
counterpointing task
    attention 124
    inhibition 167, 168
creatine (Cr) 41, 49
cytoplasmic linker 2 (Clip2) 65

day/night task
    attention 124
    inhibition 167, 168
death see mortality
declarative (explicit) memory see explicit
    (declarative) memory
deep (slow-wave) sleep (SWS) 135, 138, 139, 143
definitions task (lexical-semantic knowledge) 23–4, 25
dementia 73, 104
dental problems 86, 87, 107
dentate gyrus 67
depression 108, 109
depth processing, and stair descent 175
detour box task (attention) 124
detour-reaching task (inhibition) 167–8
detrusor instability 90
development 92
developmental coordination disorder 175, 364
developmental delay
    general 173
    severe developmental delay of unknown
        aetiology 191–2, 198
developmental dyscalculia 160, 367, 369
developmental trajectories
    challenges 29–32
    cognition 13, 17–33
    comparing linear 19–21
    figurative language development 21–9
    importance of full 5–7
diabetes mellitus 90–1, 107
diagnosing neurodevelopmental disorders 369–70
diarrhoea 91
diet 110, 111
Differential Ability Scales (DAS) 188–9, 194, 196,
    197, 225

diffuse aortic hypoplasia 87
diffusion tensor imaging (DTI) 39, 40
DiGeorge (22q) syndrome 50–1
disability living allowance 110
dissociations versus associations 366
diverticular disease 91–2
DNA methylation 73
domain-general and domain-specific developmental
    processes 339–40, 358–9
  attention
    cross-syndrome comparisons 356–7
    language and number 342–8
    literacy and numeracy 348–56
  existing evidence of interactions across
    domains 340–2
domain relevance versus domain specificity 364–6
dorsal-stream vulnerability 341, 364
  attention 120, 124–5, 248
  language skills 194, 340
  reaching 175–6
  visual domain 227–30, 237, 238, 247–51,
    257–9, 340
    form and motion coherence 249, 251, 252–4
    remembering and transforming spatial
      information 257
Down syndrome (DS)
  adulthood 112
  associations versus dissociations 366
  attention 124, 125, 126, 130
    domain-general and domain-specific processes,
      integrating 339, 342–56, 358, 359
    Early Childhood Attention Battery 126–8
    existing data 128, 129
  coeliac disease 91
  cognition
    cognitive profile 15, 16
    developmental trajectory 18, 19
    face recognition 21
    language skills 15, 105
    pattern construction 19
    pragmatics 25
    vocabulary 19
  diagnosis and remediation 369
  executive function 174
  face processing 21, 270, 274
  facial dysmorphology 368
  gait 174
  hearing loss 95
  interventions 112
  language skills 15, 105, 188, 198, 205
    grammatical development 195
    lexical abilities 210, 216
    lexical development 192, 193–4
    morphosyntactic abilities 207
    phonological abilities 212
    pragmatics 196, 213, 217
    precursors to lexical development 191–2
    vocabulary size 193–4
  literacy 313–14, 318–26, 328, 329
  memory 150–1, 152–3, 155–6, 157–8, 160
  motor planning 170, 176
  numeracy 302–3, 304–5, 309, 310
  reaching 176
  sleep 137, 142, 144–5
  social skills 169
  therapeutic advances 73
  visuospatial cognition 92, 236, 240–1
drawing skills 92, 170, 171, 172
duplicated kidney 89
dyscalculia
  brain 50
  diagnosis and remediation 369
  genes 367
  memory 160
  numeracy 310
  prevalence 299
dyslexia 217
  brain 53
  diagnosis and remediation 369
  dorsal-stream deficits 228, 253, 259
  genes 367
  literacy 313, 315, 317–29
  prevalence 299
dysthymia 108

Early Childhood Attention Battery (ECAB) 119,
    121–2, 126–8, 130
Early Learning Composite (ELC) scores 189, 196
Early Word Reading Test 349
ectopic kidney problems 89
education 106, 110, 111
  literacy 327
egocentric frames of reference 234, 256–7
electroencephalography (EEG) 39, 41–2, 43
electrophysiology of Williams syndrome brain 49
ELN gene 59, 70, 74, 85, 367
  diagnosis of Williams syndrome 86
emotional lability 93
emotional/motivational executive
    functions 165, 169
empathy 93, 280, 283, 286, 290
employment 106, 110, 112
endocrine abnormalities 90–1
endogenous attention 123
end-state comfort, motor planning for 253, 255–6
epigenetics 63–4, 68–70
  ageing 73
  environment–gene relations 5
epilepsy 91
episodic memory 104, 112
  buffer 150
ethical issues in brain studies 39
event-related potentials (ERP) 39, 40, 42
exact-number system 301, 303, 305
executive function 165–6, 176–7
  attention 120–1, 122, 130, 350
    Down syndrome 124, 130
    Williams syndrome 123–5, 130
  and dorsal-stream function 230
  emotional/motivational 165, 169
  and inhibition 169
  literacy 341, 350
  metacognitive 165
  numeracy 302, 341, 350

planning 169–70
sleep 136
task complexity and performance, interaction
between 170–1
and visuospatial cognition 226, 254–6, 258
in Williams syndrome 172–6
assessment 171–2
attention 123–5, 130
exogenous attention 123
explicit (declarative) memory 150, 156
long-term
verbal 154–5, 158, 159, 160
visuospatial 155–7, 158, 159, 160
sleep 138
expressive vocabulary 198, 205
adulthood 104–5
early language abilities as predictors of later
language and cognitive abilities 197
grammatical development 195, 196
precursors to lexical development 189
reading development 317
size 198
comparison between Williams and Down
syndromes 194
Expressive Vocabulary Test 194
eye gaze interpretation 196
eye region, face gaze directed towards
the 271–3, 274
eyes, physical appearance 86

Fabry disease 368
face processing 265, 273–4
autistic spectrum disorders 16, 21
brain 38, 42
electrophysiology 49
structural and functional atypicalities 46, 47–8
cognition
cognitive profile 14, 15, 16
developmental trajectory 20–1
communicative face skills 269–70
Down syndrome 21, 270, 274
mental state understanding 281, 282, 283, 286
multilevel analyses 4
and social interactions 270–3
structural encoding typicalities 265–9
facial dysmorphology 86–7, 367, 368–9
family support 110–11, 112
fatigue 91
feeding problems 89, 91
feeling mind 280–2
fertility 89
fetal alcohol syndrome 173, 177, 364
figurative language development 13, 21–9, 214–15
financial support for adults with Williams
syndrome 110
fine motor skills 92
fixation shift test 248, 258
fluorescence *in situ* hybridisation (FISH) 86
FMR1 gene 74
follicle-stimulating hormone 136
food refusal 109
form coherence 249, 251, 252–6

FOXP2 gene 5, 364–6
fragile X syndrome
adulthood 112
associations versus dissociations 366
attention 123, 125, 131
domain-general and domain-specific processes,
integrating 340, 356–7, 359
brain 50, 51, 364
dorsal-stream deficits 254, 259, 341, 364
cerebellar dysfunction 173, 177
cognitive and linguistic abilities 105
epigenetics 69
facial dysmorphology 368
language skills 105
memory 160
motor planning 173, 177
numeracy 310
sleep 142
therapeutic advances 64, 73–4
visuospatial perception 234
frames of reference, egocentric versus
allocentric 234, 256–7
frogs, gene expression 66
frontal lobes 45, 46
dysfunction, and hypersociability 169
lesions, and attention 122–3
frontostriatal dysfunction 48, 50
inhibition 124, 167
functional magnetic resonance imaging
(fMRI) 39, 40, 42, 43
mental health problems 109
functional near-infrared spectroscopy
(fNIRS) 39, 40, 42–3
fusiform face area (FFA) 46–7, 50
connectivity 237
face processing 269
fusiform gyrus 45, 46, 47
cross-syndrome comparisons 51
face processing 268
future directions
associations versus dissociations 366
beyond Williams syndrome 363–4
diagnosing and remediating neurodevelopmental
disorders 369–70
domain relevance versus domain specificity 364–6
facial dysmorphology 368–9
genotype–phenotype relations 367

gait 172
gamma-aminobutyric acid (GABA) 74
gamma-band activity 51
gastroesophageal reflux 92
gastrointestinal problems 91–2, 107
autism 95
sleep disturbance 141
gender, grammatical 208
general developmental delay 173
generalized anxiety disorder 72, 108
general transcription factor II-I genes 66–8, 69
genes 59–64, 74–5, 363
ageing 72–3
brain 43, 67

genes (*cont.*)
    development 49
    memory 159
  central nervous system development 64
  clinical profile 85–6
  cognitive profile 14, 16
  diabetes mellitus 91
  domain relevance versus domain
    specificity 364–6
  epigenetics 68–70
  expression 59–64
    environment–gene relations 5, 71–2
    Williams syndrome region 65–8
  facial dysmorphology 369
  genotypic and phenotypic variation 70–2
  language skills 199
  social behaviour 282, 290
  therapeutic advances in treating
    neurodevelopmental disorders 73–4
  visuospatial cognition 237–8, 239, 240, 258
genetic testing 85–6
genitourinary abnormalities 89–90, 94–5, 107
genome variation 70
Geodesic Sensor Net 42
gestalt perception 231–2
give-a-number task (numeracy) 307–8, 349
globus pallidus 158
glucose tolerance, impaired 91
glutamate receptor 5 (GRM5) signalling and
  antagonists 74
go/no-go task
  attention 124
  inhibition 166–7
grammar 188, 208–9
  early development 195–6, 198
  and memory 31, 151
grammatical errors 30, 31
greying of the hair 73, 86, 103, 107
grey-matter volume 46, 48, 52
  cross-syndrome comparisons 50
growth 89
growth hormone 136
GTF2I gene 59, 66, 69, 74
  social behaviour 282, 290
  visuospatial cognition 237
GTF2IRD1 gene 59, 66, 69, 74
  visuospatial cognition 237
GTF2IRD2 gene 66, 74

hair greying 73, 86, 103, 107
hand banging, rhythmic 190
handedness 91
head circumference 44, 69, 89
health, physical *see* clinical profile
hearing problems 73, 90, 107
  Down syndrome 95
height 89
hemiplegia 253, 254
hemispherectomy 248
herniae 89, 91
heterochromatin 70
high-density event-related potentials (HD-ERP) 42

hippocampus 49
  genes 66, 67, 68
    and stress 71, 72
  memory 158, 300
    and sleep 138
  numeracy 300
  relational knowledge 234
  spatial processing 234–5, 257, 259
histone deacetylase 3 (HDAC3) 69
home literacy environment 317, 325, 327, 329
homeobox genes 64
housing benefit 110
hygiene 94, 106, 111
hyperactivity 136
  in Williams syndrome 93
  see also attention deficit hyperactivity disorder
hyperacusis 90, 94, 107, 109
hypercalcaemia 88, 89, 91, 107
hypercalciuria 88
hypercarbia and sleep disturbance 136
hyperglycaemia 73
hyperreflexia 91
hypersociability *see* social skills
hypertension 73, 88, 90, 107
hypomania 108
hypothyroidism 90, 107
hypoxia and sleep disturbance 136–7

idiom comprehension 21, 26, 214–15, 284
illusory biases 232, 236, 238
imagery, mental
  and executive function 171
  and visuospatial construction 226, 340
impaired glucose tolerance 91
implicit (procedural) memory 104, 150, 157–8
imprinted genes 69
income support 110
independence in adult life 93–4, 105–6, 111
Infant Behaviour Questionnaire 343, 346
inferencing abilities 29
inguinal herniae 89, 91
inhibition 166–9
  brain 48
  and emotional/motivational executive
    functions 169
  motor control and planning in
    spatial tasks 254
insufficient sleep syndrome 137
integration into society *see* adult outcomes
intelligence and intellectual disability 92
  adulthood 103–4
  ageing 73
  attention 130
  brain atypicalities 46, 50
  epigenetics 69
  language skills 187, 188–9, 205
    grammatical development 195
  mental health problems 108
  mental state understanding 285
  sleep 136, 137, 141
intracranial aneurysms 70–1
intraparietal cortex 236

intraparietal sulcus (IPS) 46–7, 48
  connectivity 237
  motor planning 173
  numeracy 299, 300, 301
inversion polymorphism 85
IQ *see* intelligence and intellectual disability
irony comprehension 214, 285
  development of 25–6
  nonliteral similarity, understanding of 21
  nonspecific learning disability 26
  Prader–Willi syndrome 25–6, 214
irritable bowel syndrome 91

joint attention 189, 191–2, 196, 198, 199
jokes 25–6, 214, 284, 285
Judgement of Line Orientation Test
    (JLOT) 230

Kaufman Brief Intelligence Test 306
kidney problems 89
knee jerks 91

LacZ reporter gene 65, 67
language development, figurative 13, 21–9, 214–15
language module 206
language skills 187–8, 198–9, 205–7, 215–17
  adulthood 104–5
  attention 342–6, 359
  brain 49
  cognitive profile 14, 15
  development 92
  developmental trajectory approach, challenges
      to a 30–1
  Down syndrome *see* Down syndrome: language
      skills
  early language abilities as predictors of later
      language and cognitive abilities 197
  executive function 172
  FOXP2 gene 365
  fragile X syndrome 105
  grammatical development 195–6
  inhibition 168–9
  intellectual ability 188–9
  lexical abilities 209–11
  lexical development 192
    conceptual basis for object words 192–3
    concrete- and relational/conceptual vocabulary
        ability, relationship between 194
    precursors 189–92
    vocabulary size comparisons 193–4
  lies and jokes, distinguishing between 26
  literacy *see* literacy
  memory 150–2, 154–5, 160, 216
    grammar 31, 151
  morphosyntactic abilities 207–9
  numeracy 302, 304–8, 310, 340
  phonological abilities 211–13
  pragmatics 196–7, 213–15
  and theory of mind 284, 291
  and visuospatial cognition 236, 240–1, 340
learning
  and attention 341

  and memory 149
  and sleep 135, 136, 137, 138, 143, 145
    Down syndrome 142
    Williams syndrome 140–1
learning difficulties
  irony comprehension 26
  language skills 211
  literacy 313–14, 326, 327, 328
left angular gyrus 300
left-hand dominance 91
letter knowledge 316, 322–4, 327, 329, 341, 349,
    350, 353, 355
lexical abilities 192, 198, 199, 209–11, 216
  conceptual basis for object words 192–3
  concrete- and relational/conceptual-vocabulary
      ability, relationship between 194
  precursors to development 189–92, 199
  vocabulary size comparisons 193–4
lexical-semantic knowledge 205, 206, 210
  development of 23–5
  memory 151–2
  and receptive vocabulary, relationship
      between 14, 24
lies and jokes, distinction between 26, 214
life expectancy 94, 111
LIM domain kinase 1 (LIMK1) 65–6
LIM domain kinase 2 (LIMK2) 66
LIMK1 gene 59, 65, 367
  visuospatial cognition 237
Limk2 gene 66
linear developmental trajectories, comparing 19–21
linguistic comprehension 314, 315, 316
literacy 92, 313–14, 327–8
  and attention 341, 346–56
  reading intervention 328
  in typical development 314–17
  in Williams syndrome 318–30
living arrangements 93–4, 105–6, 112
long-sightedness 90
long-term memory (LTM) 149, 150, 159
  implicit (procedural) 157–8
  verbal explicit 154–5, 158, 159, 160
  visuospatial explicit 155–7, 158, 159, 160
lordosis 89
low birth weight, children born with 301
lumbar lordosis 89
luteinising hormone 136

macaques, ageing 72
MacArthur Communicative Development
    Inventories 343
MAGI2 gene 91
magnetic resonance imaging (MRI)
  functional 39, 40, 42, 43
    mental health problems 109
  structural 39, 43
magnetic resonance spectroscopy (MRS) 39, 41
magnetoencephalography (MEG) 39, 41
mammalian development 5
manic depression 108
MAP1B gene 237, 363
massive-modularity hypothesis 30, 31

mathematics *see* numeracy
McCarthy Scales of Children's Abilities 205
melatonin 136, 142, 144
memory 149–50, 159–60
  adulthood 104, 112
  and attention 341
  Down syndrome 150–1, 152–3, 155–6,
    157–8, 160
  episodic 104, 112
  implicit (procedural) 104, 150, 157–8
  language skills 150–2, 154–5, 160, 216
    grammar 31, 151
  neurobiological perspectives 158–9
  numeracy 300, 305
  phonological 216
  and sleep 135, 136, 137, 138, 140, 145
  spatial processing 256–7, 258, 340
  see also long-term memory, short-term
    (working) memory
mental health in adulthood 108–9, 112
mental imagery
  and executive function 171
  and visuospatial construction 226, 340
mental state understanding and social
    interaction 279, 287–91
  development 280–7
  theory of mind 280–4
metacognitive executive functions 165
metaphor comprehension 21, 26–9, 214–15, 284
methylphenidate 143
metonym comprehension 26–9, 214–15
mice studies
  ageing, genetic changes associated with 72
  central nervous system development 64
  foxp2 gene 365
  gene expression 65, 66–8, 70
microarray analysis 86
microcephaly 89
midbrain 45
middle aortic syndrome 87
migraine 71
minocycline 74
mitral valve prolapse 87
modular approach to neurodevelopmental
    disorders 1–3, 6
mood disorder 141
morphosyntactic abilities 205, 206, 207–9, 216
mortality 107
  sudden death 88, 107
motion coherence 249, 251, 252–6
motion processing 38, 48, 229, 237, 239, 341
motivational/emotional executive
    functions 165, 169
motor control in spatial tasks 254–6, 258, 259
motor milestones 92, 95, 173, 252
motor planning 165–6, 169–70, 172, 173–7
  assessment 171–2
  for end-state comfort 253, 255–6
  in spatial tasks 254–6, 259
  task complexity and performance, interaction
    between 170–1
motor skills, and sleep 138, 143

Mullen Scales of Early Learning
    (MSEL) 189, 196
multilevel analyses 4–5
music 93
myocardial infarction 88

N-acetylaspartate (NAA) 41, 49
nephrocalcinosis 88, 90
neuroconstructivist approach
  to neurodevelopmental disorders 1–4
  to remediation 7
neurological problems 91
non-Hodgkin lymphoma 107
nonliteral similarity, development of
    understanding of 21–3
nonspecific learning disability 26
number knowledge, assessment of 304–5
numeracy 92, 299, 309–10
  attention 342–56, 259
  brain 37–8
  cognitive bases
    in typical development 301–2
    in Williams syndrome 302–8
  executive function 341
  language skills 302, 304–8, 310, 340
  neural bases 299–301
  visuospatial cognition 302, 308, 309, 340

obesity 89
  obstructive sleep apnoea syndrome 142
  Prader–Willi syndrome 95
object file theory of numeracy 301, 303
object words, conceptual basis for 192–3
obsessive compulsive disorder 50, 93, 108
obstructive sleep apnoea syndrome (OSAS) 136,
    137, 142–3, 144
occipital cortex 45, 46, 48, 52
  cross-syndrome comparisons 51
  memory 158
  motor control problems 255
  visuospatial cognition 236
oculomotor nuclei 248
oral language skills in literacy 317, 324–6,
    328, 329
orbitofrontal cortex 43, 46, 48, 49, 52
  mental state understanding 282
orientation coding 230–1, 240, 253
orientation selectivity 248–9
orthographic learning 315–16
orthopaedic problems 88–9, 107
outcomes *see* adult outcomes
overweight 89
oxytocin 282

panic disorder 108
parahippocampal gyrus 47
parahippocampal place area 47–8, 237
paralogues 63, 66
parietal cortex 45, 46–7, 48, 52
  cross-syndrome comparisons 50, 51
  memory 158
  motor control problems 255

numeracy 37–8, 299–300, 301
   visuospatial cognition 236, 248
Parkinson's disease 174
passerine birds, song listening and song
      production 5
patellar dislocation/subluxation 88
pattern construction 15, 18, 29
Peabody Picture Vocabulary Test (PPVT) 188, 194
perceptual integration 232–4
perceptual segmentation 232
periodic limb movement disorder (PLMD) 137,
      139, 140
peripheral pulmonary artery stenosis 87
personal hygiene 94, 106, 111
personality 92–3, 269
phase theory of reading development 315, 317
phobias 72, 90, 93, 108, 109
phoneme awareness skills 316, 319, 321–2, 323–4,
      327, 349, 350, 355, 358
phonics reading approach 330
phonological abilities 211–13, 350
   development 189, 190
   in dyslexia 328
   in typical development 313, 314, 315, 316,
      317, 329
   in Williams syndrome 314, 318, 319–23, 326,
      327, 329
Phonological Abilities Test 349
phonological memory 216
phonological pathway 317, 327
phonological-similarity effect (working
      memory) 150, 151
phonological store 149–50
phonophobia 90
physical appearance 86–7
physical health see clinical profile
piriform cortex 67
planning see motor planning
planum temporale 158
pointing/counterpointing task
   attention 124
   inhibition 167, 168
pointing gestures, comprehension and production
      of 189, 191–2, 196, 198, 199
positron emission tomography (PET) 39, 40–1
posterior superior parietal lobule
      (PSPL) 299–300, 301
post-mortem studies of brain tissue 39
post-traumatic stress disorder 108
posture 87
Prader–Willi syndrome
   epigenetics 68
   facial dysmorphology 368
   mental state understanding 285
   obesity 95
   pragmatics 25–6, 214, 217
pragmatics 25–6, 92, 188, 213–15, 217
   early 196–7, 198, 199
      as predictor of later pragmatic abilities 197
   mental state understanding 284, 285, 291
precocious puberty 89
precuneus, medial 167

prefrontal cortex 47, 167, 176
preterm children 229, 254
primacy effect (memory) 154
procedural (implicit) memory 104, 150, 157–8
process dissociation procedure task
      (memory) 156–7
Profiling Elements of Prosody in Speech
      Communication 212
prognosis in Williams syndrome 94
prosody 206, 211–13, 215–16, 284
proverb comprehension 21
psychosis 50, 51, 108
puberty 89
pulmonary artery stenosis 87
pulmonary venous return, anomalous 87–8
pulvinar 237
Purkinje cells 67, 68
putamen 158

quality of life
   attention deficit hyperactivity disorder 143
   Williams syndrome 94, 290
      hyperacusis 90
      sleep 144
      social interaction 280, 289

radial-arm maze (RAM) task (memory) 153–4
radioulnar synostosis 88–9
raphe nucleus 67
rapid automated naming (RAN) 316, 319, 322–3,
      324, 325, 326, 327, 329
rapid eye movement (REM) sleep 135–6, 138
   attention deficit and hyperactivity syndrome 143
   Down syndrome 142
ratios (numeracy) 302
rat studies, sleep disruption 136–7
Raven's Coloured Progressive Matrices 172
reaching 175–6, 255
reading see literacy
recency effect (memory) 154
receptive vocabulary 187–8, 209
   adulthood 104–5
   attention 343
   autistic spectrum disorder 16, 19
   cognition
      cognitive profile 15, 16
      developmental trajectory 18
      figurative language development 21, 28–9
   Down syndrome 19
   and lexical-semantic knowledge, relationship
         between 14, 24
   pragmatics 215
   reading development 317, 324
   and visuospatial construction 226
rectal prolapse 91
refractive errors 252
relational/conceptual and concrete vocabulary
      ability, relationship between 194, 209–10, 216
remediating neurodevelopmental disorders 369–70
remediation, neuroconstructivist view of 7
renal agenesis 89
renal artery stenosis 87, 90

renal cysts 89
renal dysplasia 89
repetitive tasks, low tolerance for 91
residual normality assumption for
    neurodevelopmental disorders 30, 32
respite care 110
restless legs 93
Rett syndrome 64, 68, 73
rhythmic hand banging 190
rime awareness skills 321, 322, 327, 349, 350
rodents
    environment–gene relations 5, 71
    sleep disruption 136–7
    see also mice studies
route-learning tasks (visuospatial cognition) 234–6
Rubinstein–Taybi syndrome 69, 73

saccadic eye movements
    executive function 173
    triadic joint attention 192
sarcasm comprehension 25–6, 214, 285
schizophrenia 50, 108, 71, 364
scoliosis 89, 107
segmentation of words from continuous speech 189,
    190–1
selective attention 120–1, 122, 123, 130
    auditory 171
    Down syndrome 128, 130
    language and number 342
    and learning 341
    visual 171
    Williams syndrome 123, 128, 130
self-care skills 93–4, 105–6, 111
semantic skills 317, 326–7
    metaphor and metonym comprehension 29
    see also lexical-semantic knowledge
sensory-processing disorder 175
separation anxiety 108
septicaemia 107
set-shifting behaviour 172
severe developmental delay of unknown
    aetiology 191–2, 198
sexual assault 106
sexual impulse control disorders 108
short-term (working) memory (STM) 149–50, 160
    adulthood 104, 112
    attention 125
    literacy 318
    numeracy 300, 302, 304
    sleep 137–8
    verbal 150–2, 160, 187, 188–9, 216
    visuospatial 152–4
    and visuospatial construction 226
sight word reading 315–16, 323, 326, 329
sigmoid diverticulitis 92
single-copy genes 70–1
single nucleotide polymorphisms (SNPs) 70–1
sleep 135, 144–5
    architecture 135–6
    attention deficit hyperactivity disorder 136, 142–3
    autistic spectrum disorder 95, 141–2
    bladder capacity, reduced 95

cognition and 136–8
Down syndrome 142
fragmentation 137
gene expression 72
management 143–4
Williams syndrome 93, 138–41
slow-wave (deep) sleep (SWS) 135, 138, 139, 143
snoring 136, 137
social influences on literacy development 317
social phobia 108
social skills 93
    adult life 93–4, 105–6, 111
    autistic spectrum disorder 15
    brain 48, 216, 216
        cross-syndrome comparisons 50, 51
    cognitive profile 14, 15
    Down syndrome 169
    executive function 169
    and face processing 270–3
    figurative language 21, 213
    and mental state understanding 279–91
    pragmatics 213
    training 94
society, integration into *see* adult outcomes and
    integration into society
spatial cognition 247, 257–9
    dorsal-stream vulnerability 253, 254
    motor control and planning 254–6
    remembering and transforming spatial
        information 256–7
    see also visuospatial cognition
spatial reorientation 234–5
specific language impairment (SLI) 217
    dorsal-stream deficits 227
    memory 160
    morphosyntactic abilities 207, 208–9
    numeracy 310
    pragmatics 25, 213, 217
speech fragmentation 189, 190–1
squint 90
stair descent 174–5, 254, 255
standing posture 87
stooping 89
strabismus 225, 252
stress, and gene expression 71–2
striatum 51, 167
stroke 88
structural magnetic resonance imaging 39, 43
STX1A gene 65, 71
sudden death 88, 107
superior colliculus 67, 119, 248
superior longitudinal fasciculus 158
superior parietal lobule, posterior
    (PSPL) 299–300, 301
superior temporal cortex 48, 237
superior temporal gyrus 45, 158
superior temporal sulcus 229
support for adults with Williams syndrome 93–4,
    109–10, 112
supravalvular aortic stenosis 87
supravalvular pulmonary stenosis 87
sustained attention 120–1, 122, 130

auditory 127, 171
  cross-task/cross-syndrome comparisons 125–6
  Down syndrome 125, 126–8, 130
  language and number 342–5, 346
  and learning 341
  literacy and numeracy 348, 350, 353, 355, 359
  and sleep 137
  visual 127–8, 171
  Williams syndrome 125–6, 127–8, 130
syllable awareness skills 322
syntaxin 1A (STX1A) 65, 71

temporal lobe 46, 48
Test for Reception of Grammar 207
Test of Early Mathematical Ability (TEMA) 306,
  349, 353, 355
Test of Everyday Attention for Children
  (TEA-Ch) 121, 125
Test of Reglational Concepts (TRC) 194
thalamus 45
  memory 158, 159
  visuospatial cognition 237
theory of mind (ToM) 29, 280–4, 287, 290
therapeutic advances in treating neurodevelopmental
  disorders 73–4
thinking mind 282–3
thyroid hypoplasia 90
thyroid-stimulating hormones 90
thyroxine 90
time-telling 92
Tourette syndrome 50, 364
Tower of London task (planning) 171
trail-making task (executive function) 172
transcranial magnetic stimulation 39
transparent orthographies 316, 319, 320
triadic joint attention 189, 191–2, 196, 198, 199
triiodothyronine 90
tuberous sclerosis 73
Turner syndrome
  associations versus dissociations 366
  brain 50
  coeliac disease 91
  orientation coding 230, 231, 240

umbilical herniae 89
urinary tract abnormalities 89–90

valvular pulmonary stenosis 87
vascular dementia 73
Di (22q) syndrome 50–1
ventral stream 227–9, 237, 247, 249–51, 258
  form and motion coherence 249, 251, 252–3, 254
ventricular septal defect 87
verbal domain see language skills
verbal memory
  explicit long-term 154–5, 158, 159, 160
  short-term memory 150–2, 160, 187, 188–9, 216
  span, and literacy 316
vesicoureteric reflux 90
visual cortex
  in blind people 4
  visuomotor and visuospatial abilities 248, 249

in Williams syndrome 45
visual perception 225, 237–40
  dorsal visual stream and developmental
    vulnerability 227–30
  literacy 325
  orientation coding and task complexity 230–1
visual problems 90
visual processing, dorsal versus ventral stream 6
visual search tasks 234
visual selective attention 171
visual span, and literacy 316
visual sustained attention 127–8, 171–2
visuomotor action 247–8, 257–9
  brain development 248–52
  dorsal-stream vulnerability 254
visuospatial cognition 225, 226, 237–40
  attention 120, 128
  brain 47, 236–7
    development 248–52
  cognitive profile 14, 15, 16, 92
  cross-domain interactions 235–6
  dorsal-stream vulnerability 252
  Down syndrome 92, 128
    sleep apnoea 142
  gene expression 237–8
  and language skills 188, 236, 240–1, 340
  in large-scale space 234–5, 257
  memory 256–7, 258, 340
  motor planning 176
  numeracy 302, 308, 309, 340
  see also spatial cognition
visuospatial construction 225–7
visuospatial memory
  explicit long-term 155–7, 158, 159, 160
  short-term 152–4
    and visuospatial cognition 340
visuospatial perception 231–4
visuospatial scratchpad/sketchpad 150, 152, 159
vitamin D 69
vocabulary 187, 188, 198, 199, 209
  and attention 341, 342, 345, 358
  concrete- and relational/conceptual-vocabulary
    ability, relationship between 194, 209–10, 216
  expressive see expressive vocabulary
  receptive see receptive vocabulary
  size comparison between Williams and Down
    syndrome 193–4
voice 89

walking 92, 173–5, 252
Wechsler Intelligence Scale for Children
  (WISC) 225, 235, 303–4
weight disorders 89, 91, 107
white-matter volume 46, 47
  cross-syndrome comparisons 51
whole-word reading approach 330
WICH complex 69–70
Williams syndrome (WS)
  adult outcomes and integration into
    society 103–12
  ageing 73
  associations versus dissociations 366

Williams syndrome (WS) (*cont.*)
    attention 122–31
        domain-general and domain-specific processes,
            integrating 339–59
    brain 37–8, 43–53, 364
    clinical profile 85–95
    cognition 13–33
    diagnosis 85–6, 369
    executive function and motor planning 165–77
    face processing and social interaction 265–74
    facial dysmorphology 86–7, 367, 368–9
    genes 59–75, 363, 367
    later language 205–17
    literacy 313–14, 318–30
    memory 149–60
    mental state understanding and social
        interaction 279–91
    model for neuroconstructivist approach 1–8
    numeracy 299–310
    precursors to language and early language 187–99

    prognosis 94
    remediation 369
    sleep 137, 138–41, 144–5
    spatial cognition, visuomotor action and
        attention 247–59
    visual perception and visuospatial
        cognition 225–40
WINAC complex 69
Wisconsin Card Sorting Test 172
word-length effect (working memory) 150, 151
word list learning task (memory) 154–5
word recognition 314–15
word segmentation from continuous
    speech 189, 190–1
working memory *see* short-term (working) memory
writing 92

zebra finches, *foxp2* gene 365
zebrafish, gene expression 66